Testis Tumors

THIS VOLUME
IS ONE OF A SERIES

International Perspectives In Urology

EDITED BY
John A. Libertino, M.D.

NEW AND FORTHCOMING TITLES

McDougal and Persky
TRAUMATIC INJURIES OF THE GENITOURINARY SYSTEM

Javadpour
RECENT ADVANCES IN UROLOGIC CANCER

Jacobi and Hohenfellner
PROSTATE CANCER

deVere White
ASPECTS OF MALE INFERTILITY

Bennett
MANAGEMENT OF MALE IMPOTENCE

Roth and Finlayson
STONES: CLINICAL MANAGEMENT OF UROLITHIASIS

Donohue
TESTIS TUMORS

Marberger and Dreikorn
RENAL PRESERVATION

Lang
CURRENT CONCEPTS OF URORADIOLOGY

Johnston
VESICOURETERIC REFLUX
MANAGEMENT OF

McGuire
CLINICAL EVALUATION AND TREATMENT OF
NEUROGENIC VESICAL DYSFUNCTION

International Perspectives In Urology

Volume 7

John A. Libertino, M.D.
series editor

Testis Tumors

Edited by

John P. Donohue, M.D.

Professor and Chairman
Department of Urology
Indiana University
School of Medicine
Indianapolis, Indiana

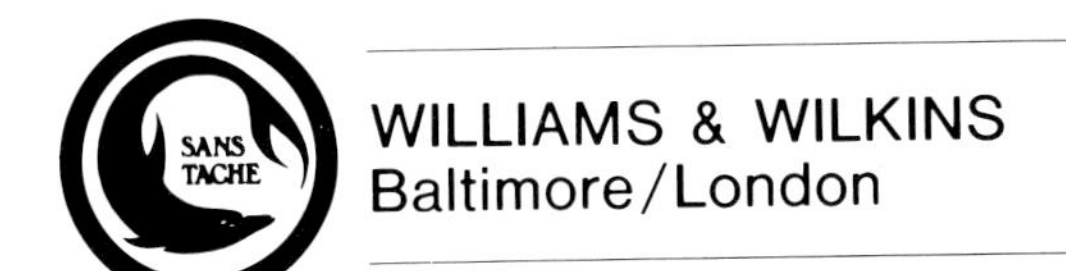

WILLIAMS & WILKINS
Baltimore/London

Williams & Wilkins
428 East Preston Street
Baltimore, MD 21202, U.S.A.

Made in the United States of America

Library of Congress Cataloging in Publication Data

Main entry under title:

Testis tumors.

(International perspectives in urology; v. 7)
Includes index.
1. Testis—Tumors. I. Donohue, John P. II. Series. [DNLM: 1. Testicular neoplasms. 2. Testicular neoplasms—Therapy. W1 IN827K v. 7 / WJ 858 T345]
RC280.T4T49 1983 616.99′463 82-17356
ISBN 0-683-02613-5

Composed and printed at the
Waverly Press, Inc.
Mt. Royal and Guilford Aves.
Baltimore, MD 21202, U.S.A.

Series Editor's Foreword

Two decades ago, when many of us were house officers, there were many patients on the urology service who were dying from metastatic nonseminomatous germ cell tumors of the testicle. The most dramatic advances in the management of any genitourinary malignancy have occurred in those patients suffering from nonseminomatous germ cell testis tumors.

During the last decade, the CAT scan and new, highly sensitive radioimmune assays for α-fetoprotein and β-HCG have significantly altered the diagnosis and treatment of testicular cancer. Likewise, combination chemotherapy, a major breakthrough, has produced excellent, long-term, complete remissions in chemosensitive tumors.

We are particularly pleased that Dr. Donohue, who has contributed many of the recent advances in the management of nonseminomatous germ cell testis tumors, has chosen to edit this monograph for the *International Perspectives in Urology* series. The monograph he has produced is the state of the art with regard to the management of testis tumors.

Though the victory over testis tumors is incomplete, we are well on our way to conquering this disease entity. My hope is that the next decade or two will yield the same degree of success with other urologic malignancies as is currently achieved in patients suffering from testis tumors.

JOHN A. LIBERTINO, M.D.

Preface

A couple of years ago, Dr. John Libertino asked me if I would edit a book in the *International Perspectives in Urology* series on testis cancer. My reaction was that such a book would be outdated by the time it was printed, so rapid have been the developments in this field. Fortunately, in the past 2 years a number of important clinical trials and laboratory studies have been completed, each providing answers to key questions. So, this text should be "in date" and reasonably timely.

If ever there was a tumor requiring international dialogue, testis cancer is one such. There have been widely varying views on tumor classification, treatment of low state disease and bulky or advanced disease on either side of the Atlantic.

One purpose of this book has been to get the leading clinicians and investigators in the field of testis cancer to "talk to each other." This has been accomplished in several settings *via* international workshops, in Minneapolis, Minnesota in June of 1980 and in London, England in May of 1981. Many contributors have continued the dialogue since then. In a real sense, these chapters contain the substance of this continuing dialogue by participants in these symposia and workshops. The reader can now join in this discussion.

Other objectives of this text are correlation of differing nomenclatures, especially that of our pathologists. Excellent contributions by Doctors Pugh and Nochomovitz accomplished this. Another goal is to examine the impact of chemotherapy on both low and high stage disease, in hopes of revealing how these advances in systemic treatment render obsolete some of our old arguments concerning local treatment options (such as radiotherapy or surgery as primary treatment for bulky metastatic non-seminomatous tumor).

Also, what insights do we have into future biologic potentials of the primary germ cell tumor? Several leading laboratories share their work with mouse and human teratocarcinoma stem cell models with provocative findings.

This is particularly a good time for an international perspective series. Today, there is much better international dialogue and an enlarging consensus; but there are still lively differences in some areas. Vive la difference.

JOHN P. DONOHUE, M.D.

Contributors

John Peter Blandy, M.A., D.M., M.Ch., F.R.C.S., F.A.C.S.
Chapter 12
Professor of Urology, University of London at the London Hospital Medical College
Consultant Urological Surgeon, St. Peter's Hospital
London, England

David L. Bronson, Ph.D.
Chapter 4
Assistant Professor and Head, Cell Biology and Urology Laboratory
Department of Urologic Surgery
University of Minnesota School of Medicine
Minneapolis, Minnesota

Judith Gann Bronson, M.S.
Chapter 4
Medical Editor
Department of Urologic Surgery
University of Minnesota School of Medicine
Minneapolis, Minnesota

John P. Donohue, M.D.
Chapter 11
Professor and Chairman, Department of Urology
Indiana University Medical Center
Indianapolis, Indiana

Lawrence H. Einhorn, M.D.
Chapters 14A and 15
Clinical Professor of Oncology
American Cancer Society
Professor of Medicine, Indiana University Medical Center
Indianapolis, Indiana

Elwin E. Fraley, M.D.
Chapters 4 and 10
Professor and Chairman
Department of Urologic Surgery
University of Minnesota School of Medicine
Minneapolis, Minnesota

John Francis Harris, Ph.D.
Chapter 3A
Assistant Professor, Department of Surgery and
Department of Medical Biophysics
University of Toronto
Toronto, Canada

H. F. Hope-Stone, M.B., B.S., D.M.R.T., F.R.C.R.
Chapter 12
Consultant Radiotherapist
Department of Urology
University of London at the London Hospital
London, England

Nasser Javadpour, M.D., F.A.C.S.
Chapter 17
Senior Investigator, National Cancer Institute
Consultant, National Naval Hospital and
Walter Reed Army Hospital
Bethesda, Maryland

Michael A. S. Jewett, M.D., F.R.C.S.(C).
Chapter 3A
Associate Professor, Department of Surgery (Urology)
University of Toronto and the Wellesley Hospital
Toronto, Ontario, Canada

Douglas E. Johnson, M.D.
Chapter 7
Professor and Head
Department of Urology
The University of Texas System Cancer Center
M. D. Anderson Hospital and Tumor Institute
Houston, Texas

Robert J. Kurman, M.D.
Chapter 5
Associate Professor, Department of Pathology and
Obstetrics and Gynecology
Georgetown University School of Medicine
Washington, D.C.

Paul H. Lange, M.D.
Chapter 6
Chief, Urology Section
Minneapolis VA Medical Center
Professor of Urologic Surgery
University of Minnesota
Minneapolis, Minnesota

Lucien E. Nochomovitz, M.B., Ch.B., M.Med. (Path.)
Chapter 2
Junior Faculty Clinical Fellow of the American Cancer Society (No. 469B)
Assistant Professor, Department of Pathology
The George Washington University Medical Center
Washington, D.C.

R. T. D. Oliver, M.D., M.C.R.P.
Chapter 12
Senior Lecturer and Honorary Consultant in Oncology
The London Hospital Medical College,
St Bartholomew's Hospital, London, and
St Peter's Hospital and Institute of Urology
London, England

M. J. Peckham, M.D.
Chapter 16
Institute of Cancer Research and
The Royal Marsden Hospital
London and Surrey, England

Roger C. B. Pugh, M.D., F.R.C. (Path.)
Chapter 1
Honorary Consulting Pathologist, St. Peter's Hospitals
and the Institute of Urology
London, England

Derek Raghavan, M.B., B.S., F.R.A.C.P.
Chapter 6
Medical Oncologist
Royal Prince Alfred Hospital
Camperdown, Australia and
Honorary Consultant
Ludwig Institute for Cancer Research
Sydney, Australia

Jerome P. Richie, M.D.
Chapter 3B
Associate Professor, Harvard Medical School
Chief of Urologic Oncology, Brigham and Women's Hospital
Consultant, Sidney Farber Cancer Center
Boston, Massachusetts

Peter Scardino, M.D.
Chapter 14B
Associate Professor of Urology
Baylor College of Medicine
Houston, Texas

William Upjohn Shipley, M.D.
Chapter 13
Associate Professor of Radiation Therapy
Massachusetts General Hospital and Harvard Medical School
Boston, Massachusetts

Donald G. Skinner, M.D.
Chapter 8
Professor and Chairman
Department of Surgery, Division of Urology
University of Southern California Medical Center
Los Angeles, California

William J. Staubitz, M.D., F.A.C.S.
Chapter 9
Emeritus Professor and Chairman
Department of Urology
State University of New York at Buffalo
Attending Urologist, Veterans Administration Medical Center
Buffalo, New York

Stephen D. Williams, M.D.
Chapters 14A and 15
Associate Professor of Medicine
Indiana University Medical Cen-
Indianapolis, Indiana

Contents

1

Pathology of Testicular Tumors—A British Perspective

R. C. B. Pugh, M.D., F.R.C. (Path.)

The main purpose of this chapter is to present the more important features of the British Testicular Tumour Panel (TTP) classification of testicular tumors[33] and where possible to relate it to the World Health Organization (WHO)[23] and AFIP classifications.[6, 22] As a first step it would perhaps be as well to consider very briefly some of the features which any classification should possess if it is to be useful and generally acceptable, though it must be recognized that the ideal scheme which will satisfy every specialist interested in the diagnosis of testicular tumors and the treatment of patients, be they surgeons, radiotherapists, oncologists, pathologists, experimentalists, embryologists or chemists, has yet to be written. The needs of the clinician are, of course, paramount—the basic requirement being simple, reliable, easily understood, pathological information which will assist in the diagnosis and assessment of prognosis in the day-to-day management of patients. In contrast the researcher and the worker in a special center or department may well require more detailed and elaborate histopathological information with which to test existing classifications and determine the value and reproducibility of new laboratory techniques and methods of tumor diagnosis. The two types of classification fulfill specific needs, and, moreover, are not mutually exclusive.

In order to maintain their validity it is essential that all histopathological classifications are reviewed from time to time to take full account of recent advances in pathology and many other related scientific disciplines. This is especially true of the four classifications under discussion here, which were published between the years 1952 and 1977 but were in the process of compilation many years before these dates. In them, tumors were grouped, and divided and subdivided, on the basis of the histological appearances with the light microscope. Hormone studies were by no means a regular procedure in every patient, and the techniques were not standardized either, so that, not surprisingly, the results were often difficult to interpret. Staging methods were very much less precise than they are today and the now familiar controversy of radiotherapy *versus* lymph node dissection in the treatment of teratomas was at its height,[45, 51] with chemotherapy reserved for the patients failing to respond to other forms of treatment. Nevertheless, despite the different treatment regimes certain tumor groups acquired prognostic significance. But all this was against a background of continual change in many fields of investigation and treatment; for instance, it was shown quite conclusively that the use of increasingly powerful radiation in the treatment of seminoma had a beneficial effect on the prognosis.[43] Also the use of chemotherapy as a primary treatment[18] and an appreciation of the fact that radiotherapy, chemotherapy and surgery may have a place in the sequential treatment of a single patient with testicular disease[9] (rather than the radiotherapy *versus* surgery arguments of earlier years), coupled with better staging techniques, are producing clinical results which are unbelievably good when judged by yesterday's standards.[7, 29] It is not yet absolutely clear where these different treatment methods are leading but it is evident that some of the follow-up information obtained in the 1960s and 1970s is virtually useless as a prognostic yardstick at the present time and, indeed, might even be considered to be in some respects apocryphal. This excludes groups of patients, for example children with yolk sac tumors, treated primarily by simple orchidectomy and for whom other forms of therapy, such as radiotherapy and chemotherapy, were reserved only for patients with late metastatic disease.[33] There have been equally dramatic changes within the last few years with the introduction of serum and tissue markers,[5, 11–13, 15–17, 26, 35] the refinement of cytohistochemical methods,[14] development of tissue culture techniques,[54] use of xenografts,[34] the identification of surface antigens[24] and numerous animal experimental models.[4, 45] Some of this work is at a relatively early stage, but already some of the ideas and concepts of what might aptly be termed the light microscope tear are being challenged by these various laboratory procedures, and some tumor groups are either being refined down or enlarged or have been shown to be in need of redefinition.

Histopathological classifications of tumors at virtually any site in the body themselves fall into two broad groups—the "splitters" and the "lumpers" and each group has its advantages and disadvantages, its advocates and its opponents, and sometimes what in practice are really quite minor points of difference and interpretation appear to prevent correlation of two different classifications. In essence the 1973 AFIP[22] and WHO groupings[23] are each an example of a splitting classification based on histological appearances whereas the 1952[6] AFIP and TTP[32] schemes are "lumpers" in which histological groups are correlated with tumor behavior and survival rate figures. Moreover, despite their nomenclatural differences, these latter two do not differ in any substantial degree so far as the broad tumor groupings are concerned except in the identification in the TTP classification of the yolk sac tumor and the spermatocytic seminoma, and the separate designation of those tumors containing teratomatous and seminomatous elements as combined tumors.

Much of the controversy over attempts to correlate the TTP and the WHO and 1973 AFIP classifications reflects differing concepts of histogenesis[21] and, while there is no denying the weight of experimental evidence supporting the germ cell theory upon which the latter two are based, a great deal of work yet remains to be done to clarify the early stages of tumor induction in the human testis.[32, 45] Evidence is accumulating that seminomas and nonseminomatous tumors may arise from a common stem cell[42] but the kinetics of the germinal epithelial cell are virtually unexplored.

GENERAL CONSIDERATIONS

In the TTP series[33] nearly 95% of the tumors proved to be seminomas, teratomas, combined tumors (*i.e.* seminoma and teratoma in the same testis) yolk sac tumors and malignant lymphomas, and the discussion here will be concerned with the first four of the five groups. So far as its general findings are concerned the TTP series does not differ significantly from other published accounts, and reference to the figures published some 5 years ago is still valid as subsequent experience has not materially altered them. A detailed account is not necessary here though several points are worthy of note.

Tumors occurred more often on the right than on the left side and were bilateral in just over 3% of patients, malignant lymphoma being the commonest and seminoma the next most common tumors to occur bilaterally. Involvement of the two sides was more often successive than simultaneous. In 6.3% of the patients there was a history of undescended testis and in nearly one-fifth of the patients the tumor developed in the normally descended testis, the majority being seminomas. Three-quarters of all tumors occurred between the ages of 20 and 49 years. Prepubertal patients were found most commonly to have malignant lymphomas, differentiated teratomas or yolk sac tumors; the mean age at orchidectomy of seminoma and teratoma patients was, respectively, 41.2 and 29.8 years, and malignant lymphoma was the commonest neoplasm in patients more than 70 years of age, though very occasionally seminomas and teratomas occurred in these older subjects.

The commonest presenting symptom was painless testicular enlargement, though some patients first sought advice for subfertility and others, less fortunate, first went to their doctors with symptoms later shown to be due to metastatic disease. Excluding the cases of bilateral tumors, just over 1% of all the patients in the series developed a second tumor subsequent to orchidectomy—carcinoma of the bronchus in 17 and carcinoma of the bowel in 6 patients. In more than half of these patients the second tumor was responsible for their death. Little useful information with regard to family history, duration of symptoms and the possible influence of trauma on tumor development could be obtained from the TTP series.

EXAMINATION OF SPECIMEN: PATHOLOGICAL STAGING

Nodularity or other deformity of the testis obviously leads the surgeon to suspect tumor when the testis is explored but another very useful indicator of neoplasm is the presence of thick ribbon-like vessels, coursing over the surface of the tunica albuginea (Fig. 1.1). These contrast with the usually much smaller reticulated pattern, not infrequently accompanied

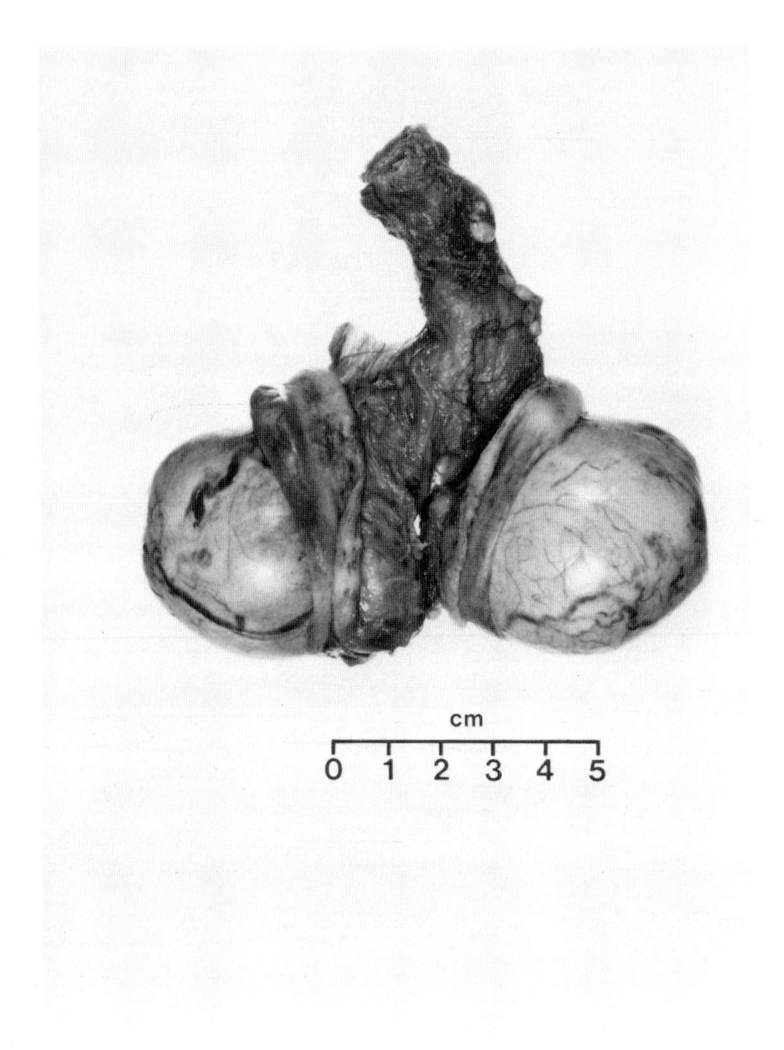

Figure 1.1. The testis has been cut into and opened out to show the prominent ribbon-like vessels on the external surface. The tumor in the body of the testis proved to be a malignant teratoma.

by adhesions, often seen when there is underlying inflammatory disease of the testis. Testicular biopsy is considered to have no place in the diagnosis of testicular tumor.[2]

The pathologist must always sample the neoplastic testis extensively and systematically and it is essential that, in addition to representative areas of tumor tissue, generous blocks are taken from the rete testis, the epididymis, lower cord, the cord at the level of surgical section and the non-neoplastic parts of the body of the testis. This will permit an assessment of the pathological stage of the tumor (Fig. 1.2). Tissue should also be preserved in appropriate fixatives if special studies, such as electron-microscopy and localization of markers, are to be undertaken. When possible fresh tissue should be placed in liquid nitrogen and banked so that it will be readily available for study at a later date as and when new marker or other techniques are developed. Once blocks have been taken, specimens must be preserved in fixative until the clinicians are fully

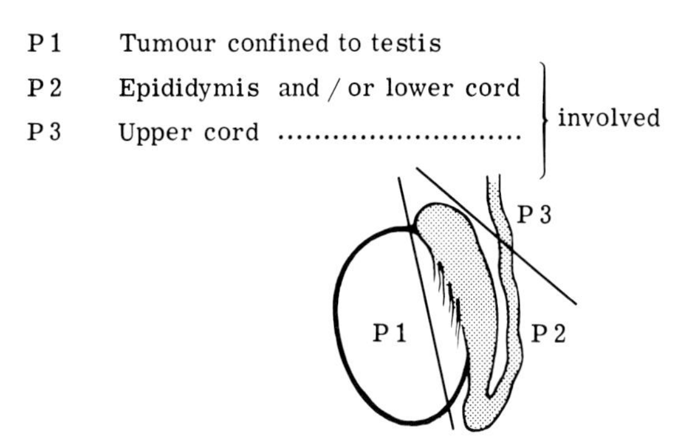

Figure 1.2. Diagrammatic representation of the pathological stages of testicular tumors.

satisfied that the postoperative course is in accord with the histopathological diagnosis.

SEMINOMA

This, the commonest single type of primary testicular tumor, occurs in two forms—the much commoner classical type and the spermatocytic variety[19] which accounts for less than 5% of all seminomas and occurs in slightly older patients, with a peak incidence in the fifth decade.

The classical seminoma usually produces a moderate, smooth or bosselated enlargement of the body of the testis and typically the cut surface is smooth, pale pinkish/white; it is usually well demarcated from the surrounding testicular tissue but sometimes replaces it entirely. Sharply outlined areas of necrosis are not uncommon.

Microscopically there is a very characteristic uniformity of the cells which are spheroidal with clear or finely granular cytoplasm and rounded nuclei, frequently with prominent nucleoli. Mitotic figures are usually relatively sparse. Cells tend to be arranged in sheets or columns; diffuse or focal lymphocytic infiltration is seen in most tumors, and in about a third of them granulomatous areas consisting of endothelioid cells with or without small giant cells are to be found (Fig. 1.3). Tumor giant cells may be seen and must always be interpreted with care and only with full information of serum marker levels, preferably coupled with marker localization studies. The giant cells which resemble mulberries (Fig. 1.4), formed by the coalescence of tumor cells, do not contain human chorionic gonadotrophin (HCG) and are not of prognostic significance.[50] Other, usually much more pleomorphic, giant cells (Fig. 1.5) resembling trophoblast may contain βHCG. Their presence is more disturbing and must prompt further sectioning of the operation specimen to see if there is an obvious nonseminomatous tumor element present. In a very few cases no teratoma can be found and the precise significance of the giant cells is as yet unresolved. Serum levels of markers[17] are of crucial value in diagnosis and, if in a patient with an apparently "pure" seminoma the serum α-fetoprotein (AFP) is raised, this must be taken to indicate the presence of a nonseminomatous germ cell tumor, provided that hepatic disease can be excluded. On the other hand, a raised serum βHCG level is consistent

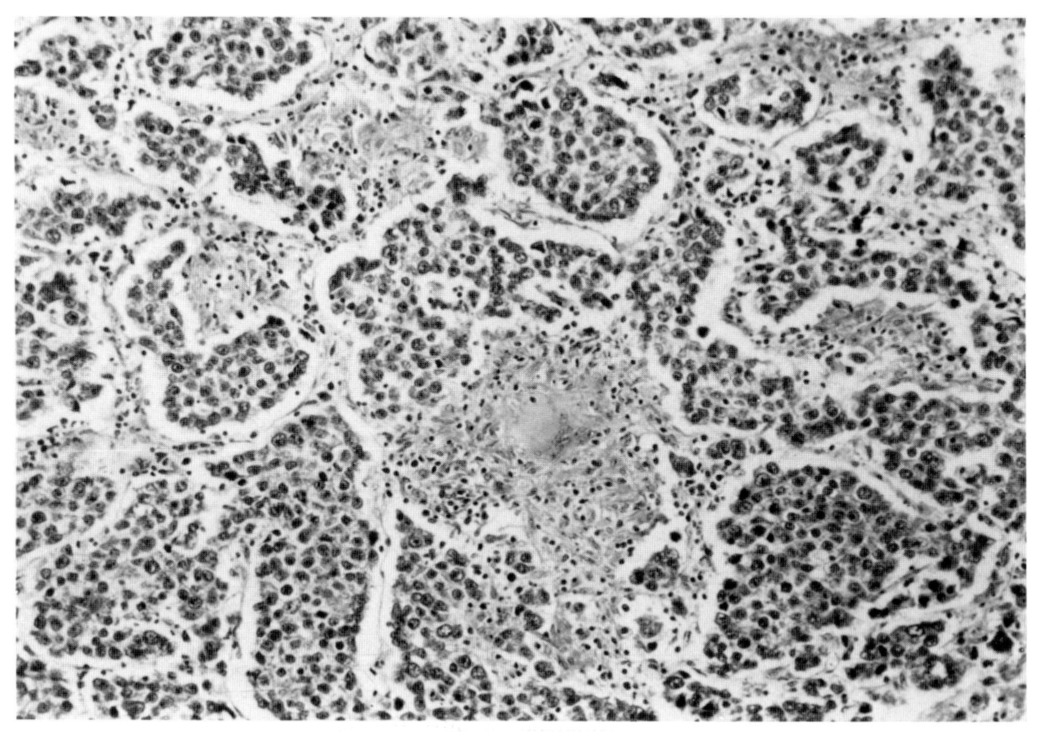

Figure 1.3. Classical type of seminoma, diffusely infiltrated with lymphocytes and with a central granulomatous area (H&E × 40; enlargement × 4.5).

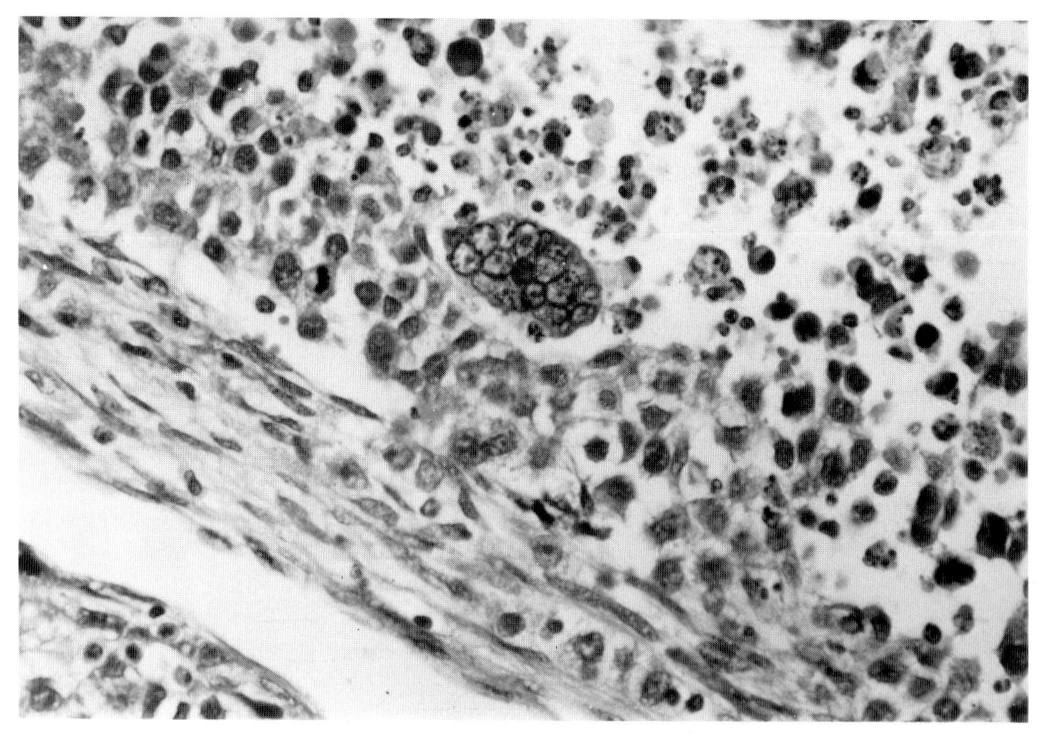

Figure 1.4. "Mulberry" cell in classical seminoma: negative staining for HCG (immunoperoxidase × 100; enlargement × 5).

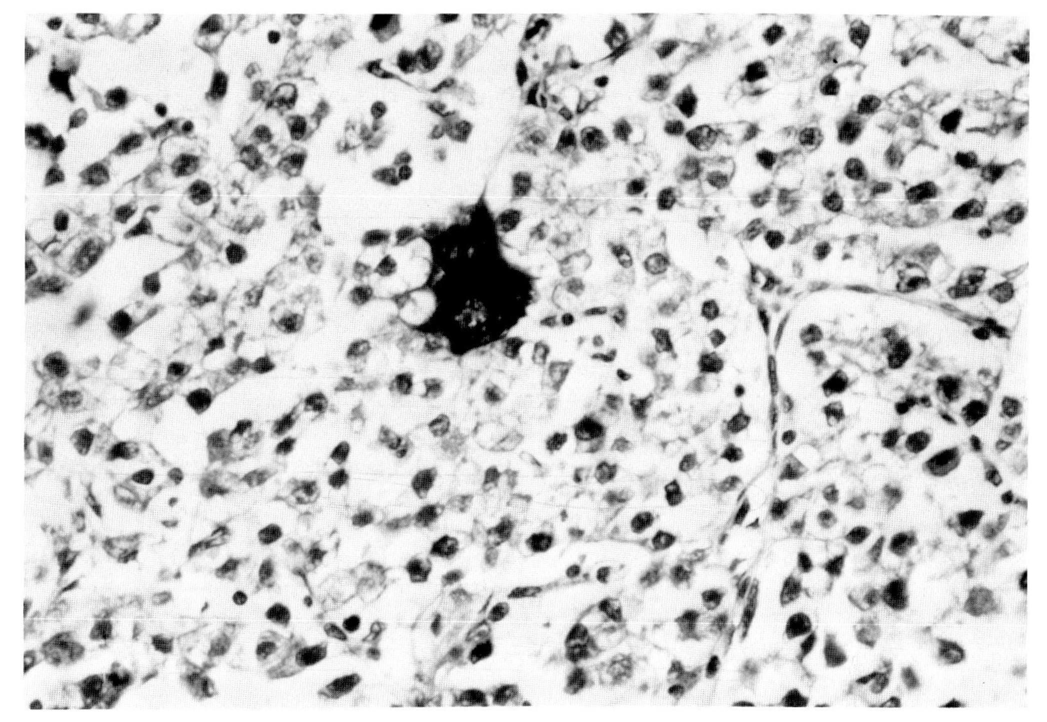

Figure 1.5. Pleomorphic giant cell in seminoma: positive staining for HCG (immunoperoxidase × 100; enlargement × 4.5).

with a diagnosis of both seminoma and nonseminomatous germ cell tumors.

Spread and Metastases

Local spread of tumor into the rete testis occurs frequently, often to be followed by extension into the epididymis and lower cord; nodular involvement of the epididymis may be mistaken clinically for a cyst and is occasionally explored as such. Involvement of the para-aortic, mediastinal and cervical lymph nodes and extralymphatic structures forms the basis of clinical staging. This is fully discussed in Chapter 3 and will not be considered further here. Tumor cells are not infrequently seen in tubules in the testicular tissue around the edge of a seminoma and, as will be described later, may represent either intratubular permeation or *in situ* neoplasia.

Prognosis

In the TTP series the factor with the greatest influence on prognosis was the presence of metastases at the time of orchidectomy—the 3-year corrected survival rates being respectively 93% and 55% in patients without and with metastatic deposits. There was no significant difference between the survival rates of patients with P1, P2 and P3 pathological stage tumors. Other factors such as the age of the patient, size of tumor and the specific histological features of lymphocytic infiltration, granulomatous response, lymphatic and vascular invasion, mitotic rate and the presence of necrosis had only a slight effect.[50]

Spermatocytic Seminoma

The spermatocytic seminoma is often larger than the classical variety and its cut surface is usually cream colored or yellow and it may be slightly gelatinous. Microscopically there are sheets of plump pleomorphic cells with large nuclei in which there is a coarse chromatin network; smaller, darker staining, cells are also seen and giant cell forms and multinucleate cells are not infrequent. Mitotic figures are usually abundant and there is a striking resemblance to active non-neoplastic spermatogenetic epithelium. Intratubular neoplastic cells are a very common feature (Fig. 1.6). Despite the somewhat bizarre histological appearances the prognosis is good and there are few authenticated examples of metastatic spread or death due to this tumor.[21, 50]

The spermatocytic seminoma does not feature in the 1952 AFIP publication while the 1973 AFIP and WHO classifications each recognizes the same two types described above. Though the TTP records that some seminomas are poorly differentiated and have a relatively poor prognosis[50] their designation as a separate group, such as the anaplastic seminoma,[22] is not considered necessary.

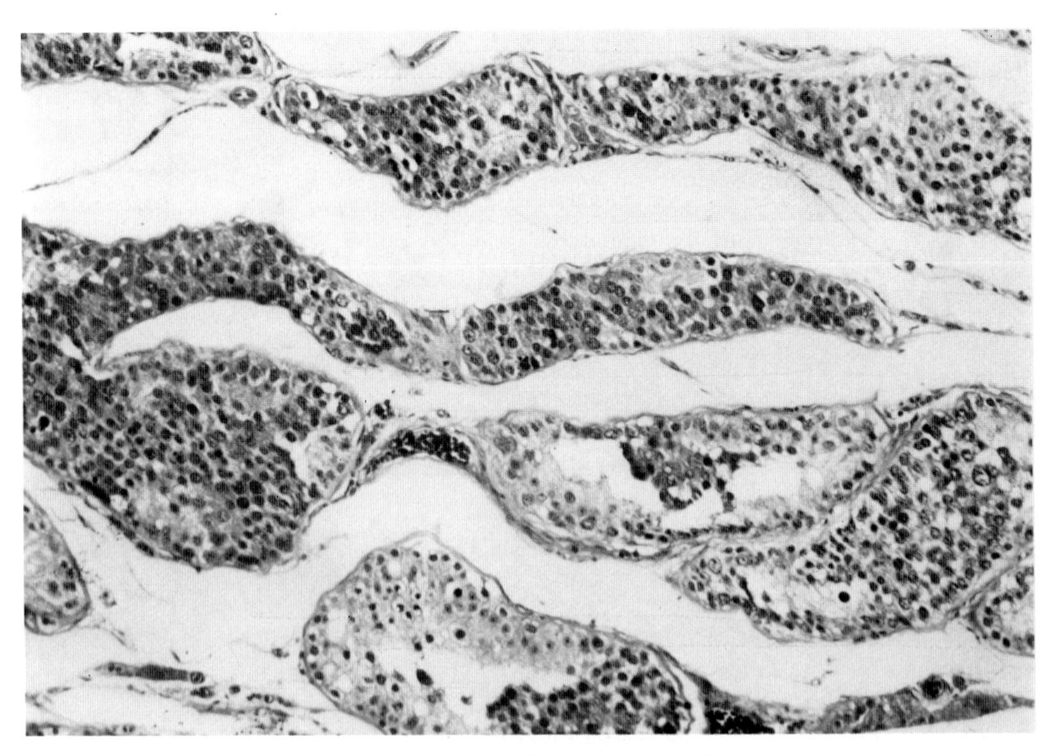

Figure 1.6. Tumor cells within spermatic tubules at the periphery of a spermatocytic seminoma (H&E × 40; enlargement × 4.5).

TERATOMA

It is in the group of teratomatous—or nonseminomatous—tumors that the major difficulties arise when attempting to integrate the British and American tumor classifications. Some of the problems relate to histological criteria and definition and others to the way in which the spectrum of histological appearances is subdivided into various groupings. Apart from differences of nomenclature the similarities between the TTP and 1952 AFIP classifications far outnumber their differences as regards both histological definition and tumor groupings, but correlation of the TTP and the WHO and later AFIP classifications is not quite so straightforward.

The external surface of the teratomatous testis differs little, if at all, from the testis containing a seminoma but on the cut surface there are varying amounts of solid tissue and cysts, often with considerable variation in different parts of the same tumor. The cysts frequently contain glairy fluid and in many tumors there are extensive areas of hemorrhage and necrosis.

Microscopically the TTP recognizes four groups of teratoma—the differentiated teratoma (TD), the malignant teratoma intermediate type (MTI), the undifferentiated malignant teratoma (MTU) and the malignant trophoblastic teratoma (MTT).

Differentiated Teratoma (TD)

The majority of these tumors occur in children and do not usually present any very great diagnostic difficulty, being predominantly cystic and composed of fully mature elements. Derivatives of all three germ layers can usually be identified and the epithelium lining the cysts may be of all types, and the surrounding mesodermal tissue is comprised of mature connective tissue in which cartilage, smooth muscle and sometimes bone may be seen. Skin with its appendages occurs occasionally. In some of these tumors in children the tissues, and especially the nonepithelial elements, are not always fully differentiated, and it is therefore important to distinguish between immature and neoplastic tissues (Fig. 1.7). In the TTP material all teratomas in children occurring below the age of 10 years, whatever their histological appearances, behaved in a benign fashion.

Tumors apparently composed of fully differentiated tissues occur occasionally in adults but their behavior is by no means so predictable. They often contain more solid tissue than do their counterparts in children and the only distinction between a differentiated teratoma in an adult and a malignant one is that no unequivocally malignant areas can be identified after extensive histological sampling. In children it is usually the nonepithelial elements which have to be examined carefully to make the distinction between immaturity and neoplastic change but in adults it is the appearances of the epithelium which tend to cause the pathologist the most difficulty. The TTP files contain records of 19 adults (with a mean age of 34 years at orchidectomy) in whom a diagnosis of differentiated testicular teratoma was made. Fifteen of these men remain alive

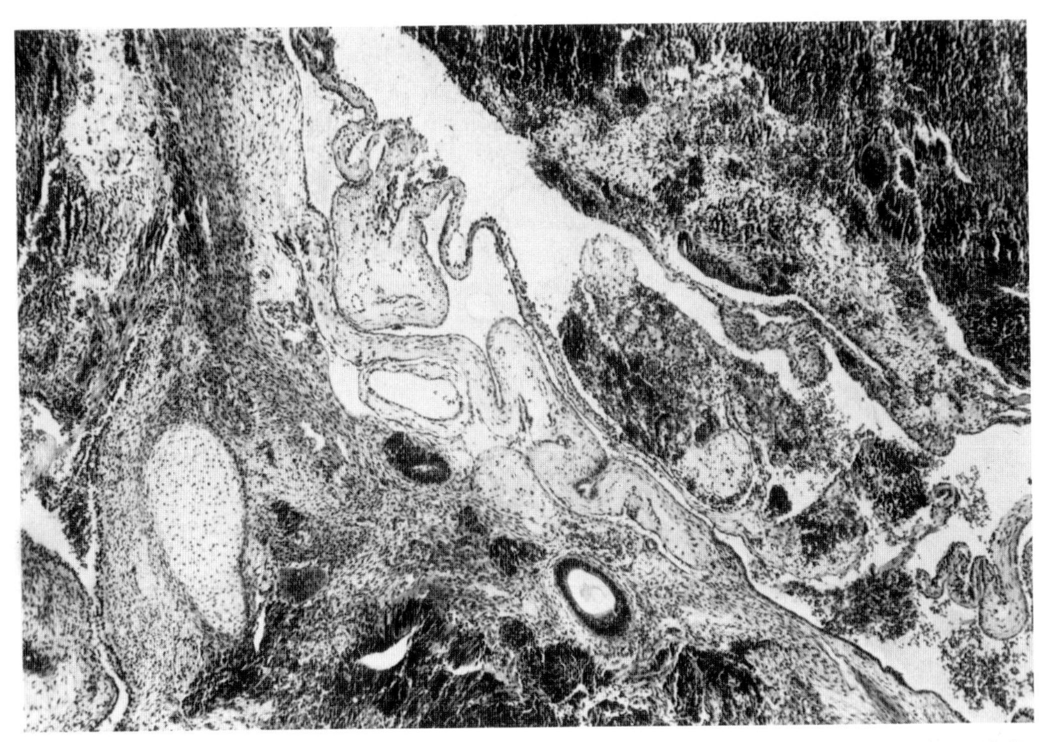

Figure 1.7. Immature teratoma in a child aged 5 years. Note the cartilage (*left*), mature epithelium (*lower center*) and the mass of incompletely differentiated, probably neural, tissue (*top right*) (H&E × 16; enlargement × 4.5).

and well for periods of from 2¾–11 years (mean 7½ years) following a simple orchidectomy, but four others died with multiple metastases and were found to have only fully differentiated testicular teratoma at autopsy. These cases were all diagnosed and treated before tumor markers became an essential feature in clinical management, but from the histological point of view the distinction between complete and incomplete differentiation may be extremely difficult.

In the 1952 AFIP classification a teratoma is described as "a chaotic arrangement of various differentiated tissues corresponding to either fetal or adult stages in development," thus making the distinction between the mature and immature without categorizing the latter. The 1973 AFIP publication uses the terms mature and immature in the same sense as the TTP, and the WHO classification includes a third group—teratoma with malignant transformation—which would seem to fall within the intermediate malignant teratoma group (MTI) of the TTP which is described below. The statement that the use of the word malignant in respect of the types of teratoma other than the differentiated teratoma implies that the differentiated teratoma is benign[22] can be dimissed as a *non sequitur*.

Malignant Teratoma Intermediate (MTI)

These tumors, which constitute the largest subgroup of teratoma, contain fully differentiated elements similar to those seen in the TD group as well as undoubtedly malignant areas, which may be entirely epithelial or a mixture of epithelial and mesenchymal elements or, least commonly, of mesenchymal type only. The distinction from TD depends on finding malignant areas and from the undifferentiated teratoma (MTU) described below by the presence of connective tissue elements such as bone, cartilage, smooth muscle bundles and areas of organoid differentiation in which mature epithelium, usually cuboidal or columnar with or without mucus secretion, connective tissue and smooth muscle are mutually orientated to reproduce structures resembling bronchioles or bowel structures (Fig. 1.8). The appearances are usually very diverse and tissues from any or all germ cell layers may be identified. Not infrequently the obviously malignant areas resemble poorly differentiated carcinoma (and are similar to the undifferentiated teratoma). Tumor giant cells occur in about one-third of tumors and yolk sac-like areas are also seen in some tumors. The MTI group is considered to be the equivalent of the 1952 AFIP teratocarcinoma and the 1973 AFIP teratoma with embryonal carcinoma. It corresponds with two groups in the WHO classification—teratoma with malignant transformation and teratoma with embryonal carcinoma.

A criticism that has been made of the TTP definition is that, contrary to usual practice in tumor pathology, the diagnosis of MTI is based on the most differentiated part of the tumor.[22] The simple answer is that if such attempts to upgrade a tumor are not made there would be, in effect, only two grades of tumor—the differentiated and the undifferentiated.

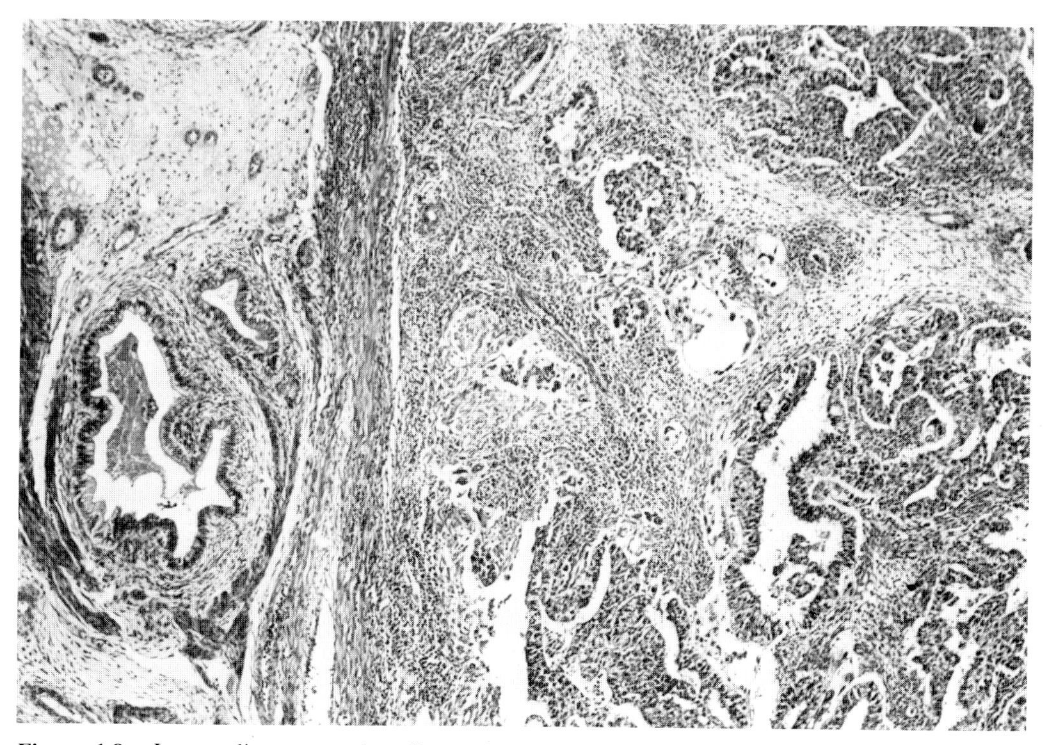

Figure 1.8. Intermediate type of malignant teratoma (MTI). Note the fully differentiated "organoid" structure on the *left*, separated by a band of smooth muscle from poorly differentiated adenocarcinomatous tumor on the right. (H&E × 16; enlargement × 4.5).

Follow-up information has demonstrated beyond all doubt the value from the prognostic point of view of defining an intermediate type.[33] Furthermore, the term teratocarcinoma[6, 8] (the equivalent of MTI) enjoys the cachet of respectability, is widely used in the world literature and would seem to have escaped similar opprobrium.

Quantitation of the various elements within a tumor is another contentious subject[21-23] but the attempt is probably of limited value unless *all* specimens are sampled in a strictly comparable fashion and in reality nothing short of serial sectioning, clearly an inpracticability in the busy routine laboratory, will provide precise information. This is not to deny the need to record the presence of unusual appearances or specific cell types.

Malignant Teratoma Undifferentiated (MTU)

In these tumors, the next largest subgroup of teratoma, there are no organoid areas or differentiated structures to be found and the appearances range from sheets of closely packed pleomorphic carcinomatous-looking cells (Fig. 1.9) to adenocarcinomatous zones in which clefts and spaces are to be seen surrounded by a variable amount of connective tissue stroma (Fig. 1.8, *right*). Mitoses are frequently very numerous, multinucleate cells occur and, in just over a third of the cases, tumor giant cells are found. Areas resembling the yolk sac tumor of children occur from time to time as well as structures not unlike embryoid bodies.

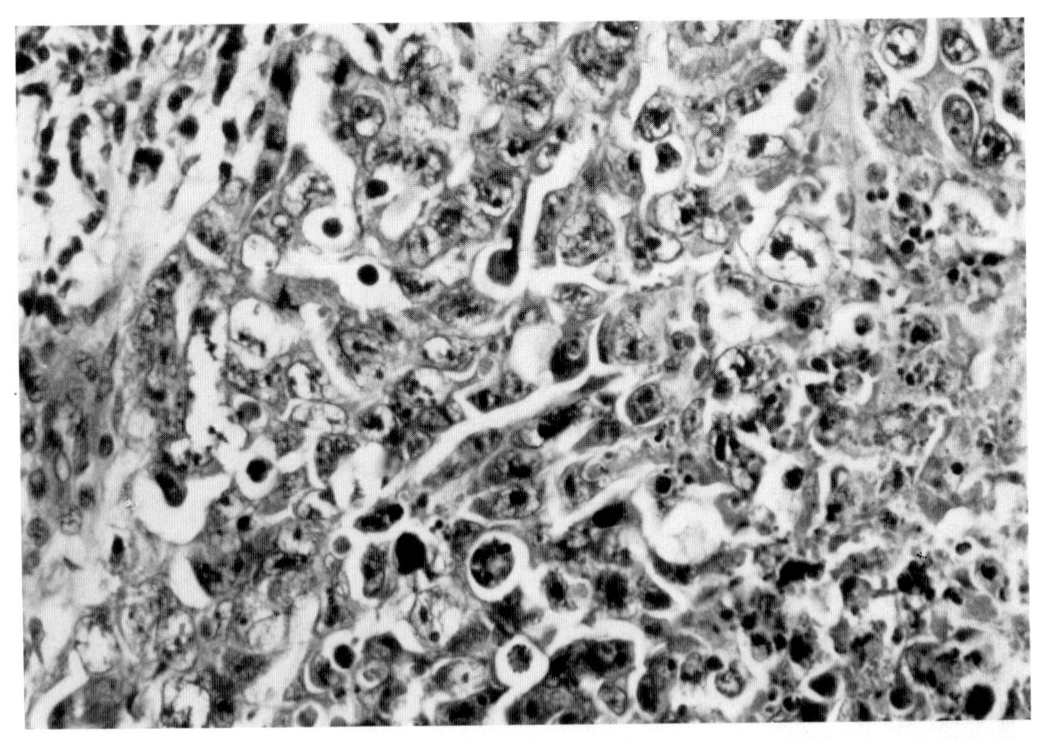

Figure 1.9. Undifferentiated malignant teratoma (MTU) consisting of sheets of closely packed pleomorphic cells with large pale vesicular nuclei (H&E × 100; enlargement × 4.5).

It is sometimes difficult to distinguish this tumor from a poorly differentiated seminoma and it is also worth recalling that problems may also occur when metastatic deposits of adenocarcinomatous type occur in the testis or adnexae. In the TTP series the majority of such tumors were found to have originated in the prostate.

The MTU group corresponds to the embryonal carcinoma in the 1952 AFIP and WHO classifications. The 1973 AFIP scheme widens the embryonal carcinoma group to comprise three separate tumors, the adult embryonal carcinoma (corresponding to MTU), the polyembryoma (a rare tumor which is composed entirely of embryoid bodies and not recognized as a separate subgroup by the TTP) and the infantile embryonal carcinoma which in the WHO and TTP classifications is designated as yolk sac tumor.

Malignant Teratoma Trophoblastic (MTT)

The majority of these, fortunately rare, tumors exhibit extensive areas of hemorrhage and necrosis on their cut surfaces and a very characteristic microscopic finding is a rim of tumor cells around a central mass of hemorrhage. In order to make the diagnosis syncytiotrophoblast and cytotrophoblast must be identified and the two should ideally be arranged in a papillary or villus pattern (Fig. 1.10). Care must be taken not to confuse "syncytiotrophoblast" with true trophoblastic tumors. What does or does not constitute a villus pattern is a matter of debate, but as the very poor prognosis in the TTP cases with and without villi is but little

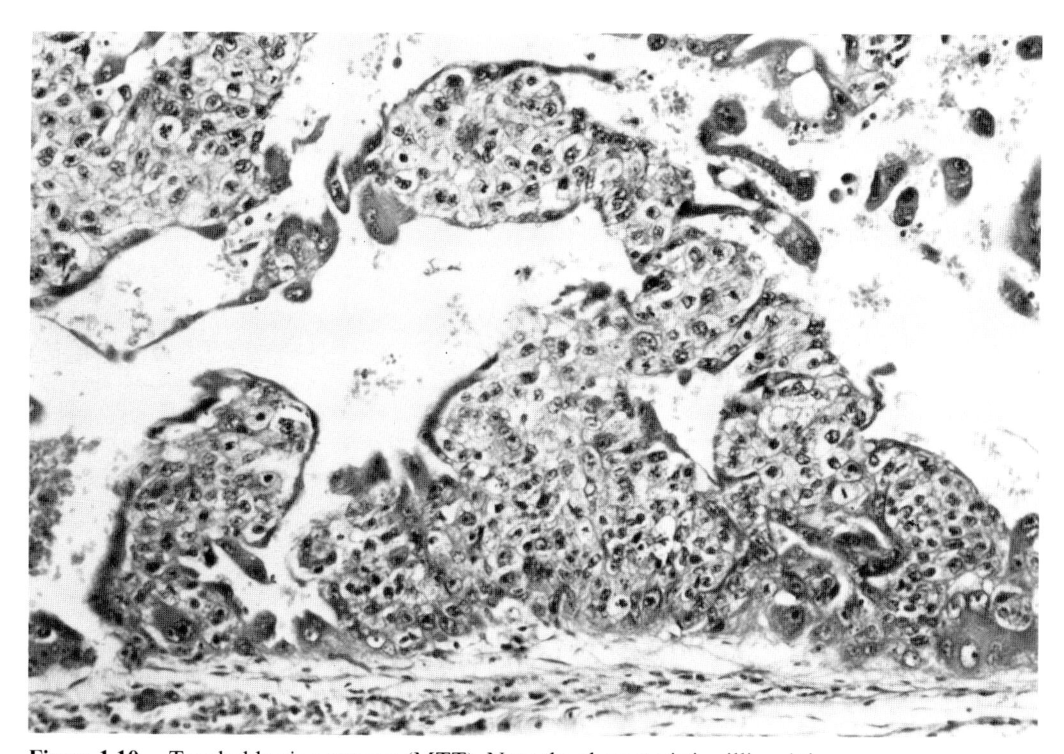

Figure 1.10. Trophoblastic teratoma (MTT). Note the characteristic villi and the two cell types (H&E × 40; enlargement × 4.5).

different,[33] it possibly may not be an absolutely essential diagnostic feature. The TTP definition differs from the ones in the 1973 AFIP and WHO classifications where the villus pattern is not a prerequisite for diagnosis, though the 1952 AFIP publication states that there is "always some formation of villus-like structures." Another, important, difference concerns the amount of trophoblastic tissue that is present. In the TTP scheme the diagnosis is made whatever the size of the trophoblastic area relative to the total amount of tumor present, whereas the 1973 AFIP and WHO classifications separate tumors composed only of choriocarcinoma (a tumor, incidentally, yet to be seen in the TTP files) from those in which other elements occur and which are diagnosed, for example, as choriocarcinoma plus embryonal carcinoma. The distinction is considered to be justified because of differences in survival.

Pulmonary metastases composed entirely of trophoblastic tumor tissue are sometimes seen in patients with apparently fully differentiated teratomas or with scars, or "burnt out" tumors, in their testis.[1]

Tumor Giant Cells

Large syncytial giant cells (syncytiotrophoblasts) occur in between one-third and one-half of all teratomas (Fig. 1.11) often in close relation to thin-walled blood vessels and must be clearly distinguished from the syncytial cells of the trophoblastic tumor described above. Using the recently introduced and technically reliable immunoperoxidase technique it has been shown that both types of giant cell contain HCG.[10] Serum levels of βHCG are raised in true trophoblastic tumor,[5, 14] and in 33–89%

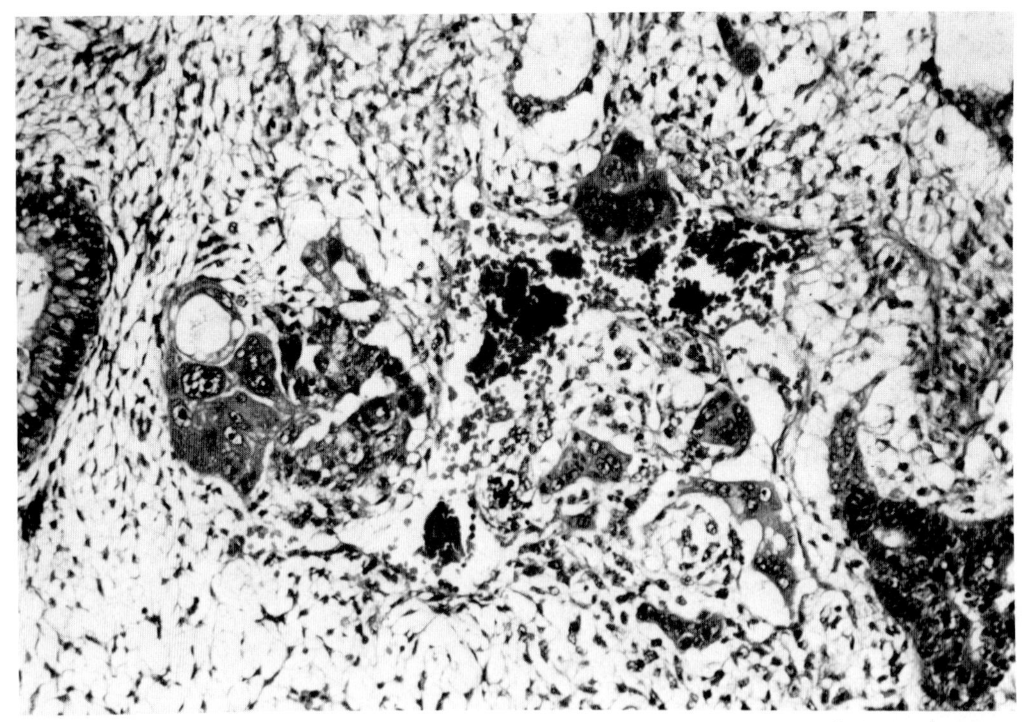

Figure 1.11. Syncytial giant cells in close relation to thin-walled vascular spaces in a malignant teratoma (H&E × 40; enlargement × 4.5).

of active teratoma,[5, 11, 16, 26, 35] as well as in 5–22% of patients with seminoma,[5, 12, 13, 16, 26, 35] leading to the suggestion that the raised serum levels were produced by the giant cells containing the HCG. In its 1976 analysis the TTP found that malignant teratoma trophoblastic (MTT) had a uniformly bad prognosis but that the presence of giant cells in MTI and MTU tumors had little effect on survival though it must be appreciated that no HCG localizing studies were carried out at that time.[33] However, recent re-examination of 86 of these MTI cases, all in P1 pathological stage, in which HCG localization studies were performed has failed to demonstrate any difference in survival at 3 years between patients with HCG-positive giant cells and those without giant cells.[20] This contrasts with an earlier report that MTIs with HCG-positive giant cells had a worse prognosis than similar tumors in which the hormone could not be localized.[25]

Several questions arise—is a villus pattern one of the morphological criteria essential for the diagnosis of MTT?; should the relative amounts of trophoblast and other elements determine the categorization of a trophoblastic tumor?; should the diagnosis of trophoblastic tumor be based only on morphological grounds or must βHCG localization be taken into account, and if so how? And, finally, do syncytial giant cells and true trophoblastic tumors represent the two extremes of a single spectrum?[31] These are all fundamental questions which must await answer until more truly comparable control studies have been carried out.

Yolk Sac Elements in Teratoma

Though there is usually little difficulty in making the diagnosis of yolk sac tumor in children, much the same sort of problems as those relating to giant cells arise with the identification and import of yolk sac elements in teratomatous tumors in adults (Fig. 1.12). These areas are referred to very briefly in the TTP monograph and in the 1973 AFIP and WHO publications, but there are widely differing views regarding their incidence, figures from 37–89% being quoted in the literature.[30, 46, 53] There are also differences with respect to their prognostic significance, some authors believing that they do not affect the outlook,[53] whereas others believe the prognosis to be worsened[46] or to be dismal.[30] As some of the differences in incidence are obviously due to varying interpretations of the histological appearances it was hoped that tissue localization of AFP would help to establish a firm morphological/cytohistochemical basis for diagnosis, but unfortunately the immunoperoxidase technique is not yet sufficiently refined or accurate to have the necessary reliability.[21] Until a firm tissue diagnosis of yolk sac elements can be made their prognostic significance obviously cannot be established. Moreover, once satisfactory criteria are laid down the problem of categorizing the tumors containing them remains and there is an urgent need for prospective studies correlating morphological appearances, serum AFP levels and clinical behavior.[31]

Atypical Intratubular Cells

Considerable interest has centered recently on the finding of atypical cells in testicular tubules and there has been much speculation as to their

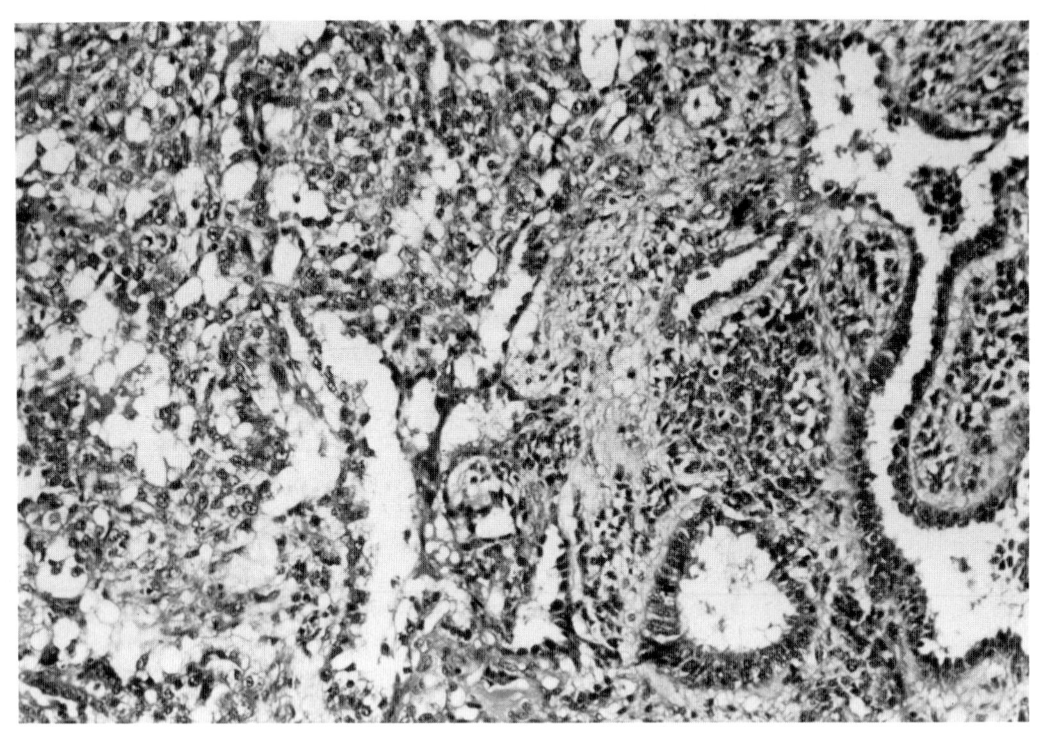

Figure 1.12. Yolk sac element (*left*) in an undifferentiated malignant teratoma—MTU (*right*)—in a 32-year-old patient (H&E × 40; enlargement × 4.5).

significance.[42] Pathologists have long been familiar with unusual, often hyperchromatic, cells in the tubules around the periphery of a testicular tumor[36] and while some clearly resulted from degenerative changes in the spermatic epithelium or to direct intratubular spread of tumor cells others appear to be arising from the epithelium itself suggesting *in situ* neoplastic change (Fig. 1.13). The finding of cells of this type in the atrophic testis of between 0.5–1.0% of infertile men in Denmark,[37, 38, 40] later confirmed from Switzerland,[28, 36] has focused attention on to the problem anew. Eight of the 16 infertile subjects studied by the Danish and Swiss workers developed testicular tumors; three were seminomas, one an embryonal carcinoma, two were teratocarcinomas and in two patients atypical cells were seen infiltrating the interstitial tissues of the testis. Though these cells had all the characteristics of malignancy it has not so far been possible to identify them more precisely and to establish whether they are truly totipotential primordial cells or if they are to some extent differentiated and already have been programmed to develop into a seminoma or teratoma. Similar atypical intratubular cells have been seen in between 2–8% of undescended testes,[36, 42] in the contralateral testis in 4–5% of patients with testicular tumor[39] and in an as yet undetermined proportion of patients of ambiguous sex.[41] In Denmark the finding of these cells in the infertile patient warrants immediate orchidectomy, but the Swiss[36] workers have so far preferred to adopt a watch-and-wait policy. The management of the patients in the other three "risk" groups has yet to be decided.

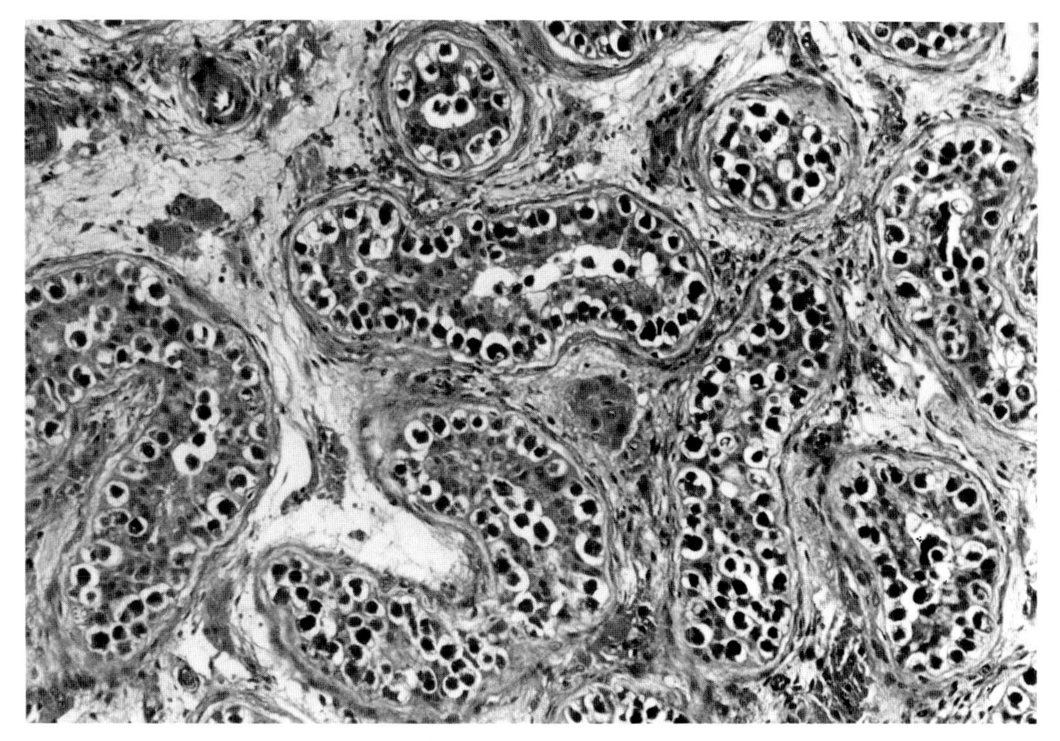

Figure 1.13. Atypical germ cells in spermatic tubules at the periphery of an adenocarcinomatous (MTU) tumor. Similar atypical cells were found deep to the epithelium lining the rete testis (H&E × 40; Enlargement × 4.5).

Once these malignant intratubular cells can be fully characterized, for example by the techniques already referred to such as tissue culture, transplantable xenografts, determination of cell surface molecules and DNA measurements, there will be a very much greater understanding of the earlier stages of tumor development.

Spread and Metastases

Teratoma spreads in the same manner as seminoma though direct extension into the epididymis is less often encountered. As a generalization the metastases are usually less well differentiated than the primary from which they arise with the exception, already referred to, of the rare cases in which pulmonary trophoblastic deposits are found in patients with a differentiated testicular primary.

Prognosis

In the "premarker" days when the TTP series was being collated, the majority of patients were treated by orchidectomy and radiotherapy, and the factors influencing prognosis were the histological type of the tumor, the presence or absence of metastatic disease at the time of orchidectomy and the pathological stage of the tumor. The 3-year corrected survival rate was considered to be a useful prognostic yardstick and was shown to be 47% for all teratomas; the figures for TD, MTI, MTU and MTT being, respectively, 92%, 52%, 38% and 19% (this last figure being based on very small numbers and therefore of doubtful significance). In the whole group the survival rate in those patients without metastases at orchidectomy rose to 59% compared with a drop to 3% in those with demonstrable secondaries; the MTI patients without metastases had a 62% 3-year survival rate and no patient with metastases at orchidectomy survived beyond the first year. Similar trends were seen in the other subgroups. The adverse effect of rising pathological stage is exemplified in the MTI group whose overall 62% 3-year survival rate fell to 44% and 11% in P2 and P3 cases, respectively.

The histological type of the tumor and its pathological stage are still of importance in the assessment of prognosis but the current very much more accurate techniques of clinical staging, with improved lymphography and scanning methods, and the serial determination of serum levels of tumor markers must hold pride of place in this respect. The effects of new treatment measures, and in particular the influence that primary chemotherapy is likely to have, remain to be determined.

COMBINED TUMORS

In essence these tumors are composed of a teratomatous moeity of any of the types described above and a seminomatous element which is usually smaller than the teratomatous one and is invariably of classical type. The age at orchidectomy of patients with combined tumors lies between the ages of maximum incidence of teratoma and seminoma. The presence of seminoma slightly improves the survival rate when it is combined with MTI but it had no obvious effect on the survival of the MTU patient. Aside from this the factors influencing prognosis are the same as those in the teratoma group.

YOLK SAC TUMOR

The yolk sac tumor, the commonest primary testicular tumar in children, has been known for many years under a variety of different names, such as adenocarcinoma of the infant's testis, orchioblastoma[33] and prepubertal variety of embryonal carcinoma[22, 23] to cite but a few. Similarity to the malignant ovarian tumor in girls,[47, 48] believed to be of extraembryonic origin, lead to its present designation.

In the TTP series of 53 cases[3] the mean age at orchidectomy was 17 months and though at the time of that publication yolk sac-like foci were noted in some teratomas (see above) a pure form had not been encountered in an adult. However, one such specimen has recently been added to the Registry, arising in a 24-year-old mentally retarded epileptic who, on routine physical examination, was found to have an enlarged testis. The swelling was painless and had been present for about 3 months. Extensive sectioning failed to reveal any features which might suggest that a teratomatous element was present.

Macroscopically the childhood tumor is either firm or soft with some cystic areas and sometimes has a mucoid cut surface.

Microscopically there is a characteristic pattern[30] with Schiller-Duval bodies, microcystic, acinopapillary and solid nodular areas; there is a

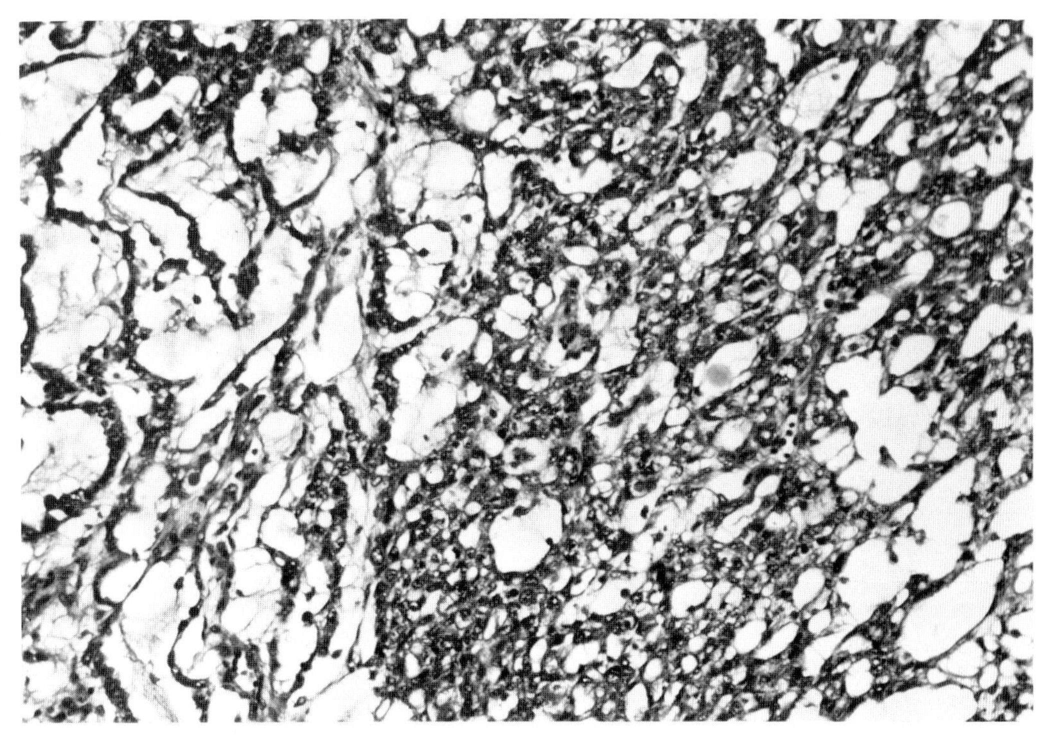

Figure 1.14. Yolk sac tumor in a child aged 10 months (H&E × 40; enlargement × 4.5).

variable amount of faintly basophilic mesenchymal stroma and many of the cells have a vacuolated cytoplasm and are actively secreting mucus (Fig. 1.14). Mitoses are frequent in some tumors. Using the immunoperoxidase technique AFP can be located without any difficulty in the tumor cells,[27, 49] a situation strikingly different from that obtaining when yolk sac-like areas are found in the teratomatous tumor of the adult.

The TTP patients were treated by orchidectomy and unless, and until, metastatic disease was evident, postorchidectomy radiotherapy or salvage chemotherapy were withheld. With this regime there was a 64% 3-year survival rate[3] which accorded well with a 60% rate found in a survey of the world literature.[52] Cellular pleomorphism, mitotic activity, vascular and lymphatic invasion were of little help in making a judgement regarding the probable behavior of a tumor, though a short history and the age of the patient were useful guides. All these patients were seen and treated in the premarker era; nowadays serial estimations of serum levels of AFP are mandatory and in the postoperative period a sustained rise may precede clinical detection of metastatic deposit by weeks or months.[43]

The yolk sac tumor does not feature in the 1952 AFIP classification. The WHO and 1973 AFIP classifications include it as a subgroup of embryonal carcinoma.

CONCLUSION

Any pathologist dealing today with the problem of classifying a testicular tumor might be forgiven for believing that clinicians often appear to have little patience with the intricacies and subtleties of this or that classification, seemingly being content with a simple distinction between seminoma and nonseminomatous tumor, thereafter concentrating their efforts on determining the site and bulk of the tumor deposits in the retroperitoneal tissues and elsewhere. This trend will surely continue until such time as pathologists are able to devise a classification which accords with histogenetic fact and theory and groups the tumors on the basis of their light microscopical appearances, histochemical affinities and prognostic significance coupled preferably with, in certain groups at any rate, an indication of those tumors which are likely to respond to particular chemotherapeutic regimes. None of the four classifications considered here fulfills all of these very demanding criteria and they are, therefore, in need of revision, though they should probably continue in use until some of the current problems are resolved. The areas which require particular attention are the precise identification of the trophoblastic and yolk sac tumors and the incorporation in a working tumor classification of information relating to serum levels and tissue localization of marker substances.

REFERENCES

1. Azzopardi, J. G., Mostofi, F. K., and Theiss, E. A. Lesions of testes observed in certain patients with widespread choriocarcinoma and related tumors. *Am. J. Pathol. 38:*207–225, 1961.
2. Blandy, J. P., Hope-Stone, H. F., and Dayan, A. D. *Tumours of the Testicle.* Heinemann, London, 1970.
3. Brown, N. J. Yolk sac tumour (orchioblastoma and other testicular tumours of childhood. In *Pathology of the Testis,* edited by R. C. B. Pugh. Blackwell, Oxford, 1976.
4. Cochin, E. Spontaneous and experimentally-produced tumours in animals. In *Pathology of the Testis,* edited by R. C. B. Pugh. Blackwell, Oxford, 1976.
5. Cochran, J. S., Walsh, P. C., Porter, J. C., Nicholson, T. C., Madden, J. D., and Peters, P. C. The endocrinology of human chorionic gonadotrophin-secreting testicular tumors: new methods in diagnosis. *J. Urol. 114:*549–555, 1975.
6. Dixon, F. J., and Moore, R. A. Tumors of the Male Sex Organs. Fascicle 31b and 32, Atlas of Tumor Pathology, Armed Forces Institute of Pathology, Washington, D.C., 1952.
7. Einhorn, L. H., and Donohue, J. *Cis*-diamminedichloro-platinum, vinblastine and bleomycin combination chemotherapy in disseminated testicular cancer. *Ann. Intern. Med. 87:*293–298, 1977.
8. Friedman, N. B., and Moore, R. A. Tumors of the testis: a report on 922 cases. *Milit. Surg. 99:*573–593, 1946.
9. Hendry, W. F., Barrett, A., McElwain, T. J., Wallace, D. M., and Peckham, M. J. The role of surgery in the combined management of metastases from malignant teratomas of the testis. *Br. J. Urol. 52:*38–44, 1980.
10. Heyderman, E., and Neville, A. M. Syncytiotrophoblasts in malignant testicular tumours. *Lancet 2:*103, 1976.
11. Javadpour, N. Biologic tumor markers in management of testicular and bladder cancer. *Urology 12:*177–183, 1978.
12. Javadpour, N., McIntire, K. R., and Waldmann, T. A. Human chorionic gonadotrophin (HCG) and alpha-fetoprotein (AFP) in sera and tumor cells of patients with testicular seminoma. *Cancer 42:*2768–2772, 1978.
13. Javadpour, N., McIntire, K. R., Waldmann, T. A., and Bergman, M. The role of alpha-fetoprotein and human chorionic gonadotrophin in seminoma. *J. Urol. 120:*687–690, 1978.
14. Kurman, R. J., Scardino, P. T., McIntire, K. R., Waldmann, T. A., and Javadpour, N. Cellular localization of alpha-fetoprotein and human chorionic gonadotrophin in germ cell tumors of the testis using an indirect immunoperoxidase technique: a new approach to classification utilizing tumor markers. *Cancer 40:*2136–2151, 1977.

15. Lange, P. H. Serum and tissue markers of testicular tumours. In *Early Detection of Testicular Cancer*, pp. 191–199, edited by N. E. Skakkebaek, J. G. Berthelsen, K. M. Grigor and J. Visfeldt Scriptor, Copenhagen, 1981. *Also published* in *Int. J. Andrology Suppl. 4*, 1981.
16. Lange, P. H., McIntire, K. R., Waldmann, T. A., Hakala, T. R., and Fraley, E. E. Alpha-fetoprotein and human chorionic gonadotrophin in the management of testicular tumors. *J. Urol. 118:*593–596, 1977.
17. Lange, P. H., Nochomovitz, L. E., Rosai, J., Fraley, E. E., Kennedy, B. J., Bosl, G., Brisbane, J., Catalona, W. J., Cochran, J. S., Comisarow, R. H., Cummings, K. B., de Kernion, J. B., Einhorn, L. E., Hakala, R., Jewett, M., Moore, M. R., Scardino, P. T., and Streitz, J. M. Serum alpha-fetoprotein and human chorionic gonadotrophin in patients with seminoma. *J. Urol. 124:*472–478, 1980.
18. Li, M. C., Whitmore, W. F., Golbey, R., and Grabstald, H. Effects of combined drug therapy on metastatic cancer of the testis. *JAMA 174:*1291–1299, 1960.
19. Masson, P. Étude sur le seminome. *Rev. Can. Biol. 5:*361–387, 1946.
20. Masters, J. R. W., and Parkinson, M. C. Personal observation, 1981.
21. Mostofi, F. K. Pathology of germ cell tumors of testis. A progress report. *Cancer 45 (Suppl.):*1735–1754, 1980.
22. Mostofi, F. K., and Price, E. B. Tumors of the male genital system. *Atlas of Tumor Pathology, Second Series, Fascicle 8.* Armed Forces Institute of Pathology, Washington, D.C., 1973.
23. Mostofi, F. K., and Sobin, L. H. Histological typing of testis tumours. *International Histological Classification of Tumours, No. 16.* World Health Organization, Geneva, 1977.
24. McIlhinney, R. A. J. Cell surface molecules of human teratoma cell lines. In *Early Detection of Testicular Cancer*, pp. 93–106, edited by N. E. Skakkebaek, J. G. Berthelsen, K. M. Grigor and J. Visfeldt. Scriptor, Copenhagen, 1981. *Also published* in *Int. J. Androl., Suppl. 4*, 1981.
25. Neville, A. M., Grigor, K. M., and Heyderman, E. Biological markers and human neoplasia. In *Recent Advances in Histopathology*, edited by P. P. Anthony and N. Woolf. Churchill-Livingstone, Edinburgh, 1978.
26. Newlands, E. S., Dent, J., Kardana, A., Searle, F., and Bagshawe, K. D. Serum α_1-fetoprotein and HCG in patients with testicular tumours. Lancet *2:*744–745, 1976.
27. Nøgaard-Pedersen, B., Albrechtsen, R., and Teilung, G. Serum alpha-foetoprotein as a marker for endodermal sinus tumour (yolk sac tumour) or a vitelline component of "teratocarcinoma". *Acta Pathol. Microbiol. Scand.[A] 83:*573–589, 1975.
28. Nüesch-Bachmann, J. H., and Hedinger, Chr. Atypische Spermatogonien als Präkanzerose. *Schweiz. Med. Wochenschr. 107:*795–801, 1977.
29. Oliver, R. T. D., Ama Rohatiner, A., Wrigley, P. F. M., and Malpas, J. S. Chemotherapy of metastatic testicular tumours. *Br. J. Urol. 52:*34–37, 1980.
30. Parkinson, M. C., and Beilby, J. O. W. Features of prognostic significance in testicular germ cell tumours. *J. Clin. Pathol. 30:*113–119, 1977.
31. Parkinson, M. C., and Beilby, J. O. W. Testicular germ cell tumours: should current classifications be revised? *Invest. Cell Pathol. 3:*135–140, 1980.
32. Pierce, G. B., and Abell, M. A. Embryonal carcinoma of the testis. In *Pathology Annual*, edited by S. C. Sommers. Butterworth, London, 1970.
33. Pugh, R. C. B. (ed). *Pathology of the Testis.* Blackwell, Oxford, 1976.
34. Raghavan, D. The application of xenografts in the study of human germ cell tumours. In *Early Detection of Testicular Cancer*, pp. 79–89, edited by N. E. Skakkebaek, J. G. Berthelsen, K. M. Grigor and J. Visfeldt. Scriptor, Copenhagen, 1981. *Also published* in *Int. J. Androl., Suppl. 4*, 1981.
35. Scardino, P. T., Cox, H. D., Thomas, A., Waldmann, K., McIntire, K. R., Mittemeyer, B., and Javadpour, N. The value of serum markers in the staging and prognosis of germ cell tumors of the testis. *J. Urol. 118:*944–999, 1977.
36. Sigg, Chr., and Hedinger, Chr. Atypical germ cells in testicular biopsy in male sterility. In *Early Detection of Testicular Cancer*, pp. 163–169, edited by N. E. Skakkebaek, J. G. Berthelsen, K. M. Grigor and J. Visfeldt. Scriptor, Copenhagen, 1981. *Also published* in *Int. J. Androl., Suppl. 4*, 1981.
37. Skakkebaek, N. E. Possible carcinoma *in situ* of the testis. *Lancet 2:*516–517, 1972.
38. Skakkebaek, N. E. Abnormal morphology of germ cells in two infertile men. *Acta Pathol. Microbiol. Scand.[A] 80:*374–378, 1972.

39. Skakkebaek, N. E. Atypical germ cells in the adjacent "normal" tissue of testicular tumours. *Acta Pathol. Microbiol. Scand.[A] 83:*127–130, 1975.
40. Skakkebaek, N. E. Carcinoma *in situ* of the testis: frequency and relationship to invasive germ cell tumours in infertile men. *Histopathology 2:*157–170, 1978.
41. Skakkebaek, N. E. Carcinoma *in situ* of testis in testicular feminization syndrome. *Acta Pathol. Microbiol. Scand.[A] 87:*87–89, 1979.
42. Skakkebaek, N. E., Berthelsen, J. G., and Visfeldt, J. Clinical aspects of testicular carcinoma *in situ.* In *Early Detection of Testicular Cancer,* pp. 153–159, edited by N. E. Skakkebaek, J. G. Berthelsen, K. M. Grigor and J. Visfeldt. Scriptor, Copenhagen, 1981. *Also published* in *Int. J. Androl., Suppl. 4,* 1981.
43. Smith, I. E., Eckstein, H. B., Kohn, J., and McElwain, T. J. Metastatic orchioblastoma: $alpha_1$-fetoprotein in diagnosis and combination chemotherapy in treatment: a case report. *Br. J. Urol. 49:*427–430, 1977.
44. Smithers, D. W. The management of patients with tumours of the testis. K. M. Grigor and J. Visfeldt. Scriptor, Copenhagen, 1981. *Also published In Pathology of the Testis,* edited by R. C. B. Pugh. Blackwell, Oxford, 1976.
45. Stevens, L. C. Experimental production of testicular tumours in the mouse. In *Early Detection of Testicular Cancer,* pp. 54–59, edited by N. E. Skakkebaek, J. G. Berthelsen, K. M. Grigor and J. Visfeldt. Scriptor, Copenhagen, 1981. *Also published* in *Int. J. Androl., Suppl. 4,* 1981.
46. Talerman, A. The incidence of yolk sac tumor (endodermal sinus tumor) elements in germ cell tumors of the testis in adults. *Cancer 36:*211–215, 1975.
47. Teilum, G. Endodermal sinus tumor of ovary and testis. Comparative morphogenesis of the so-called mesonephroma ovarii (Schiller) and extra embryonic (yolk sac allantoic) structures of the rat placenta. *Cancer, 12:*1092–1105, 1959.
48. Teilum, G. Classification of endodermal sinus tumor (mesoblastoma vitellinum) and so-called "embryonal carcinoma" of the ovary. *Acta Pathol. Microbiol. Scand.[A] 64:*407–429, 1965.
49. Teilum, G., Albrechtsen, R., Nørgaard-Pedersen, B. Immunofluorescent localization of alpha-fetoprotein synthesis in endodermal sinus tumor (yolk sac tumor). *Acta Path. Microbiol. Scand.[A] 82:*586–588, 1974.
50. Thackray, A. C., and Crane, W. A. J. Seminoma. In *Pathology of the Testis,* edited by R. C. B. Pugh. Blackwell, Oxford, 1976.
51. Whitmore, W. F., Jr. Germinal tumors of the testis, In *Sixth National Cancer Conference Proceedings.* J. B. Lippincott, Philadelphia, 1970.
52. Woodtli, W., and Hedinger, Chr. Endodermal sinus tumor or orchioblastoma in children and adults. *Virchows Archiv Pathol. Anat. 364:*93–110, 1974.
53. Wurster, K., Hedinger, C., and Meienberg, O. Orchioblastomatige Herde in Hodenteratomen von erwachsenen zur Frage der Eigenstandigkeit des Orchioblastomas. *Virchows Arch. Pathol. Anat. 357:*231–242, 1972.
54. Zeuthen, J. Human teratocarcinoma cell lines: a review. In *Early Detection of Testicular Cancer,* pp. 61–746, edited by N. E. Skakkebaek, J. G. Berthelsen, K. M. Grigor and J. Visfeldt. Scriptor, Copenhagen, 1981. *Also published* in *Int. J. Androl., Suppl. 4,* 1981.

2

The Pathology of Germ Cell Tumors of the Testis

Lucien E. Nochomovitz, M.B. Ch.B., M. Med. (Path.)

The standard approach to the pathologic diagnosis of germ cell tumors of the testis has changed comparatively little since the identification of the yolk sac tumor a few years ago.[1-3] Histologic diagnosis depends upon separating these lesions into two broad groups, seminomatous or nonseminomatous, with further classification into more specific types. Although the application of tumor markers has added a functional dimension to the morphologic approach, the basic diagnostic guidelines remain, in general, fairly stable. Much of the recent movement and impetus in the field of germ cell testicular cancer results from a broad interest in the histogenesis and biologic attributes of these tumors and in the formulation of optimal modes of therapy. The fascinating implications of testicular tumor model systems, the role of oncofetal proteins in patient management and the striving for advanced survival for men affected by these tumors, affords the pathologist ample opportunity to engage the related disciplines. The field of testicular cancer appears to be a profitable staging ground for the study of cancer in general and it is an area in which the fruits of the experimentalist are constantly borne to the clinician and pathologist for their avid consumption. In this spirit, an International Symposium on Human Testis Cancer, incorporating the basic and clinical sciences, was recently held in Minneapolis.[4] Some of the data presented at that meeting have been published elsewhere.[5]

There have been at least six major attempts since 1940[6-11] to classify testicular tumors along clinically meaningful lines. The American terminology was devised by Friedman and Moore[6] and Dixon and Moore,[7] and later modified by Mostofi and Price,[9] to be eventually embodied in the scheme of the World Health Organization (WHO) International Reference Centre for the Definition and Classification of Testicular Tumors (Table 2.1).[12] The British system,[10] which uses a different nomenclature, was recently compared to other classifications and discussed by Mostofi[13] (Table 2.1). In this chapter, I shall use the Dixon and Moore[7]

Table 2.1.
Comparison of Classifications of Testicular Germ Cell Tumors.[a]

Dixon and Moore[7]	Mostofi and Price[9]	WHO[12]	British Testicular Tumour Panel[10]
	TUMORS OF ONE HISTOLOGICAL TYPE	TUMORS OF ONE HISTOLOGICAL TYPE	
Seminoma	Seminoma (typical) Spermatocytic seminoma Anaplastic seminoma[b]	Seminoma Spermatocytic seminoma	Seminoma Spermatocytic seminoma
Embryonal carcinoma	Embryonal carcinoma Adult Polyembryoma[c]	Embryonal carcinoma Polyembryoma	Malignant teratoma, undifferentiated (MTU)
Teratoma Adult	Teratoma Mature Immature With malignant change[d]	Teratoma Mature Immature With malignant transformation	Teratoma, differentiated (TD)
	Embryonal carcinoma Juvenile	Yolk sac tumor (Embryonal carcinoma, juvenile type, endodermal sinus tumor)	Yolk sac tumor
Choriocarcinoma	Choriocarcinoma[e]	Choriocarcinoma[e]	
	TUMORS OF MORE THAN ONE HISTOLOGICAL TYPE	TUMORS OF MORE THAN ONE HISTOLOGICAL TYPE	
Teratoma with embryonal carcinoma (teratocarcinoma)	Embryonal carcinoma with teratoma (teratocarcinoma)	Embryonal carcinoma and teratoma (teratocarcinoma)	Malignant teratoma, intermediate (MTI)
	Specifies types	Choriocarcinoma and any other types (specify type)	Malignant teratoma, trophoblastic (MTT)
	Specifies types	Other combinations (specify)	"Combined tumour," when seminoma present

[a] Excluding intratubular germ cell neoplasia (see Table 2.2).
[b] This term has been discarded in a more recent formulation.[13]
[c] Rare tumor consisting mainly of embryoid bodies, *i.e.* structures resembling the early embryo.
[d] Refers to malignant areas independent of seminoma, embryonal carcinoma or choriocarcinoma.[13]
[e] In the pure form.[13]

terminology and will discuss the gross and microscopic criteria that enable one to identify the different germinal tumors of the testis.

SEMINOMA

Classical Seminoma

Among the seminomas, the classical type is the one with which pathologists are the most familiar. Although this tumor occurs in younger men as well, it most frequently presents in the fourth and fifth decades of life,[14, 15] accounting for about 30–40% of testicular neoplasms. It is unfortunate that symptoms in the early stages of the disease tend to be relatively mild, so that patient- and even physician-delay diminish what would otherwise be an outstanding prognosis.[9,16,17] The large number of individuals who have metastatic disease when first examined attests to the fact that most adult males are as yet unaware of the importance of self-examination of the testes. Seminoma, like other germinal tumors, appears to proceed through an intratubular *in situ* stage, detectable only upon biopsy. The subject of carcinoma *in situ* of the testis is considered, however, toward the end of this chapter.

The gross tumor may be situated anywhere within the organ and usually forms a sharply demarcated mass which, through expansion, compresses the uninvolved testis (Fig. 2.1). The cut surface is whitish tan

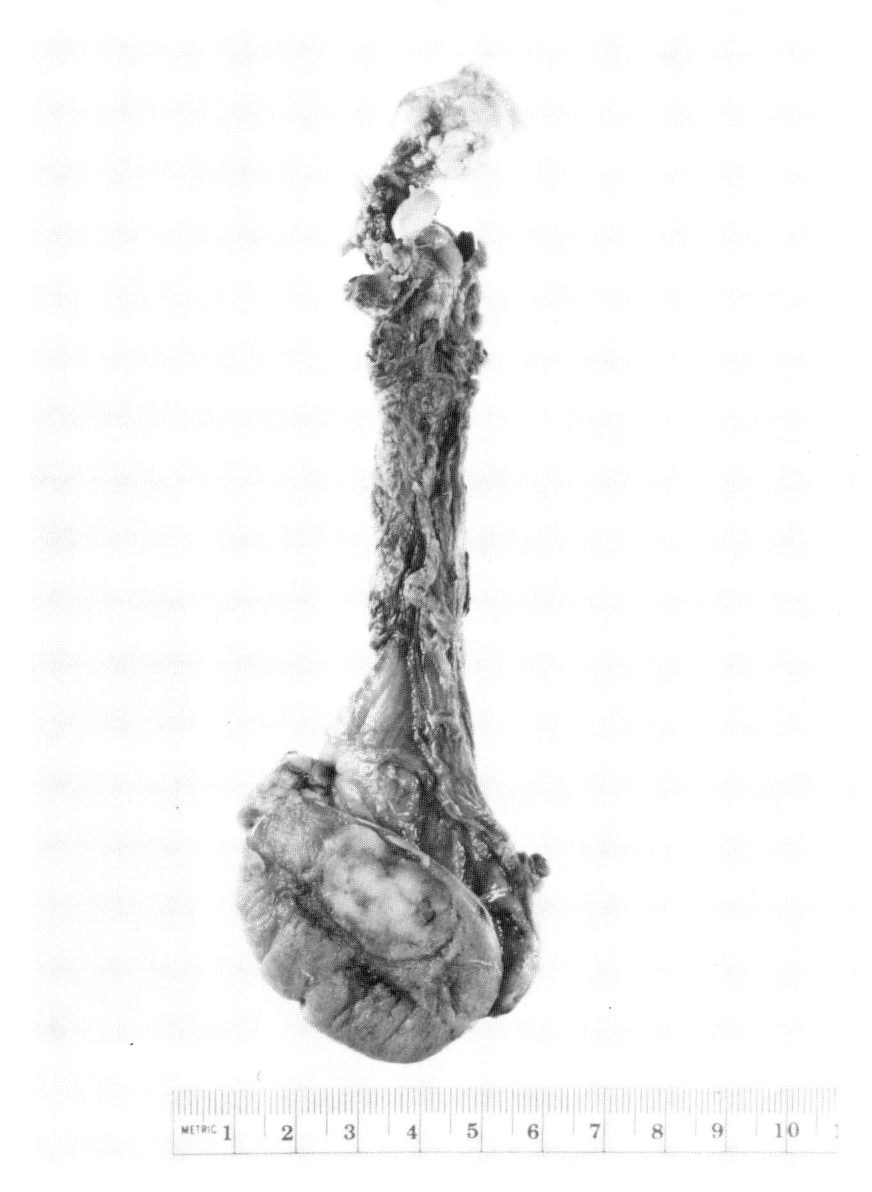

Figure 2.1. Seminoma. Well circumscribed, expansile tumor compresses adjacent testis.

to pink and characteristically shows well defined areas of infarct-like necrosis. In order to obtain maximal information from a given specimen, it is imperative that the excised scrotal contents be handed to the pathologist for immediate fixation. I would advocate a suitably stained touch-preparation from the longitudinally cut fresh surface and the collection of material for eventual ultrastructural study when it is desired. Fixation of a few thin slices of tumor tissue in Bouin's solution and/or in B-5 will prevent the artefacts associated with formalin. Samples should be widely taken for paraffin sections (to avoid overlooking a nonseminomatous component) and should include a generous area of uninvolved testicular tissue. The epididymis, spermatic cord and margin of resection must be carefully examined microscopically, since tumor in any one of these locations would render the lesion beyond stage 1.

When optimally fixed, the classical seminoma is composed of sheets of polyhedral cells segregated into compartments by slender fibrous septa that ramify through the tumor (Fig. 2.2). This fibrous component will occasionally predominate, obscuring the tumor cells, which can then be identified singly or as small clusters within the connective tissue matrix (Fig. 2.3). An infiltrate of mature lymphocytes usually impregnates the septa and may actually form lymphoid follicles.[15] It is likely that these lymphocytes fulfill an immunologic role, although their influence upon prognosis is open to question.[10, 18] Tumor cell nuclei tend to be large, round and centrally situated within a clear-to-thready cytoplasm that is enclosed by a well-defined, almost penciled cell border and which contains stainable glycogen (Fig. 2.4). It is the presence of this cell border that is

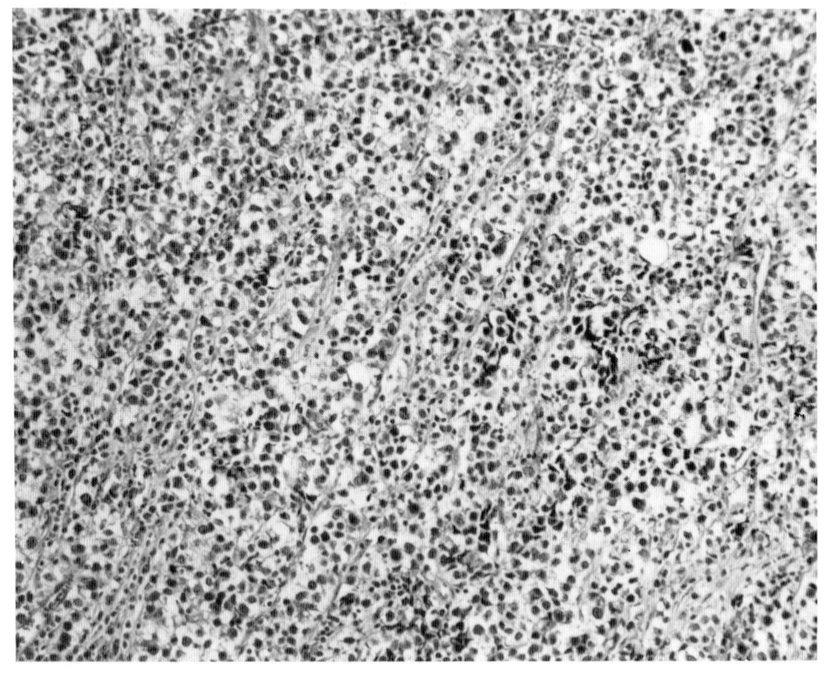

Figure 2.2. Seminoma. Tumor cells segregated into compartments by fibrous stroma (H&E × 140).

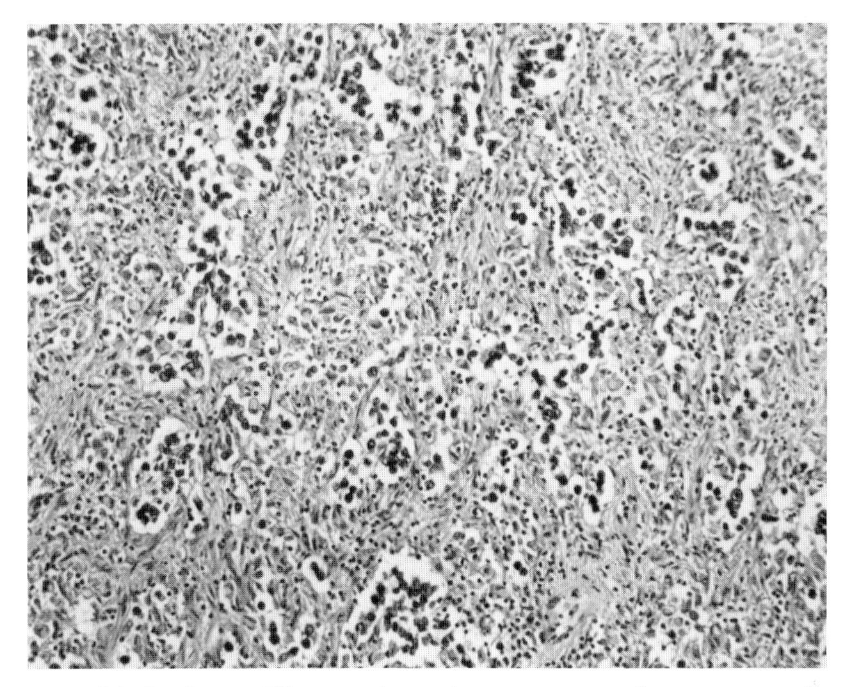

Figure 2.3. Seminoma. Fibrous and granulomatous stroma obscures tumor cells (H&E × 130).

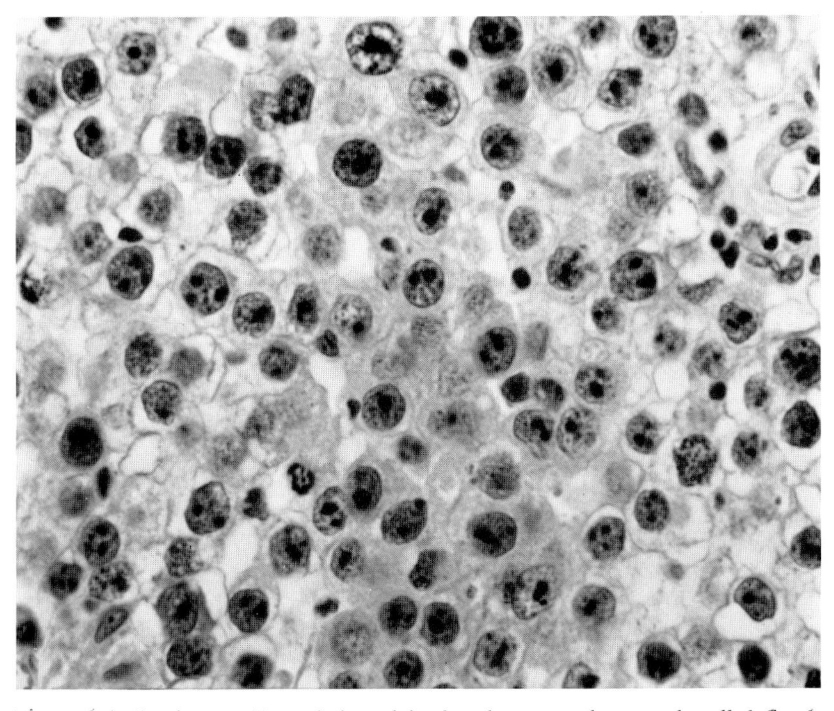

Figure 2.4. Seminoma. Rounded nuclei, abundant cytoplasm and well-defined cell borders (H&E × 600).

sometimes helpful in distinguishing seminoma from embryonal carcinoma. One or several prominent eosinophilic nucleoli, possibly representing nucleolonemal dispersion, are found in most of the tumor cells. One will quite frequently observe individual tumor cells infiltrating the interstitium of the adjacent, apparently uninvolved testis (Fig. 2.5). These represent either direct extension from the main tumor mass or migration from an *in situ* component nearby. Of some interest is the fact that germ cells have been observed to migrate from the seminiferous tubules into the interstitium of the newborn rabbit testis,[19] a finding that may lead toward an explanation of the manner in which neoplastic cells emerge from the tubule, where they appear to be under some form of Sertoli cell control.[20, 21]

In the classical seminoma, mitoses are infrequent and in the opinion of Mostofi and Price[9] should number less than three per 10 high power fields (HPF). In areas that correspond to the macroscopic zones of infarction, the tumor cells appear necrotic and "ghost-like." Giant cells of two types may occur: the Langhans' giant cell, participating in the formation of granulomas, and a multinucleated tumor giant cell that mimics syncytiotrophoblast in appearance and which contains intracytoplasmic human chorionic gonadotropin (HCG) (Fig. 2.6). Seminomas possessing the latter type of giant cell were referred to as "seminoma with trophocarcinoma" and were believed to be aggressive variants.[22] The yield of these cells is increased if one pays particular attention to minute hemorrhagic foci around which the trophoblast tends to group. The occurrence of raised serum levels of HCG (without classical choriocarcinoma) is probably explained by the secretion of hormone from these isolated trophoblastic cells,[23] which account for hormonal elevations in patients with nonseminomatous tumors as well.[24]

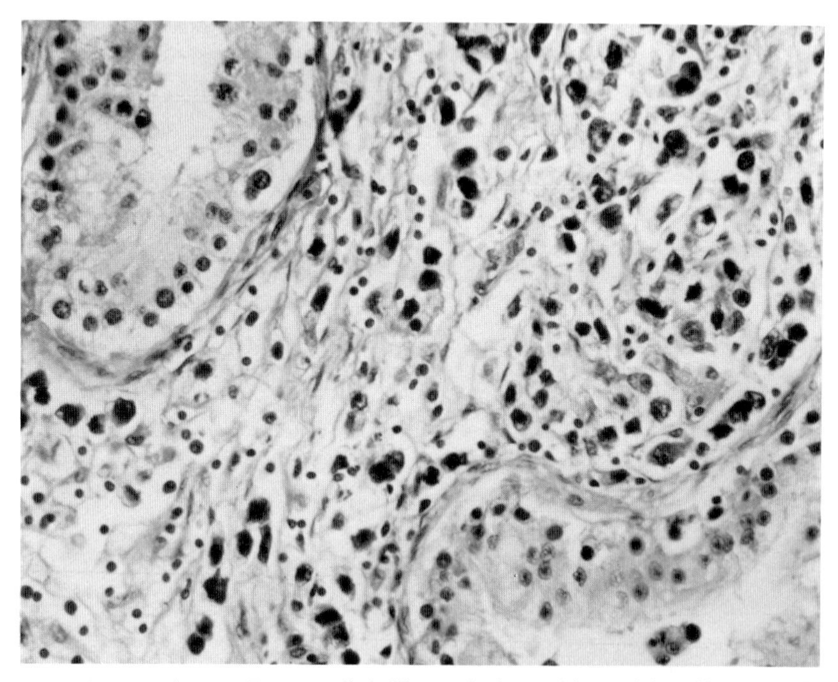

Figure 2.5. Seminoma. Tumor cells infiltrate the interstitium of the adjacent testis (H&E × 300).

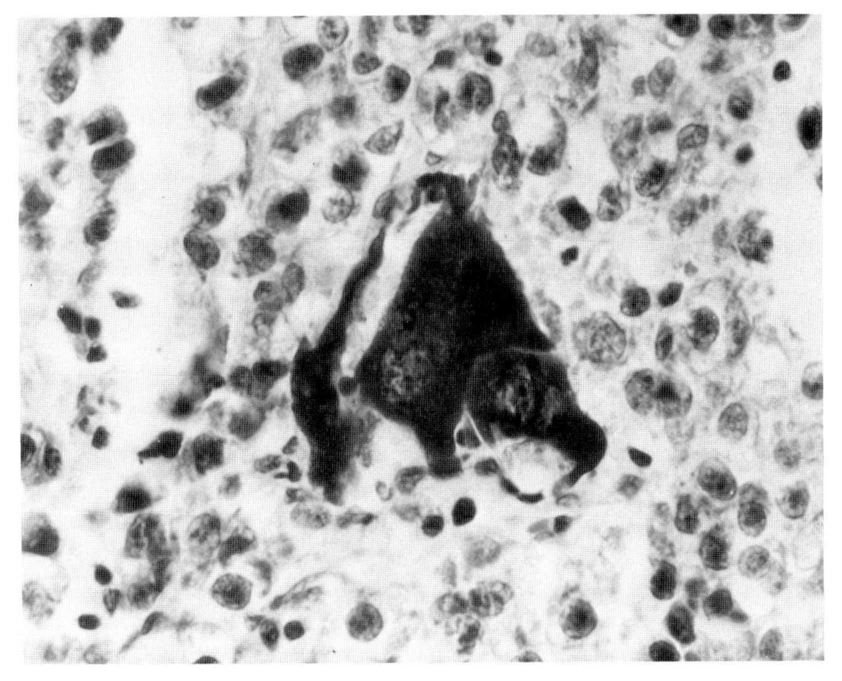

Figure 2.6. Seminoma. Syncytiotrophoblast with granular deposit of intracytoplasmic HCG (immunoperoxidase, × 600).

Placental proteins other than HCG may also be demonstrated in tumors that contain isolated syncytiotrophoblast or genuine choriocarcinoma.[25] These include pregnancy-specific glycoprotein (SP1) and placental-specific tissue proteins such as PP5.[26] SP1 occurs in two forms (α and β) of differing electrophoretic mobility[27] and can be demonstrated by the indirect immunoperoxidase technique in formalin-fixed, paraffin-embedded testicular tumor tissue. Its serum level tends to parallel that of HCG and its elevation may be used to advantage in certain cases in which, for some reason, HCG levels are not elevated.[26] PP5 has a very short half-life[28] and does not as yet appear to have a promising role as a serum marker in testicular cancer, although it is also stainable immunohistochemically in tumor tissue. The presence of human placental lactogen (HPL) appears to have been demonstrated many years ago in trophoblastic cells in testicular germ cell cancer[29] and more recently Heyderman[25] effected the staining of HPL in several choriocarcinomas.

An ultrastructural range, from poorly differentiated cells with a paucity of cytoplasmic organelles to more differentiated cells which, in addition to having well-developed Golgi complexes, cytoplasmic cysternae with electron-dense granular inclusions and cytoplasmic glycogen, also possessed material resembling proacrosomal granules, characterizes the classical seminoma (Fig. 2.7).[30]

The prognosis for patients with classical seminoma when confined to the testis and without capsular invasion or spread to the spermatic cord (stage 1) is excellent, with cure rates of over 90%.[14, 18] As with germ cell testicular tumors in general, seminomas spread mainly *via* lymphatics to the common iliac and para-aortic lymph nodes. Mediastinal and supraclavicular nodes may also, however, become involved. Although semi-

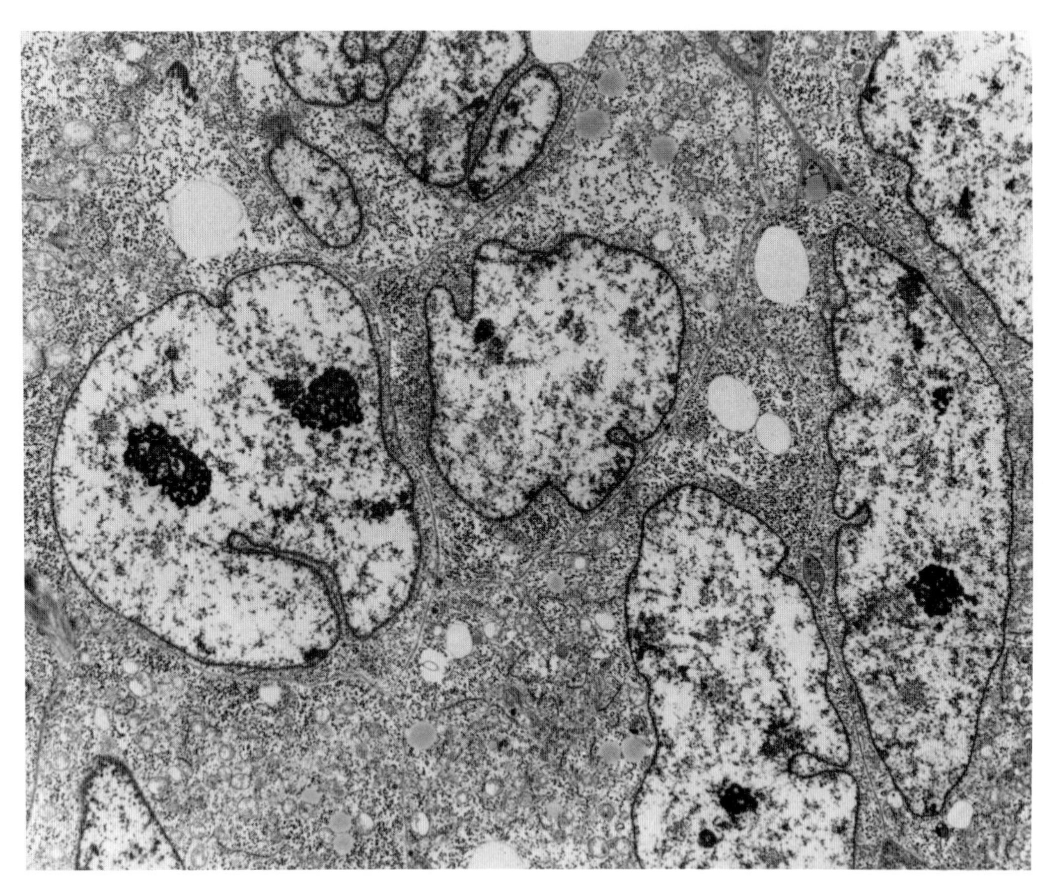

Figure 2.7. Seminoma. Intracytoplasmic glycogen is the predominant intracellular constituent. (× 4000).

nomas are exquisitely radiosensitive, some centers have employed chemotherapy in the treatment of advanced disease in an effort to obtain better patient survival.[31, 32]

There is a recognition among pathologists that while most seminomas conform histologically to what has been described as the classical lesion, one will now and again meet a tumor that contains more cytologic anaplasia and mitotic activity than one would expect from the typical seminoma (Figs. 2.8 and 2.9). Although histologically more disturbing, there are no gross characteristics that reliably distinguish this variety from the classical type. Since it originally appeared that this "atypical" seminoma was more prone to metastasize than the classical, it was identified separately as an "anaplastic" variant whenever certain microscopic criteria, *i.e.* elevated mitotic figures with nuclear and cytoplasmic abnormalities, were satisfied. The quantity of three or more mitoses per 10 HPF, suggested by Mostofi and Price,[9] has been used to determine the relative incidence of this tumor over the last few years by many, but not all, pathologists. However, whether the so-called anaplastic seminoma is truly distinct and intrinsically more aggressive than its classical counterpart is by no means certain. There have been several contradictory reports in the recent literature,[13, 33–35] the number of patients studied has been, on the whole, quite small and the marked improvement in modern forms of

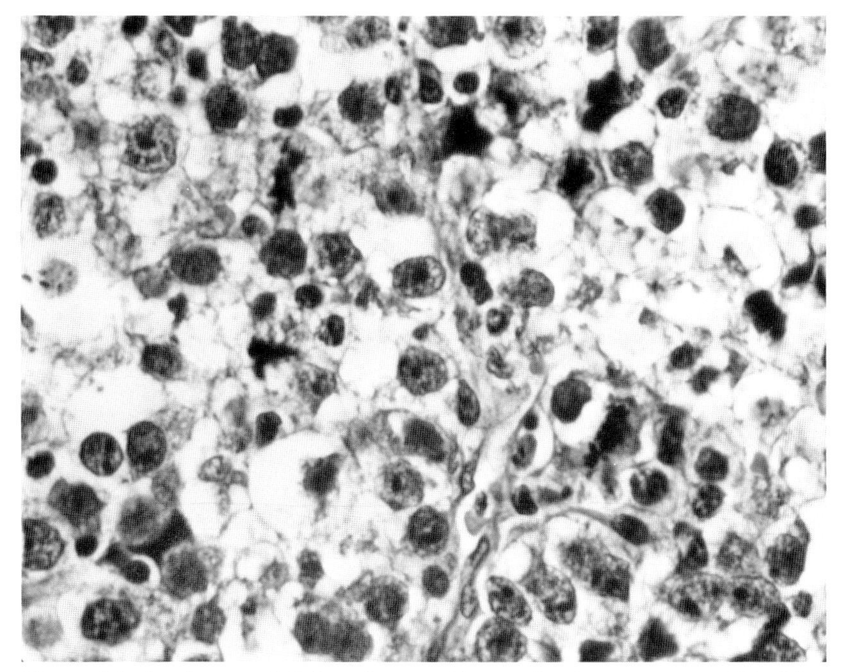

Figure 2.8. Seminoma. Cellular pleomorphism and mitoses create a disturbing impression in this lesion (H&E × 680).

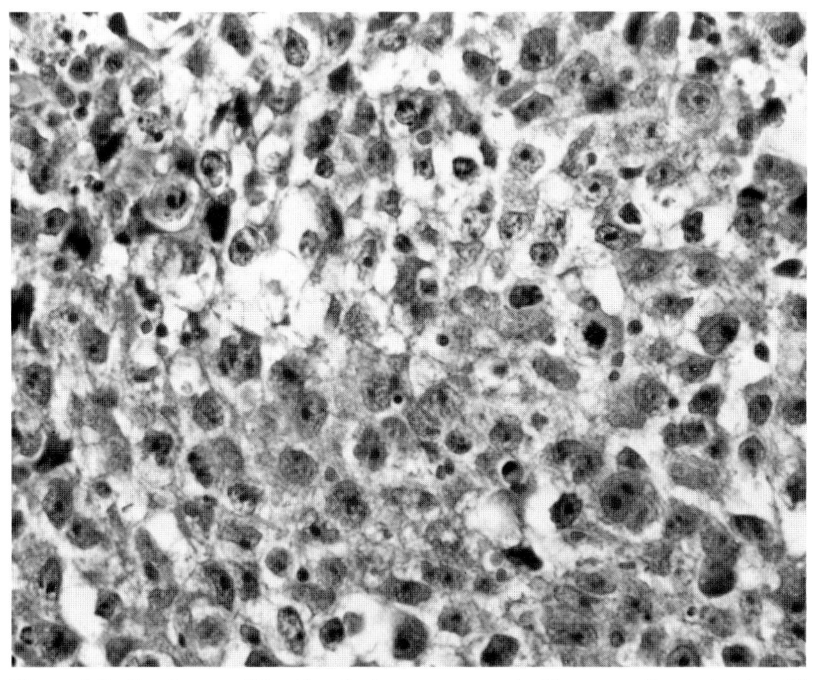

Figure 2.9. Seminoma. The disorderly arrangement of tumor cells contrasts with the appearance in Figure 2.4 (H&E × 375).

therapy has also tended to obscure the meaning of histologic variation within a given tumor type. Since the term "anaplastic seminoma" is imprecise and because it is difficult to consistently assign the majority of seminomas to a given category, some pathologists prefer to draw attention to the atypical features and designate the tumor as a "high grade" lesion. As a result of the uncertainty surrounding the diagnosis and specific clinical behavior of the so-called anaplastic seminoma, a panel of pathologists* at the International Symposium on Human Testis Cancer[4] recently recommended that the term be used with caution. They stressed the importance of developing a standard approach to the preparation of testicular tumor tissue, including a uniform method of assessing mitotic activity. Some of the inconsistencies that I experienced when examining a relatively small group of atypical seminomas have recently been discussed elsewhere.[5]

The meaning of trophoblastic cells in an otherwise pure seminoma still requires resolution. Some authors believe that the presence of these cells implies a more aggressive tumor that may require additional therapy.[36, 37] In a study of 31 patients with seminoma and elevated serum HCG,[38] Lange *et al.* concluded that the response to irradiation is good with low stage disease, but that abnormal HCG levels in the presence of metastatic disease is a poor prognostic sign when conventional treatment is administered. They emphasized too that, while patients with pure seminoma may display abnormally high levels of serum HCG, it remains important to exclude frank nonseminomatous spread by all available means.

Parkinson and Beilby,[39] in a recent evaluation of the classification of testicular germ cell tumors, have correctly pointed out that seminomas that contain individual syncytiotrophoblastic cells do not exhibit the highly aggressive characteristics of choriocarcinoma and should not be classified as such. It is quite possible therefore that the malignant potential of trophoblast may be determined in some way by its amount.[9, 40] From a histogenetic point of view, the occurrence of trophoblast in seminomas suggests that perhaps these neoplasms ought not to be as sharply separated from the nonseminomatous germ cell tumors, which has long been the case (Fig. 2.10). It is therefore of interest to note that Raghavan *et al.*[41] recently succeeded in obtaining a stable cell line derived from a patient with a histologically pure seminoma but with elevated serum levels of α-fetoprotein (AFP). Following serial xenograft passages, the "seminoma-like" histologic pattern remained constant, although yolk sac features were also recognized. Both patterns contained immunohistochemically demonstrable AFP and there was ultrastructural evidence of several cell types, *i.e.* classical seminoma, yolk sac tumor and combinations of the two. These authors suggested that their findings may indicate a continuum in differentiation between seminoma and yolk sac tumor.

Spermatocytic Seminoma

Spermatocytic seminoma is a rare but distinct clinicopathologic variant that deserves complete separation from the usual forms of seminoma. Described originally by Masson[42] (*séminome spermatocytaire*), this tumor accounts for about 7% of all seminomas.[15, 43] It is likely, however, that many were misdiagnosed as classical seminoma in the past. The spermatocytic seminoma occurs as a gradual testicular enlargement in older

*Drs. E. Heyderman, R. Kurman, F. Mostofi, L. Nochomovitz, J. Rosai (Chairman) and R. Scully.

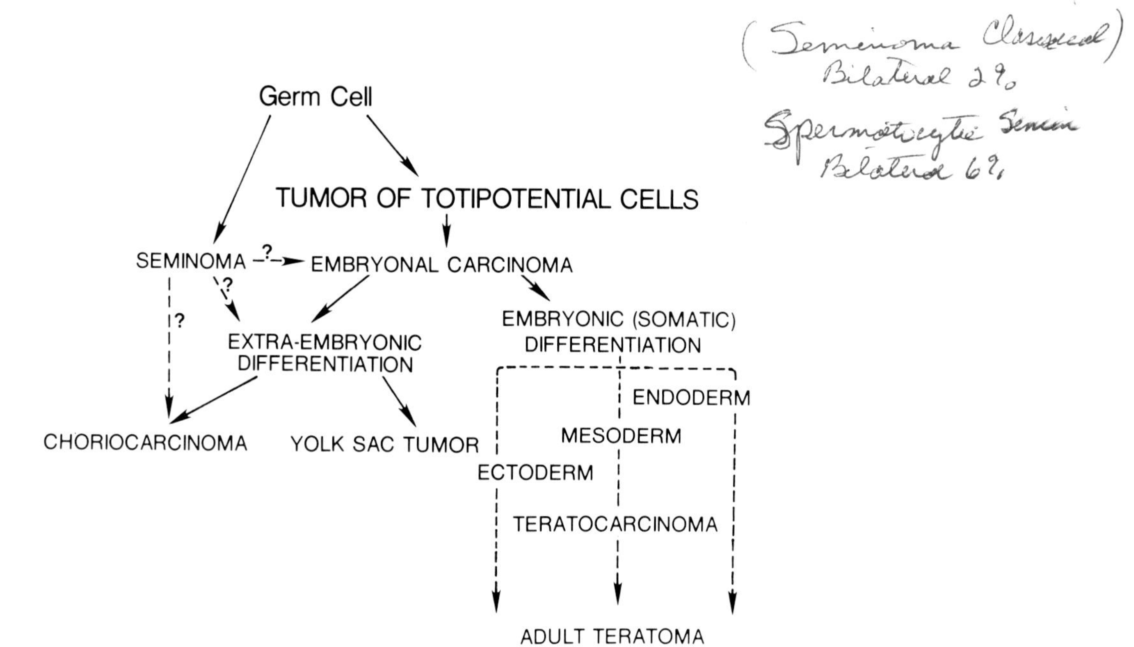

Figure 2.10. Interrelationships of testicular germ cell tumors. (Adapted from F. J. Dixon and R. A. Moore: Tumors of the male sex organs. *Atlas of Tumor Pathology, Section 8, Fascicles 31b and 32*, 1952. (Courtesy of the Armed Forces Institute of Pathology, Washington, D.C.)

males and in the series of Rosai *et al.*[43] the average age was 65 years. It is an extremely indolent tumor, rarely metastasizes, and men with this lesion have an outstanding prognosis. Only 2 of the 50 patients reviewed by Rosai *et al.* died from the disease, which suggests that its malignant potential is rather limited. Bilateral tumors occur somewhat more frequently (6%)[43, 44] than with the classical seminoma (2%).[15] In Rosai's series, the average tumor diameter was 3.5 cm. The cut surface is usually soft, with a gelatinous or mucoid appearance. Cystic degeneration, particularly toward the center of the lesion, is common but necrosis and hemorrhage are almost always absent.

Microscopically, the tumor forms a solid mass of cells without the nesting pattern of the classical seminoma (Fig. 2.11). From a diagnostic point of view, there are roughly three tumor cell populations, divided primarily on the basis of size: (1) the commonest, medium-sized cell (15–18 μ) with a round nucleus and finely granular chromatin pattern; (2) the small cells (6–8 μ) that superficially resemble lymphocytes and which are probably degenerate; (3) the conspicuous giant cells (50–100 μ) that display irregular shapes, abundant eosinophilic cytoplasm and either single or multiple nuclei (Figs. 2.12 and 2.13). These giant cells are obviously neoplastic and differ from the Langhans' giant cell seen in classical seminoma. Their nuclear chromatin offers a clue as to the cell of origin, since it appears to simulate the *spirémes* of the normal meiotic prophase in primary spermatocytes. Spermatocytic seminoma usually contains frequent and often atypical mitoses, a fact that does not imply malignancy. The accumulation of edema fluid results in a microcystic and pseudoglandular pattern which explains the gelatinous, mucoid appearance of the cut surface. Unlike the classical seminoma, the spermatocytic

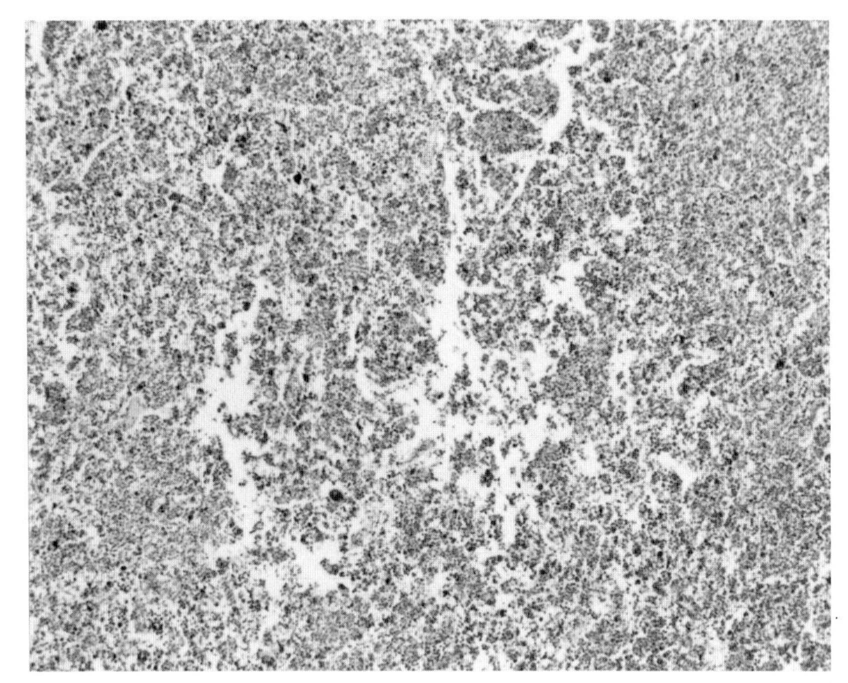

Figure 2.11. Spermatocytic seminoma. Solid sheets, absence of fibrous septa and deeply stained larger tumor cells (H&E × 60).

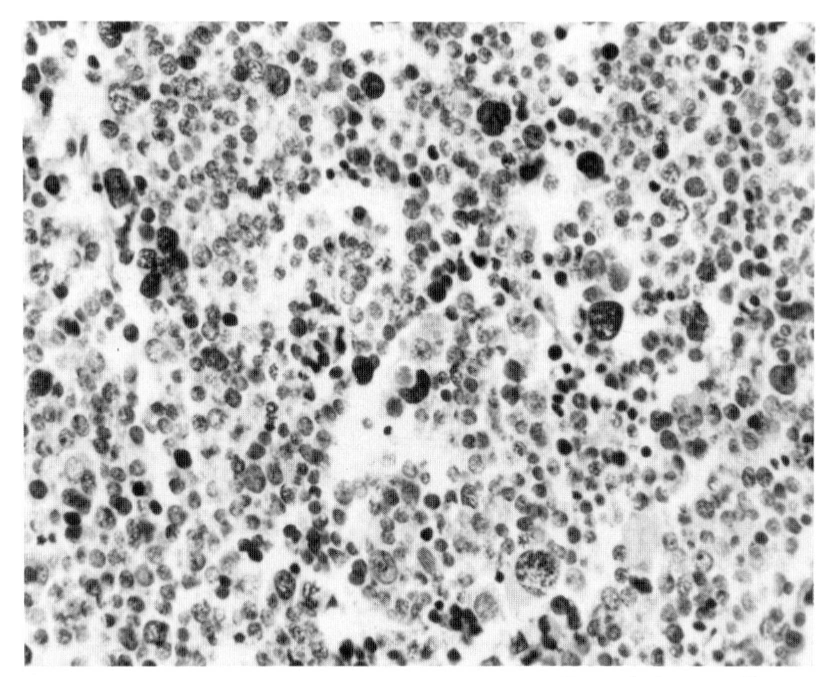

Figure 2.12. Spermatocytic seminoma. Three tumor cell populations are discernible (H&E × 360).

variant lacks a lymphocytic infiltrate or a granulomatous reaction. It does, however, show a marked disposition toward intratubular growth at the edge of the lesion. There is no association with other neoplastic germ cell elements and it is of interest that no homologous counterpart exists, either

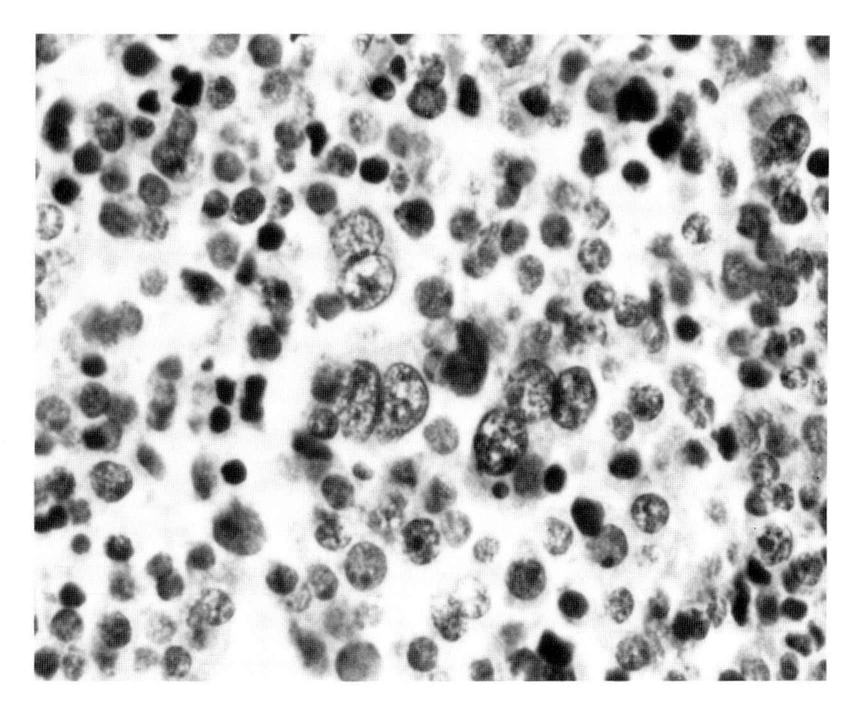

Figure 2.13. Spermatocytic seminoma. Multinucleated tumor giant cells (H&E × 770).

in the ovary or in other sites in which germinal tumors are commonly found.[44] This has been adduced as evidence that the spermatocytic seminoma is a tumor derived from spermatogonia, which are found only in the testis.

This theory was confirmed following the ultrastructural study of two such tumors by Rosai *et al.*[45] The spermatocytic seminoma bore nuclei that closely resembled the leptotene stage of meiotic prophase, thus corroborating Masson's[42] light microscope impression that the threads of nuclear chromatin he had observed represented the *spirémes* of meiosis. Other cytoplasmic components similar to those seen in normal spermatocytes and spermatids were reported, *i.e.* basal bodies and striated rootlets, suggesting development toward spermatozoon tails. There were also intercellular bridges, virtually identical to those seen in seminiferous epithelium.

NONSEMINOMATOUS GERM CELL TUMORS

There are several experimental studies that support the idea that nonseminomatous germ cell tumors of the testis arise from an undifferentiated cellular progenitor that retains an ability to express a wide range of malignancy.[46, 47] Embryonal carcinoma represents the most primitive form of nonseminomatous germinal cancer that we are able to recognize, whereas the teratocarcinoma reflects the occurrence of organoid differentiation and a less aggressive mode of behavior. At the opposite, mature end of this morphologic spectrum lies the adult teratoma, from which all traces of histologic malignancy are, by definition, absent. An additional variant is referred to as immature teratoma and will be described in the following text.

Nonseminomatous germ cell tumors of the testis are the subject of considerable interest among urologists and those concerned with fundamental research upon these neoplasms. On one hand, one would like to offer more patients with this disease reasonable prospects of absolute cure. Therapy directed toward this end depends upon early diagnosis, chemotherapeutic advances, the refinement of tumor markers and the development of more suitable staging techniques. On the other hand lie the intriguing relationships between normal embryogenesis, gene expression and malignant transformation. In this regard, the role of the murine teratocarcinoma model has been amply reviewed[48–51] and several important experiments in this field have contributed to our present understanding of the nonseminomatus forms of testicular cancer.[52–54]

Embryonal Carcinoma

Embryonal carcinoma is a highly malignant tumor that usually presents as a gradual testicular swelling, with or without pain, most frequently in the third decade of life. According to the large series of Friedman and Moore,[6] it accounts for about 20% of all testicular tumors. It is said that the primary lesion may be small and that widespread metastases may originate from a comparatively minute tumor. The embryonal carcinomas that I have seen have tended to be somewhat large, replacing most of the testis. The cut surface, unlike that of seminoma, is quite variegated as a result of focal hemorrhage and necrosis. It is important that these hemorrhagic foci be sampled and studied histologically in the event that they represent frank choriocarcinoma, an extraembryonal derivative.

The tumor is characterized histologically by a variety of patterns that include anaplastic and solid primitive zones with acinar and tubular configurations, necrosis and hemorrhage (Fig. 2.14). Typically, the embryonal carcinoma possesses embryonic and anaplastic cells with poorly defined cell boundaries (Fig. 2.15). This distinguishes the lesion from seminoma in which the tumor cells are usually defined by a crisp cell border. Pathologists who have examined many testicular tumors recognize that in some cases it can be very difficult to draw a distinction between embryonal carcinoma and an atypical disturbing seminoma. Embryonal carcinoma is comparatively fast growing and contains many mitoses, but a granulomatous reaction of the kind seen in seminoma appears to be exceptional. Since the embryonal carcinoma cell can evolve into a range of tissue types analogous morphologically to the developing embryo,[55] this type of tumor constititues an invaluable source of experimental material for those studying the biologic events concerned with tissue differentiation.[56]

It is not surprising, considering the versatility of embryonal carcinoma, that it frequently contains histologic evidence of yolk sac differentiation. Although the yolk sac patterns are more fully discussed in the section on yolk sac tumor itself, it is worth mentioning here that when the typical lacy, reticular network occurs only focally within a nonseminomatous germ cell tumor, it is still frequently misinterpreted or ignored. The presence of the yolk sac pattern in embryonal carcinoma can usually be correlated with abnormal levels of AFP in the serum of the patient.[57–60]

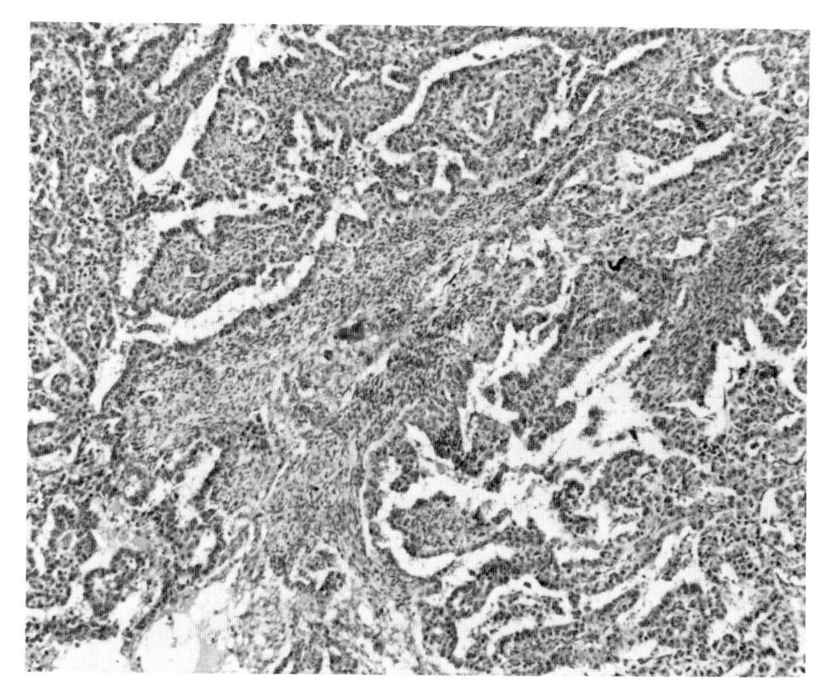

Figure 2.14. Embryonal carcinoma. Tubulopapillary glandular pattern (H&E × 60).

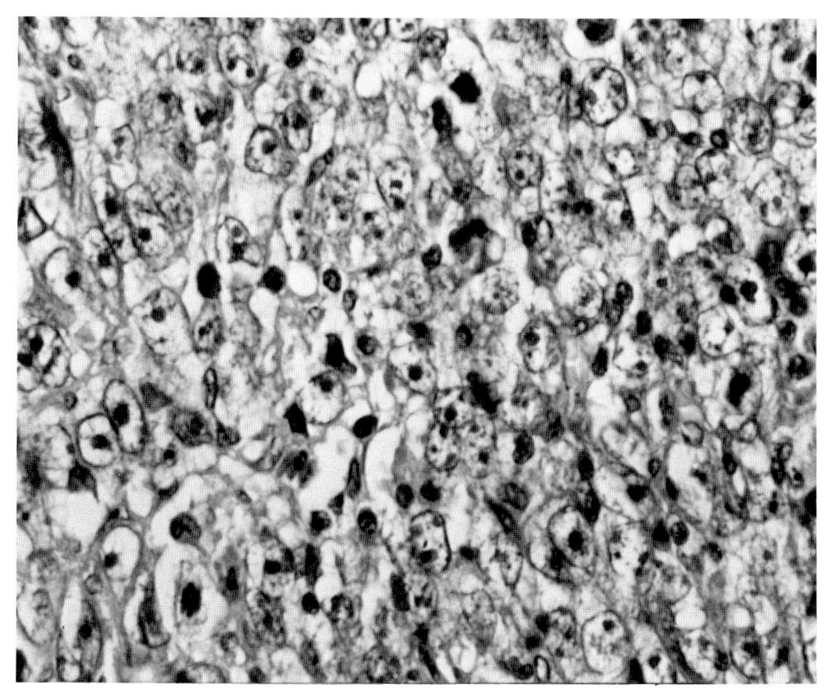

Figure 2.15. Embryonal carcinoma. Closely packed, overlapping tumor cells (H&E × 600).

This protein is now a well established marker for monitoring clinical progress and its elevation is taken to indicate the presence of nonseminomatous germ cell components in patients with testicular cancer. It is noteworthy that yolk sac elements can be detected immunohistochemically before the characteristic histologic patterns are actually recognizable.[24] Therefore, accurate classification of testicular germ cell tumors may require immunologic staining of representative tumor tissue and Kurman *et al.*[24] have proposed a tentative scheme using histologic and immunohistochemical techniques to evaluate yolk sac (AFP) and trophoblastic (HCG) differentiation. However, Parkinson has cautioned against the uncritical acceptance of AFP as an unequivocal marker of the yolk sac since this protein has been demonstrated in other tissues, such as immature gut and fetal liver.[39]

One should mention, of course, that embryonal carcinoma is also frequently associated with trophoblastic differentiation and the production of HCG, which explains the heightened serum levels of this hormone in many patients with this tumor.[60, 61] A point of interest is that nonseminomatous human testicular tumors frequently demonstrate nonrandom abnormalities in chromosome 1, but the precise meaning of this finding is unclear.[62]

In the United States, the extended retroperitoneal dissection is the established form of treatment of patients with nonseminomatous germ cell testicular tumors in clinical stages 1 and 2.[63–64] When the disease is more extensive, however, adjuvant chemotherapy is usually indicated.[65–67] This operative procedure has effected a dramatic improvement in survival, and it is claimed that "the overall cure rate in these tumors... now approaches 90%."[68] A comprehensive review on this subject was recently published.[63, 64] Several European centers employ radiotherapy following orchidectomy and, while apparently obtaining high cure rates, also appear to avoid the problems of aspermia and infertility associated with surgery.[69] On the other hand, it is well to note that many patients with testicular cancer already have abnormal spermatocytes and oligospermia when first operated upon.

Teratocarcinoma

Teratocarcinoma, according to the terminology of Dixon and Moore,[7] is a term that describes a germinal tumor that theoretically occupies a position somewhere between the highly malignant embryonal carcinoma and the histologically benign adult (mature) teratoma. Its behavior, accordingly, lies between these extremes. Teratocarcinoma occurs most frequently in the third decade of life and usually causes testicular enlargement and/or pain. The cut surface of the tumor displays a mixture of solid areas and cystic spaces. The solid zones, often containing soft, hemorrhagic and necrotic material, represent the poorly differentiated components of the lesion, whereas the cystic spaces, often interspersed with grossly visible cartilaginous tissue, reflect mature elements.

Corresponding to the gross appearance is a histologic admixture of frankly malignant tissue (identical to embryonal carcinoma) intermixed with fully differentiated cartilage, muscle or nests of squamous epithelium (Fig. 2.16). I have occasionally seen distorted and dilated epididymal ducts interpreted as differentiated neoplastic epithelial structures in what was otherwise an embryonal carcinoma. Extraembryonal components, such as yolk sac tumor and choriocarcinoma are also frequently found in these tumors and may be demonstrated using immunohistochemical techniques.[24] These elements are believed to arise from the extraem-

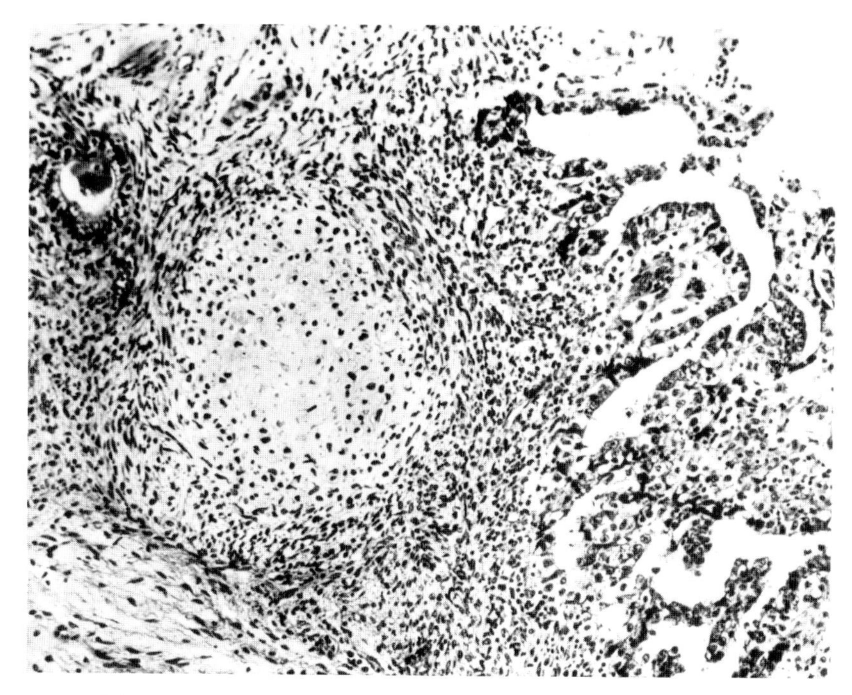

Figure 2.16. Teratocarcinoma. Admixture of mature cartilage with embryonal carcinoma (H&E × 137).

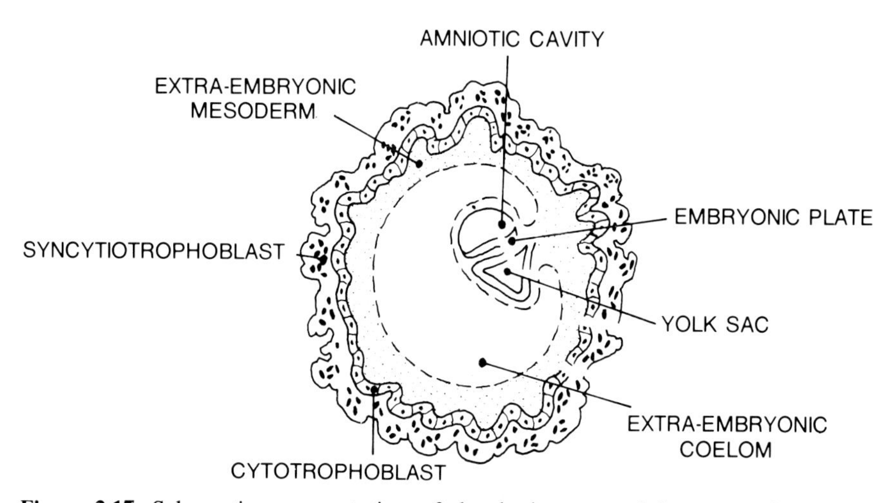

Figure 2.17. Schematic representation of developing normal human embryo. Yolk sac, synctio- and cytotrophoblast constitute extraembryonal components; somatic elements arise from the embryonic plate.

bryonal structures (yolk sac, synctio- and cytotrophoblast) that correspond to the developing fetus (Fig. 2.17). It is also possible to find carcinoembryonic antigen (CEA) in those areas of teratocarcinoma that show an apparent differentiation towards intestinal mucosa.[25] Of some interest, too, is the fact that when the HLA antigen frequency in patients with testicular cancer is studied, those with teratocarcinoma express a significantly increased incidence of HLA-Dw7 by comparison to normal controls and men with choriocarcinoma, seminoma or embryonal cell carcinoma. DeWolf *et al*[70] have recently suggested that this finding may indicate a region in the human genome that influences the development of teratocarcinoma.

As in the case of pure embryonal carcinoma, isolated collections of synctiotrophoblastic cells lining hemorrhagic cystic spaces do not themselves constitute choriocarcinoma. The common iliac and para-aortic lymph nodes are again the usual metastatic sites although hematogenous dissemination to other organs and tissues occurs too.

Adult (Mature) Teratoma

The adult teratoma expresses the fulfillment of complete histologic maturity and, by definition, contains no malignant tissue. In order to establish this diagnosis, it is therefore necessary to sample the tumor as widely as is practically possible to exclude undifferentiated foci. Although the mature teratoma is the least aggressive of the nonseminomatous germ cell tumors of the testis, it is quite capable of metastasizing in the adult patient and cannot be regarded as biologically benign. However, it has been pointed out that, when occurring in childhood, the mature teratoma does not spread.[71, 72]

Grossly, the body of the testis is distorted and partially or wholly replaced by the tumor, which on cut section is frequently cystic and multiloculated. The cysts vary in size and contain serous, viscid or blood-stained fluid. Solid and/or hemorrhagic areas are likely to represent foci of immaturity or frankly malignant tumor and should be sampled. Microscopically there is usually no difficulty in making the diagnosis. Mature cartilage, smooth muscle and epithelial-lined cysts (alimentary, respiratory, squamous) are frequent (Fig. 2.18). It has been often stated that neuroblastic differentiation does not confer malignancy and is of no prognostic significance.[71]

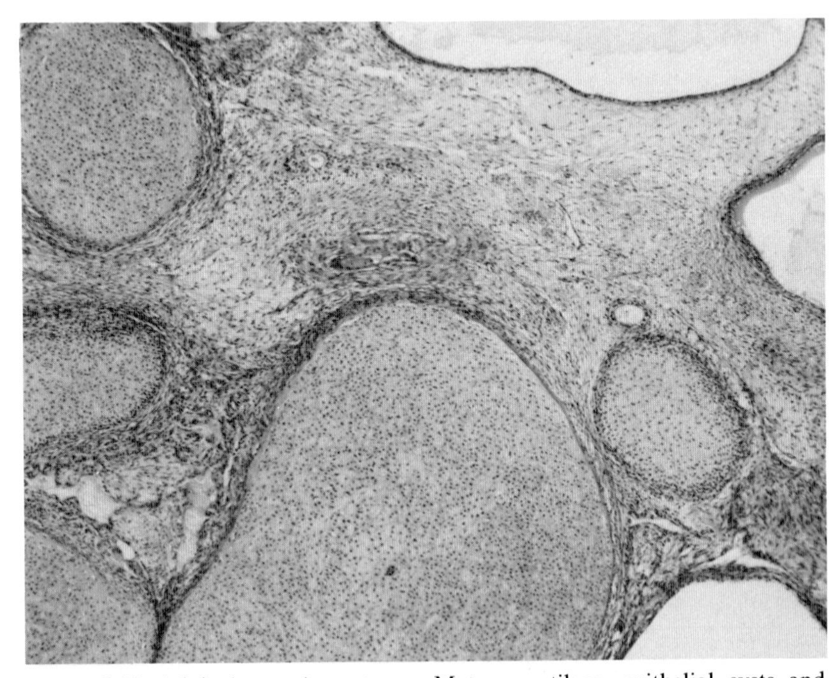

Figure 2.18. Adult (mature) teratoma. Mature cartilage, epithelial cysts and connective tissue stroma (H&E × 50).

When a germinal testicular tumor, otherwise resembling an adult teratoma, possesses a rather cellular and active stroma with mitotic figures, the lesion is referred to as an *immature teratoma* (Figs. 2.19 and 2.20). One also encounters adult teratomas in which the glandular epithelium is

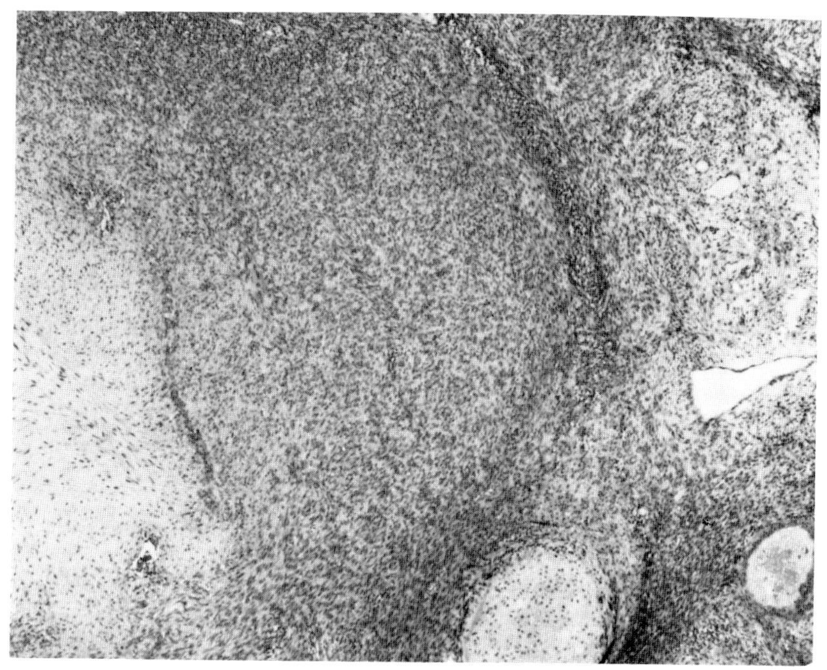

Figure 2.19. Immature teratoma. A solid and cellular stroma admixed with mature cartilage (H&E × 40).

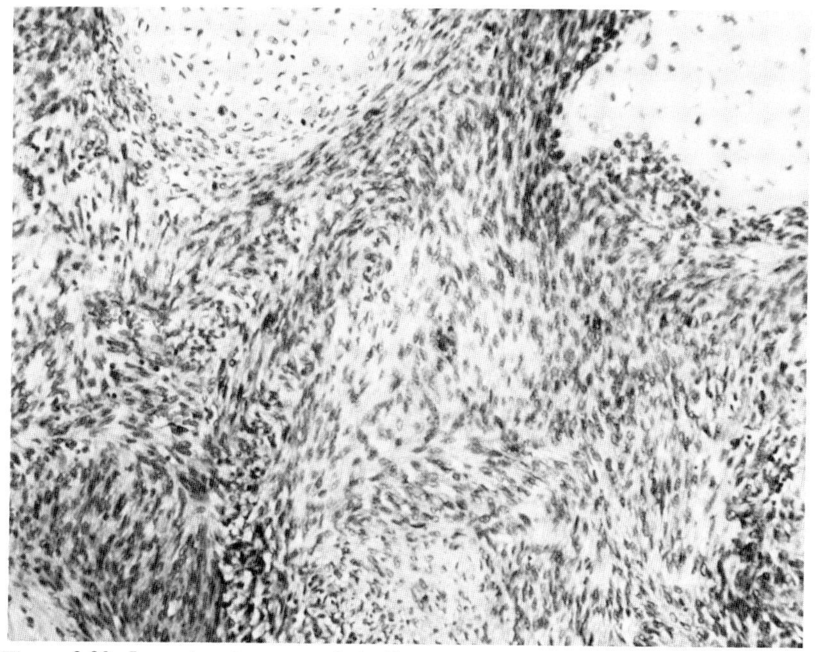

Figure 2.20. Immature teratoma. Spindled stromal cells appear plump and active (H&E × 132).

cytologically abnormal, suggesting that these lesions also be considered immature. There appears to be no reliable means yet of determining the likely behavior of this variant of teratoma and no grading system of the kind used to evaluate immature teratoma of ovary[73] has been applied to comparable tumors of the testis.

Patients with adult teratoma, particularly in stage 1, have an excellent prognosis. In a series of 18 patients with stage 1 adult teratoma treated by radical inguinal orchidectomy and retroperitoneal lymphadenectomy, Johnson *et al.*[74] reported a 5-year survival of 100%. Several interesting theories as to why the ovarian teratomas (dermoid cysts) are usually benign while the mature testicular teratomas in adults tend to be malignant have been proposed elsewhere.[75, 76]

Yolk Sac Tumor

The yolk sac tumor pattern has been recognized for many years but its histogenetic derivation was established quite recently through the careful work of Teilum[1–3] and others. Terms that have been used to describe the lesion include *distinctive adenocarcinoma of infant testis,*[77] *orchioblastoma,*[78] *testicular adenocarcinoma with clear cells,*[79] and *infantile embryonal carcinoma.*[10, 78] However, the term *yolk sac tumor*[80] appears to be now most widely used. Among the nonseminomatous germ cell tumors of the testis, the yolk sac pattern occurs in one of two contexts, *i.e.* either as a pure yolk sac tumor in infants and young children or as focal differentiation within embryonal carcinoma or teratocarcinoma in later life. Pure yolk sac tumor of the adult testis is rare but when it occurs in males under the age of 3½ years, it presents as a fairly rapid testicular enlargement. The cut surface is yellowish and may be cystic.

Microscopic recognition of yolk sac tumor should not be difficult when the pattern is extensive. The morphology may vary considerably within the same lesion. The most common and well known pattern is that of a loose meshwork of small spaces and cysts lined by either flattened cells or by vacuolated cells with nuclei that tend to protrude in a "hobnail" fashion (Figs. 2.21 and 2.22). This loose arrangement blends with solid areas that occasionally assume a nodular distribution (Fig. 2.23). A helpful clue to the diagnosis is the so-called endodermal sinus, a structure that resembles the renal glomerulus but which is composed of a mesodermal core, a central capillary and a "visceral" and "parietal" layer of cells that are epithelial in appearance (Fig. 2.24). There is a loose mesenchymal stroma with a variable amount of mucin.

α-Fetoprotein, a substance known to be synthesized by the human yolk sac,[81, 82] can be demonstrated by immunohistochemical[24, 83, 84] and immunofluorescent[85, 86] means within neoplastic mononuclear cells of the yolk sac tumor. Another technique for the detection of AFP is that of tissue immunoelectophoresis using cryostat-cut tumor tissue, smears or tumor imprints. This method appears to detect large amounts of AFP in as little as 0.5 μg of tumor tissue, even when the preoperative serum levels of AFP are only marginally elevated.[87]

Ultrastructurally, the most notable features of the yolk sac tumor appear to be intra- and extracellular aggregates of basement membrane-like material and deep grooving of the tumor cell nuclei.[49, 88]

The occurrence of yolk sac elements within nonseminomatous germ

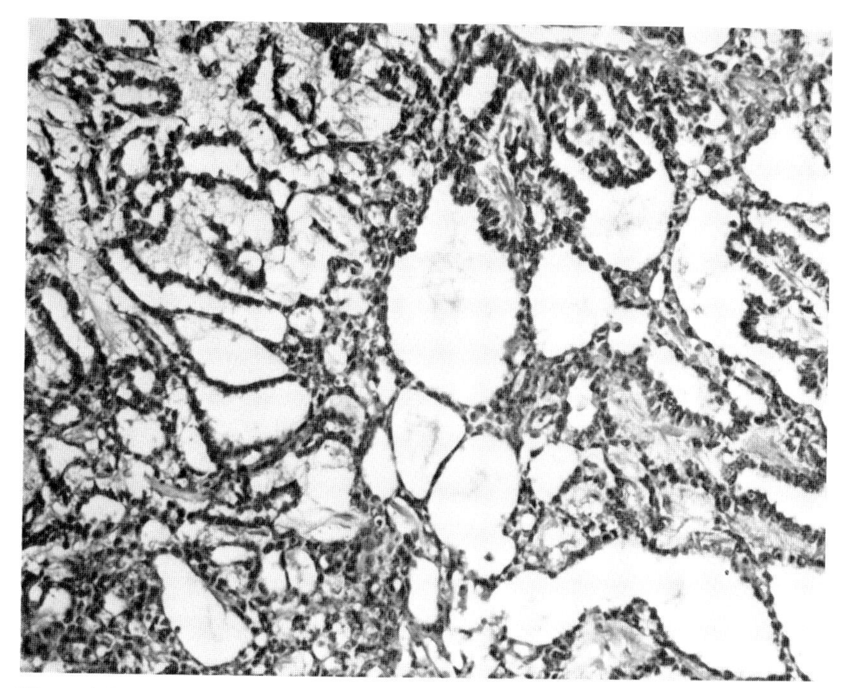

Figure 2.21. Yolk sac tumor. Typical sieve-like spaces with inwardly protruding lumenal tumor cells (H&E × 140).

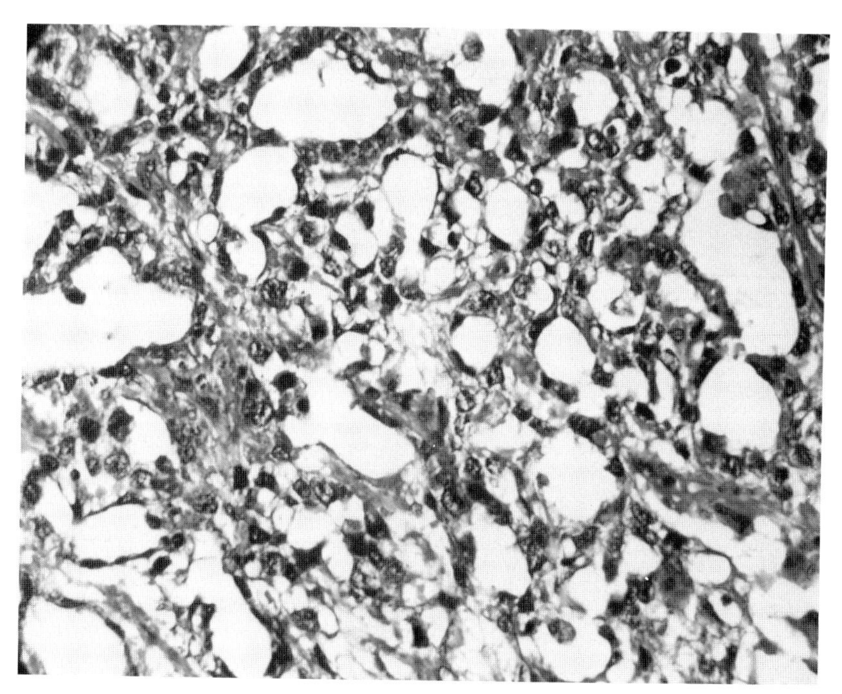

Figure 2.22. Yolk sac tumor. Spaces lined by flattened and protruding (hobnailed) tumor cells (H&E × 290).

cell testicular tumor appears to worsen the prognosis.[89] In one recent study, patients whose tumors contained yolk sac derivatives were more prone to develop central nervous system metastases than when the pattern was absent.[90] In young children and infants with the pure lesion there is

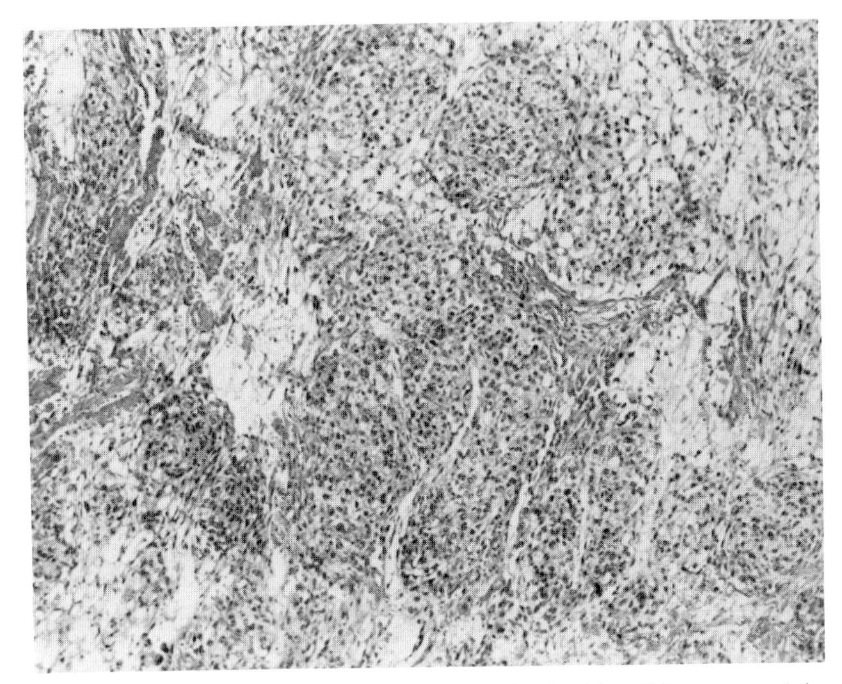

Figure 2.23. Yolk sac tumor. Latticework admixed with solid tumor nodules (H&E × 70).

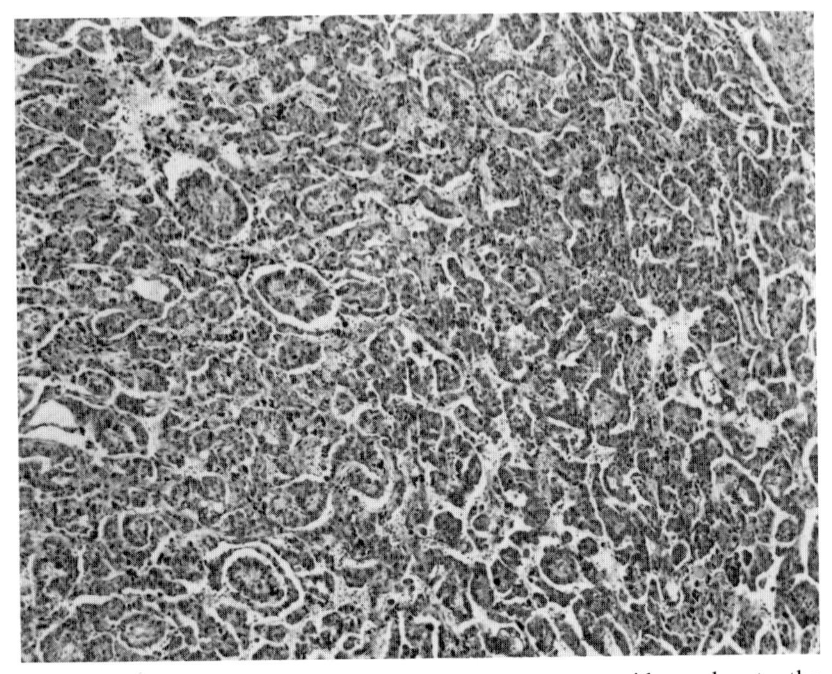

Figure 2.24. Yolk sac tumor. Glomeruloid structures provide a clue to the diagnosis (H&E × 60).

a definite prospect of cure, provided that surgical intervention is early and prompt. It has been claimed that cure is more likely if the tumor is removed before the child is 2 years of age.[80] Fifty-three cases of yolk sac tumor were reviewed by the British Testicular Tumour Panel. Twenty-five percent of the patients died with widespread disease between 2 and 24 months of orchidectomy but 24 patients were alive and well, seven for 5–10 years and five for more than 10 years postoperatively.[10]

The discovery of AFP within the yolk sac tumor clarified the source of the elevated serum marker, which is now widely used to measure the progress of testicular cancer patients after surgery and chemotherapy.[91, 92] Elevation of serum AFP means that the primary tumor or metastasis almost certainly contains nonseminomatous elements. Its elevation in the postorchidectomy patient indicates that tumor is still present somewhere in the body, but the latter determination has to, of course, take account of the half-life of AFP when measurements are made in the immediate postoperative phase. Since the level of AFP does not always parallel that of HCG, the measurement of only one marker may prove unreliable in detecting tumor recurrence.[93] It should be pointed out, too, that circumstances other than germinal testicular cancer can be responsible for elevations of serum AFP, but here the clinical context is quite different.[94–99]

Choriocarcinoma

One of the most aggressive and lethal of human tumors is the choriocarcinoma, an extraembryonal neoplasm that may occur in relation to pregnancy (gestational choriocarcinoma), independent of pregnancy (nongestational choriocarcinoma) in the testis or ovary or, rarely, as a primary extragenital tumor. Pure choriocarcinoma of the testis is rare and there are only a few reported examples.[9, 11] In the pure form, the tumor tends to occur in the second and third decades of life. It is more frequently seen, however, admixed with other germ cell elements such as embryonal carcinoma and teratocarcinoma, and may be recognized grossly by the focal hemorrhages on the cut surface of the tumor.

The microscopic diagnosis of choriocarcinoma depends upon recognition of synctiotrophoblastic giant cells with multiple, often hyperchromatic nuclei and voluminous eosinophilic cytoplasm in intimate relationship to cytotrophoblast, *i.e.* sheets of cells with single nuclei, abundant clear cytoplasm and well defined cell borders (Fig. 2.25). The synctial cells often contain intracytoplasmic lumina filled with erythrocytes and are frequently closely applied to small blood vessels. Small and large blood-filled spaces lined by syncytiotrophoblastic cells alone are not unusual in embryonal carcinoma or teratocarcinoma (Fig. 2.26). One should, however, resist the temptation to regard these foci as choriocarcinoma since they lack cytotrophoblast and because these tumors are not usually associated with the extraordinarily high levels of serum HCG and the widespread dissemination of true choriocarcinoma.

When a male presents with distant choriocarcinomatous metastases, the testes, even though apparently normal to palpation, should be considered as a possible primary source since choriocarcinoma has a well known propensity toward systemic spread when still very small. Serial section of the testes at autopsy may even reveal a fibrous scar, regarded by some authors as representing a regressed or "burned out" primary tumor. In these testes one may also encounter small hematoxylin-staining deposits, which may originate from necrotic germinal tumor cells.[100]

Human chorionic gonadotropin has long been employed as a diagnostic

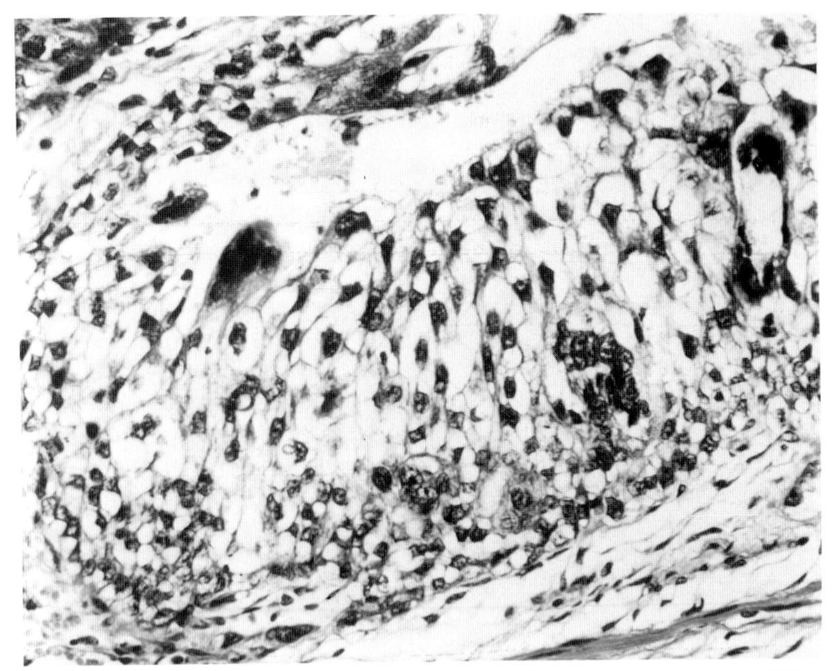

Figure 2.25. Choriocarcinoma. Closely related synctio- and cytotrophoblast (H&E × 275).

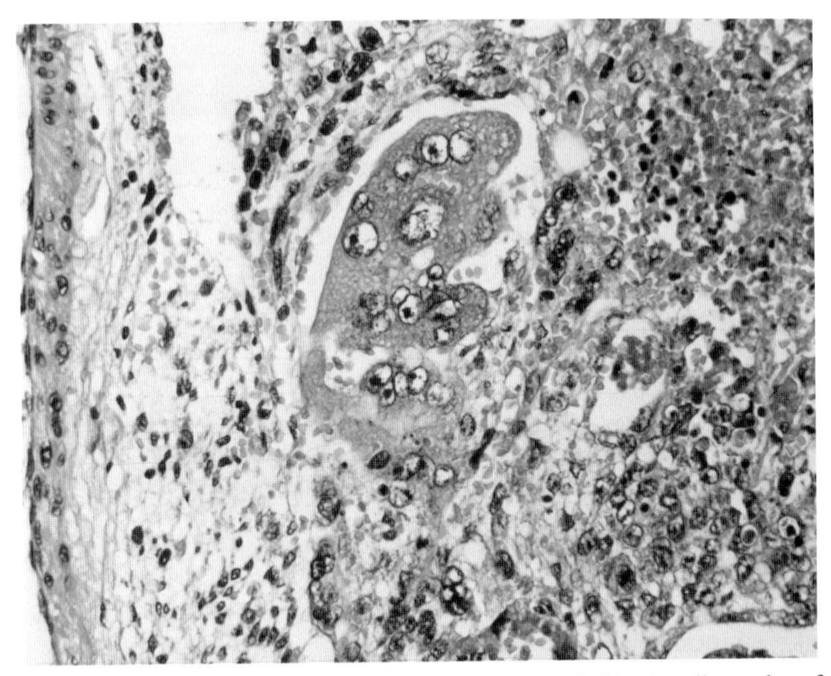

Figure 2.26. Embryonal carcinoma. Isolated synctiotrophoblastic cells at edge of blood-filled cyst do not constitute choriocarcinoma.

marker of trophoblastic neoplasia, but since it is structurally similar to the pituitary counterpart, luteinizing hormone (HL,HLH), it was relatively difficult to discriminate one hormone from the other by the older available techniques, *e.g.* agglutination-inhibition. However, when the subunits of

HCG[101] and HLH[102] were eventually characterized, it was discovered that, of the two units (α, β) in each molecule, immunologic specificity resided in the β segment.[103] This paved the way for the development of a radioimmunoassay that could measure small quantitites of β-HCG without interference from HLH present in the sample.[104] Nonetheless, a certain amount of cross-reactivity does still occur, depending upon the type of assay used. For this reason, caution should be exercised with borderline elevations of serum HCG, particularly when the circumstances are such that the patient is already prone to high levels of HLH, *e.g.* postoperative or post-therapeutic hypogonadism. The determination of serum HCG *via* measurement of the β-subunit now forms an indispensable part of the management of patients with germ cell tumors of the testis. The clinical applications of this marker have been presented elsewhere in detail.[91]

INTRATUBULAR GERM CELL NEOPLASIA

The early detection of preneoplastic change is perhaps one of the most important means of improving survival from a wide range of tumors and the prognosis for patients with germinal tumors of the testis is no doubt best when these lesions are discovered at an early stage. It would be most desirable to detect germ cell tumors of the testis in their infancy, when they are still confined within the boundary of the seminiferous tubule (Fig. 2.27). Such an approach to premalignant alterations within the seminiferous epithelium has, through the work of Skakkebaek and his coworkers yielded fruitful results. In several articles, they have described the occurrence of atypical intratubular germ cells in testicular biopsy

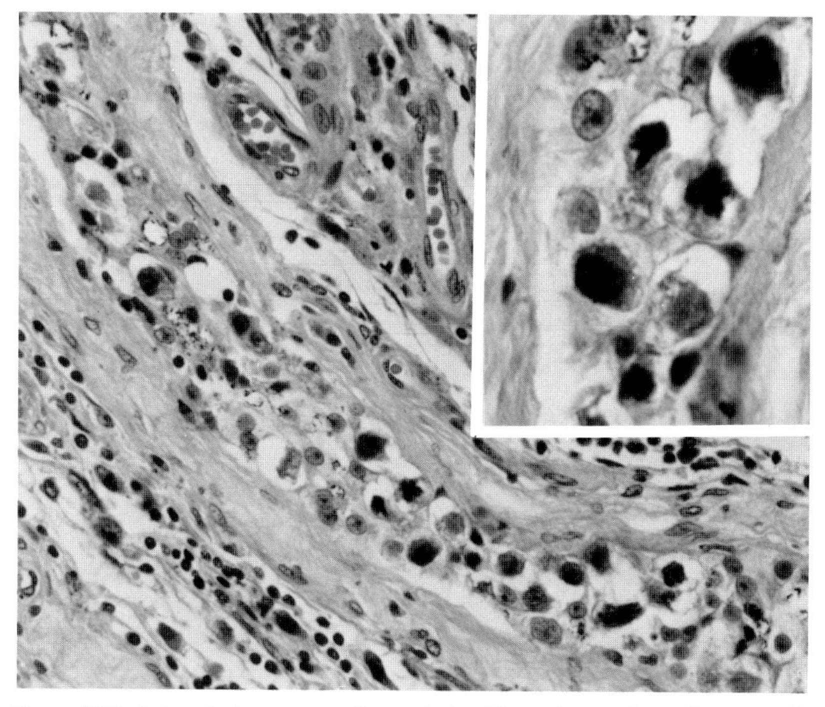

Figure 2.27. Intratubular germ cell neoplasia. Hyperchromatic malignant cells occupy the seminiferous tubules (*see inset*) (H&E × 375, 800).

samples from infertile men.[105, 106] In one series, four of their six patients with intratubular germ cell neoplasia developed an invasive tumor between 1 and 5 years after initial biopsy, while the remaining 449 men in the study were unaffected.[107] A different group in Switzerland reported the testicular findings in 1635 infertile men; of nine patients with cytologic abnormalities, five developed malignant tumors within 6 years.[108] The evidence therefore strongly suggests that intratubular malignancy precedes invasive germ cell tumors of the testis in infertile men. Precancerous changes have also been observed in the adjacent, apparently uninvolved areas of testes that contain germinal tumors,[109] and this poses the difficult question of how to manage the opposite gonad, particularly since there is a known tendency for a second germ cell tumor to develop in the contralateral testis of men who have already had testicular cancer.[110] At a practical level, Skakkebaek[107] has suggested the use of testicular biopsy in patients with cryptorchidism, previous unilateral testicular cancer, and infertility. Among the latter, those with intratubular cytologic abnormalities stand an approximately 70% chance of developing an invasive germ cell tumor within 5 years of the recognition of germinal dysplasia.[111, 112]

It is apparent from recent studies that the atypical cells that characterize intratubular germinal neoplasia of the testis may form seminoma, spermatocytic seminoma, embryonal carcinoma and even yolk sac tumor.[13] Rarely may syncytiotrophoblast be observed to take origin within the seminiferous tubular epithelium.[13] Based upon this diverse potential, Scully has proposed a systematic approach that takes account of the range of morphologic expression in carcinoma *in situ* of the testis (Table 2.2).[4, 71]

MALDESCENT

Most authors agree that maldescent of the testis definitely incurs a greater risk of eventual malignant change than in the male population in general.[10, 113–115] The probability of such a development appears to be about 20–40 times greater in the cryptorchid than in the normally descended (eutopic) organ[113, 116] and the risk of cancer seems to be higher when the testis lies intra-abdominally.[4] However, in about 20% of cases, patients with unilateral cryptorchidism actually develop a neoplasm in the contralateral eutopic testis.[10, 117] While the most likely tumor to occur in the maldescended testis is a seminoma, other germ cell tumors such as embryonal carcinoma and teratocarcinoma have also been reported.[113]

Table 2.2.
Classification of Intratubular Germ Cell Neoplasia[a]

1. Intratubular germ cell neoplasia, unclassified
2. Intratubular germ cell neoplasia, unclassified, with extratubular infiltration
3. Intratubular seminoma, typical
4. Intratubular seminoma, spermatocytic
5. Intratubular embryonal carcinoma
6. Other forms of intratubular germ cell tumor (*e.g.* with syncytiotrophoblast, yolk sac tumor or teratoma)[13]

[a] Presented at the International Symposium on Testis Cancer, Mouse Teratocarcinoma and Oncofetal Proteins. University of Minnesota Medical School, Minneapolis, Minn., June 26–28, 1980.

There appears to be no guarantee that orchiopexy, even when performed before a child is 10 years of age, will prevent subsequent tumor formation.[114, 118, 119] It is therefore important to observe these individuals well beyond the occurrence of spontaneous late descent or orchiopexy. Since histologic changes representing carcinoma *in situ* have been reported as occurring in the cryptorchid testis,[115] it would appear that testicular biopsy should assume a role in the management of patients with this condition.

It is now apparent that, in addition to its effect upon the female genital system, prenatal exposure to diethylstilbestrol produces anatomic changes in the male reproductive organs as well, including cryptorchidism as a possible sequel.[120] In the series of 308 men exposed to the drug *in utero*, Gill *et al.*[120] found that 31.5% of this group had hypoplastic testes and/or epididymal cysts. Of the 26 diethylstilbestrol-exposed men with testicular hypoplasia, 65% had a history of cryptorchidism.

The interruption of the spermatic cord lymphatics necessitated by orchiopexy probably explains the high incidence of ilioinguinal metastases when cancer occurs in the testis at some time after such an operation.[4] Germ cell tumors occurring under such circumstances may consequently

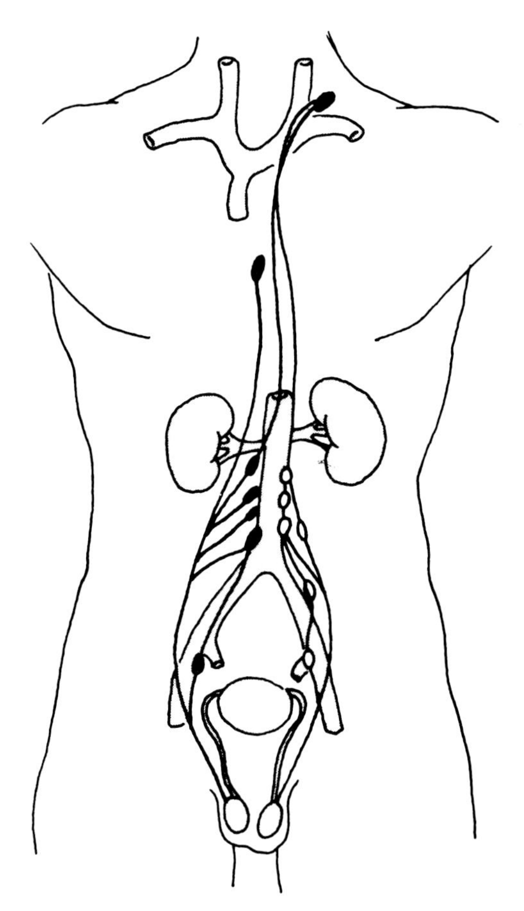

Figure 2.28. Lymphatic spread of germ cell testicular tumors to the retroperitoneum and mediastinum. (Reproduced by permission from L. E. Nochomovitz and J. Rosai. Pathology of germ cell tumors of the testis. *Urological Clinics of North America 4:*374, 1977.)

be more difficult to treat. The 5-year survival from seminoma developing in the cryptorchid testis was reported in one series as 78% after orchidectomy and regional lymph node irradiation.[113]

METASTATIC DISEASE PATTERNS

The spread of germ cell tumors of the testis usually occurs *via* lymphatics that drain toward the common iliac and para-aortic lymph nodes (Fig. 2.28). Supradiaphragmatic disease (*i.e.* tumorous mediastinal and supraclavicular nodes) may occasionally be found in the absence of detectable abdominal or scrotal involvement, in which case both testes must be carefully sectioned should an autopsy be performed, before concluding that the lesion is primarily extragonadal. However, the anterior mediastinum is a most unlikely site for spread from a testicular tumor and, in the absence of other evidence of disease, a germinal tumor in that location is most probably of primary mediastinal origin.[121] Epididymal disease drains to the external iliac lymph nodes, with possible spread to the obturator node in the internal iliac group. Scrotal exploration is not warranted for testicular tumors since the interruption of lymphatics then invites drainage to the inguinal lymph nodes. Tumor recurrence, when it occurs in a cutaneous scrotal scar, may eventually involve the latter group of nodes as well. Embryonal carcinoma frequently spreads to the liver, lungs, and bones of the trunk.[8] Similarly, adult teratoma involves the abdominal and mediastinal lymph nodes, lungs, liver, brain and other miscellaneous sites.[9] The classical seminoma usually spreads as such, while the metastases arising from teratocarcinoma frequently consist of embryonal carcinoma alone.[11]

REFERENCES

1. Teilum, G. Gonocytoma; homologous ovarian and testicular tumors; I; with discussion of "mesonephroma ovarii." *Acta Pathol. Microbiol. Scand. 23:*242, 1946.
2. Teilum, G. "Mesonephroma ovarii" (Schiller)—an extra-embryonic mesoblastoma of germ cell origin in the ovary and the testis. *Acta Pathol. Microbiol. Scand. 27:*249, 1950.
3. Teilum, G. Special Tumors of Ovary and Testis. *Comparative Pathology and Histological Identification*, Ed. 2. Lippincott, Philadelphia, 1977.
4. International Symposium on Human Testis Cancer, Mouse Teratocarcinoma and Oncofetal Proteins. University of Minnesota Medical School, Minneapolis, Minnesota, June 26–28, 1980.
5. Nochomovitz, L. E. Seminoma of the testis. *World Urology Update Series*, Vol. 1, Lesson 24 (In press) 1982.
6. Friedman, N. B., and Moore, R. A. Tumors of the testis. A report on 922 cases. *Milit. Surg. 99:*573, 1946.
7. Dixon, F. J., and Moore, R. A. Tumors of the male sex organs. In *Atlas of Tumor Pathology, Section 8, Fascicles 31b, 32.* Armed Forces Institute of Pathology, Washington, D.C., 1952.
8. Collins, D. H., and Pugh, R. C. B. (eds). *The Pathology of Testicular Tumours.* Livingstone,Edinburgh, 1964.
9. Mostofi, F. K., and Price, E. B., Jr. Tumors of the male genital system. *Atlas of Tumor Pathology, 2nd series, Fascicle 8,* Armed Forces Institute of Pathology, Washington, D.C., 1973.
10. Pugh, R. C. B. (ed). *Pathology of the Testis.* Blackwell, Oxford, 1976.
11. Bär, W., and Hedinger, C. Comparison of histologic types of primary testicular germ cell tumors—consequences for the WHO and the British nomenclatures? *Virchows Arch. [Pathol. Anat.] 370:*41, 1976.

12. Mostofi, F. K., and Sobin, L. H. *International Histological Classification of Tumors of Testes (No. 16)*, World Health Organization, Geneva, 1977.
13. Mostofi, F. K. Pathology of germ cell tumors of the testis. A progress report. *Cancer 45:*1735, 1980.
14. Mostofi, F. K. Testicular tumors. Epidemiologic, etiologic and pathologic features. *Cancer 32:*1186, 1973.
15. Thackray, A. C. Seminoma. In *The Pathology of Testicular Tumours*, edited by D. H. Collins, and R. C. B. Pugh. Livingstone, Edinburgh, 1964, pp. 12–27.
16. Fraley, E. E. The testicular mass: an approach to diagnosis and treatment. In *Advances in Cancer Surgery*, edited by J. S. Najarian and J. P. Delaney. Symposia Specialists, Miami, 1976.
17. Lindsey, C. M., and Glenn, J.F. Germinal malignancies of the testis: experience, management and prognosis. *J. Urol. 116:*59, 1976.
18. Johnson, D. E., Gomez, J. J., and Ayala, A. G. Histologic factors affecting prognosis of pure seminoma of the testis. *South. Med. J. 69:*1173, 1976.
19. Gould, R. P., and Haddad, R. Extratubular migration of gonocytes in the foetal rabbit testis. *Nature 273:*464, 1978.
20. McGinley, D., Posalaky, Z., and Porvaznik, M. Intercellular junctional complexes of the rat seminiferous tubules: a freeze-fracture study. *Anat. Rec. 189:*211, 1977.
21. Dunia, I., Nicholas, J., Jakob, H., Benedetti, E., and Jacob, F. Junctional modulation in mouse embryonal carcinoma cells by Fab fragments of rabbit antiembryonal carcinoma cell serum. *Proc. Natl. Acad. Sci.* USA *76:*3387, 1979.
22. Friedman, M., and Pearlman, A. W. "Seminoma with trophocarcinoma." A clinical variant of seminoma. *Cancer 26:*46, 1970.
23. Heyderman, E., and Neville, A. M. Syncytiotrophoblasts in testicular tumours. *Lancet 2:*103, 1976.
24. Kurman, R. J., Scardino, P. T., McIntire, K. R., Waldmann, T. A., and Javadpour, N. Cellular localization of alpha-fetoprotein and human chorionic gonadotropin in germ cell tumors of the testis using an indirect immunoperoxidase technique. A new approach to classification using tumor markers. *Cancer 40:*2136, 1977.
25. Heyderman, E. Multiple tissue markers in human malignant testicular tumours. *Scand. J. Immunol. 8 (Suppl 8):*119, 1978.
26. Lange, P. H., Bremner, R. D., Horne, C. H. W., Vessella, R. L., and Fraley, E. E. Is SP1 a marker for testicular cancer? *Urology 15:*251, 1980.
27. Teisner, B., Westergaard, J. G., Folkersen, J., Husby, S., and Svehag, S. E. Two pregnancy-associated serum proteins with pregnancy-specific β1-glycoprotein determinants. *Am. J. Obstet. Gynecol. 131:*262, 1978.
28. Obiewke, B. C., Grudzinskas, J. G., Gordon, Y. B., Chard, T., and Bohn, H. Circulating levels of placental protein 5 (PP5) in third trimester. In *Carcino-Embryonic-Proteins: Chemistry, Biology, Clinical Applications*, Vol. 2, pp. 629–632, edited by F. G. Lehmann. Elsevier/North-Holland Biomedical Press, New York, 1979.
29. Porteous, I. B., Beck, J. S., and Pugh, R. C. B. Localization of human placental factor in malignant teratoma of the testis. *J. Pathol. Bacteriol. 95:*527, 1968.
30. Pierce, G. B., Jr. Ultrastructure of human testicular tumors. *Cancer 19:*1963, 1966.
31. Whitmore, W. F., Smith, A., Yagoda, A., Cvitkovic, E., and Golbey, R. Chemotherapy of seminoma. *Recent Results Cancer Res 60:*244, 1977.
32. Einhorn, L. H., and Donohue, J. Combination chemotherapy in disseminated testicular cancer: the Indiana University experience. *Semin. Oncol. 6:*87, 1979.
33. Percarpio, B., Clements, J. C., McLeod, D. G., Sorgen, S. D., and Cardinale, F. S. Anaplastic seminoma. An analysis of 77 patients. *Cancer 43:*2510, 1979.
34. Kademian, M., Bosch, A., and Caldwell, W. L. Anaplastic seminoma. *Cancer 40:*3082, 1977.
35. Johnson, D. E., Gomez, J. J., and Ayala, A. G. Anaplastic seminoma. *J. Urol. 114:*80, 1975.
36. Scardino, P. T., Cox, H. D., Thomas, A., Waldmann, K., McIntire, K. R., Mittemeyer, B., *et al.* The value of serum tumor markers in the staging and prognosis of germ cell tumors of the testis. *J. Urol. 118:*994, 1977.
37. Javadpour, N., McIntire, K. R., Waldmann, T. A., and Bergman, M. The role of alpha-fetoprotein and human chorionic gonadotropin in seminoma. *J. Urol. 120:*687, 1978.
38. Lange, P. H., Nochomovitz, L. E., Rosai, J., Fraley, E. E., Kennedy, B. J., Bosl, G., *et al.* Serum alpha-fetoprotein and human chorionic gonadotropin in patients with seminoma. *J. Urol. 124:*472, 1980.

39. Parkinson, C., and Beilby, J. O. W. Testicular germ cell tumours: should current classification be revised? *Invest. Cell Pathol. 3:*135, 1980.
40. Pugh, R. C. B., and Cameron, K. M. Teratoma. In *Pathology of the testis*, edited by R. C. B. Pugh, Blackwell, Oxford, 1976.
41. Raghavan, D., Heyderman, E., Monaghan, P., Gibbs, J., Ruoslahti, E., Peckham, M. J., *et al.* Hypothesis: when is a seminoma not a seminoma? *J. Clin. Pathol* (In press).
42. Masson, P. Étude sur le séminome. *Rev. Can. Biol. 5:*361, 1946.
43. Rosai, J., Silber, I., and Khodadoust, K. Spermatocytic seminoma. I: Clinicopathologic study of six cases and review of the literature. *Cancer 24:*92, 1969.
44. Talerman, A. Spermatocytic seminoma. Clinicopathologic study of 22 cases. *Cancer 45:*2169, 1980.
45. Rosai, J., Khodadoust, K., and Silber, I. Spermatocytic seminoma. II: Ultrastructural study. *Cancer 24:*103, 1969.
46. Kleinsmith, L. J., and Pierce, G. B., Jr. Multipotentiality of single embryonal carcinoma cells. *Cancer Res 24:*1544, 1964.
47. Stevens, L. C. The development of teratomas from intratesticular grafts of tubal mouse eggs. *J. Embryol. Exp. Morphol. 20:*329, 1968.
48. Damjanov, I., and Solter, D. Experimental teratoma. *Curr. Top. Pathol. 59:*69, 1974.
49. Nochomovitz, L. E., and Rosai, J. Current concepts on the histogenesis, pathology, and immunochemistry of germ cell tumors of the testis. *Pathol. Annu. 13:*327, 1978.
50. Illmensee, K., and Stevens, L. C. Teratomas and chimeras. *Sci. Am. 240:*120, 1979.
51. Martin, G. R. Teratocarcinomas and mammalian embryogenesis. *Science 209:*768, 1980.
52. Mintz, B., and Illmensee, K. Normal genetically mosaic mice produced from malignant teratocarcinoma cells. *Proc. Natl. Acad. Sci. USA. 72:*3585, 1975.
53. Brinster, R. L. The effect of cells transferred into the mouse blastocyst on subsequent development. *J. Exp. Med. 140:*1049, 1974.
54. Papaioannou, V. E., McBurney, M. W., Gardner, R. L., and Evans, M. J. Fate of teratocarcinoma cells injected into early mouse embryos. *Nature 258:*70, 1975.
55. Nicolas, J. F., Avner, P., Gaillard, J., Guénet, J. L., Jakob, H., and Jacob, F. Cell lines derived from teratocarcinoma. *Cancer Res. 36:*4224, 1976.
56. Kemler, R., Babinet, C., Eisen, H., and Jacob, F. Surface antigen in early differentiation. *Proc. Natl. Acad. Sci. USA. 74:*4449, 1977.
57. Talerman, A., and Haije, W. G. Alpha-fetoprotein and germ cell tumors: a possible role of yolk-sac tumor in production of alpha-fetoprotein. *Cancer 34:*1722, 1974.
58. Nørgaard-Pedersen, B., Albrechtsen, R., and Teilum, G. Serum alpha-foetoprotein as a marker for endodermal sinus tumour (yolk sac tumour) or a vitelline component of "teratocarcinoma." *Acta Pathol. Microbiol. Scand. [A] 83:*573, 1975.
59. Lange, P. H., McIntire, R. K., Waldmann, T. A., Hakala, T. R., and Fraley, E. E. Serum alpha-fetoprotein and human chorionic gonadotropin in the diagnosis and management of nonseminomatous germ cell testicular cancer. *N. Eng. J. Med. 295:*1237, 1976.
60. Lange, P. H., and Fraley, E. E. Serum alpha-fetoprotein and human chorionic gonadotropin in the treatment of patients with testicular tumors. *Urol. Clin. North. Am. 4:*393, 1977.
61. Keogh, B., Hreshchyshyn, M. M., Moore, R. H., Merrin, C. E., and Murphy, G. P. Urinary gonadotropins in management and prognosis of testicular tumor. *Urology 5:*496, 1975.
62. Wang, N., Trend, B., Bronson, D. L., and Fraley, E. E. Nonrandom abnormalties in Chromosome 1 in human testicular cancers. *Cancer Res. 40:*796, 1980.
63. Fraley, E. E., Lange, P. H., and Kennedy, B. J. Medical Progress: germ cell testicular cancer in adults. *N. Engl. J. Med. 301:*1370, 1979.
64. Fraley, E. E., Lange, P. H., and Kennedy, B. J. Medical Progress: germ cell testicular cancer in adults. *N. Engl. J. Med. 301:*1420, 1979.
65. Bosl, G. J., Lange, P. H., Fraley, E. E., Nochomovitz, L. E., Rosai, J., Vogelzang, N. J., *et al.* Vinblastine, bleomycin, and *cis*-diamminedichloroplatinum in the treatment of advanced testicular carcinoma. Possible importance of longer induction and shorter maintenance schedules. *Am. J. Med. 68:*492, 1980.
66. Einhorn, L. H., and Donohue, J. P. *Cis*-diamminedichloroplatinum, vinblastine and bleomycin combination chemotherapy in disseminated testicular cancer. *Ann. Intern. Med. 87:*293, 1977.
67. Einhorn, L. H., and Williams, S. D. Chemotherapy of disseminated testicular cancer:

a random prospective study. *Cancer, 46:*1339, 1980.

68. Fraley, E. E., Kedia, K., and Markland, C. The role of radical operation in the management of nonseminomatous germinal tumors of the testicle in the adult. In *Controversy in Surgery*, pp. 479–488, edited by J. P. Delaney and R. Varco, Saunders, Philadelphia, 1976.
69. Van der Werff-Messing, B. Radiotherapeutic treatment of testicular tumors. *Int. J. Radiat. Oncol. Biol. Phys. 1:*235, 1976.
70. DeWolf, W. C., Lange, P. H., Einarson, M. E., and Yunis, E. J. HLA and testicular cancer. *Nature 277:*216, 1979.
71. Ackerman, L. V., and Rosai, J. (eds). Male reproductive system—testis. In Surgical Pathology Ed. 6, Mosby, St. Louis, 1981.
72. Parkinson, C., Beilby, J. O. W. Features of prognostic significance in testicular germ cell tumours. *J. Clin. Pathol. 30:*113, 1977.
73. Norris, H. J., Zirkin, H. J., and Benson, W. L. Immature (malignant) teratoma of the ovary. A clinical and pathologic study of 58 cases. *Cancer 37:*2359, 1976.
74. Johnson, D. E., Bracken, R. B., Blight, E. M. Prognosis for pathologic stage I nonseminomatous germ cell tumors of the testis managed by retroperitoneal lymphadenectomy. *J. Urol. 116:*63, 1976.
75. Riley, P. A., and Sutton, P. M. Why are ovarian teratomas benign whilst teratomas of the testis are malignant? *Lancet 1:*1360, 1975.
76. Erickson, R. P., and Gondos, B. Alternative explanations of the differing behaviour of ovarian and testicular teratomas. *Lancet 1:*407, 1976.
77. Teoh, T. B., Steward, J. K., and Willis, R. A. The distinctive adenocarcinoma of the infant's testis: an account of 15 cases. *J. Pathol. Bacteriol. 80:*147, 1960.
78. Hessl, J. M. Orchioblastoma or infantile embryonal carcinoma. *Urology 5:*265, 1975.
79. Magner, D., Campbell, J. S., Wiglesworth, F. W. Testicular adenocarcinoma with clear cells occurring in infancy. *Cancer 9:*165, 1956.
80. Pierce, G. B., Bullock, W. K., and Huntington, R. W., Jr. Yolk-sac tumors of the testis. *Cancer 25:*644, 1970.
81. Gitlin, D., and Perricelli, A. Synthesis of serum albumin, prealbumin, α-foetoprotein, α_1-antitryspin and transferrin by the human yolk sac. *Nature 228:*995, 1970.
82. Gitlin, D., Perricelli, A., and Gitlin, G. M. Synthesis of α-fetoprotein by liver, yolk sac and gastrointestinal tract of the human conceptus. *Cancer Res. 32:*979, 1972.
83. Kurman, R. J., and Norris, H. J. Endodermal sinus tumor of the ovary: a clinical and pathologic analysis of 71 cases. *Cancer 38:*2404, 1976.
84. Palmer, P. E., Safaii, H., and Wolfe, H. J. Alpha$_1$-antitrypsin and alpha-fetoprotein. Protein markers in endodermal sinus (yolk sac) tumors. *Am. J. Clin. Pathol. 65:*575, 1976.
85. Itoh, T., Shirai, T., Naka, A., and Matsumato, S. Yolk sac tumor and α-fetoprotein: clinicopathologic study of four cases. *Gan 65:*215, 1974.
86. Teilum, G., Albrechtsen, R., and Nørgaard-Pedersen, B. Immunofluorescent localization of alpha-fetoprotein synthesis in endodermal sinus tumor (yolk-sac tumor). *Acta Pathol. Microbiol. Scand. [A] 82:*586, 1974.
87. Nørgaard-Pedersen, B., Toftager-Larsen, K., Nørcgaard-Hansen, K., Albrechtsen, R. Radioimmunoelectrophoretical detection of alpha-fetoprotein in tumor tissue specimens. *Invest. Cell. Pathol. 3:*147, 1980.
88. Nogales-Fernandez, F., Silverberg, S. G., Bloustein, P. A., Martinez-Hernandez, A., and Pierce, G. B. Yolk sac carcinoma (endodermal sinus tumor). Ultrastructure and histogenesis of gonadal and extragonadal tumors in comparison with normal human yolk sac. *Cancer 39:*1462, 1977.
89. Talerman, A. The incidence of yolk sac tumor (endodermal sinus tumor) elements in germ cell tumors of the testis in adults. *Cancer 36:*211, 1975.
90. Williams, S. D., and Einhorn, L. H. Brain metastases in disseminated germinal neoplasms. Incidence and clinical course. *Cancer 44:*1514, 1979.
91. Lange, P. H., McIntire, K. R., and Waldmann, T. A. Tumor markers in testicular tumors: current status and future prospects. In *Testicular Tumors: Management and Treatment*, edited by L. H. Einhorn. Masson, New York, 1980.
92. Sell, S. (ed). *Cancer Markers: Diagnostic and Developmental Significance.* Humana Press, Clifton, N.J., 1980.
93. Braunstein, G. O., McIntire, K. R., and Waldmann, T. A. Discordance of human chorionic gonadotropin and alpha-fetoprotein in testicular teratocarcinomas. *Cancer 31:*126, 1979.

94. Alpert, E., Pinn, V. W., and Isselbacher, K. J. Alpha-fetoprotein in a patient with gastric carcinoma metastatic to the liver. *N. Eng. J. Med. 285:*1058, 1971.
95. Nørgaard-Pedersen, B., Dabelsteen, E., and Edeling, C-J. Localisation of human α-foetoprotein synthesis in hepatoblastoma cells by immunofluorescence and immunoperoxidase methods. *Acta Pathol. Microbiol. Scand. [A] 82:*169, 1974.
96. Purves, L. R., and Purves, M. Serum alpha-fetoprotein. VI. The radioimmunossay evidence for the presence of AFP in the serum of normal people during pregnancy. *S. Afr. Med. J. 46:*1290, 1972 (abstract).
97. Ruoslahti, E., and Seppälä, M. α-Foetoprotein in normal human serum. *Nature 235:*161, 1972.
98. Nayak, N. C., Malaviya, A. N., Chawla, V., and Chandra, R. K. α-Fetoprotein in Indian childhood cirrhosis. *Lancet 1:*68, 1972.
99. Waldmann, T. A., and McIntire, K. R. Serum alpha-fetoprotein levels in patients with ataxia-telangiectasia. *Lancet 2:*1112, 1972.
100. Azzopardi, J. G., Mostofi, F. K., and Theiss, E. A. Lesions of the testes observed in certain patients with widespread choriocarcinoma and related tumors. *Am. J. Pathol. 38:*207, 1961.
101. Swaminathan, N., and Bahl Om P. Dissociation and recombination of the subunits of human chorionic gonadotropin. *Biochem. Biophys. Res. Commun. 40:*422, 1970.
102. Reichert, L. E., and Ward, D. N. Studies on subunits of human pituitary luteinizing hormone (H-LH). *Fed. Proc. 28:*505, 1977, (abstract).
103. Pierce, J. G., Bahl, Om P., Cornell, J. S., and Swaminathan, N. Biologically active hormones prepared by recombination of the α-chain of human chorionic gonadotropin and the hormone-specific chain of bovine thyrotropin or of bovine luteinizing hormone. *J. Biol. Chem. 246:*2321, 1971.
104. Vaitukaitis, J. L., Braunstein, G. D., and Ross, G. T. A radioimmunoassay which specifically measures human chorionic gonadotropin in the presence of human luteinizing hormone. *Am. J. Obstet. Gynecol. 113:*751, 1972.
105. Skakkebaek, N. E. Possible carcinoma *in situ* of the testis. Lancet *2:*516, 1972.
106. Skakkebaek, N. E. Abnormal morphology of germ cells in two infertile men. *Acta Pathol. Microbiol. Scand. [A] 80:*374, 1972.
107. Skakkebaek, N. E. Carcinoma *in situ* of the testis: frequency and relationship to invasive germ cell tumours in infertile men. *Histopathology 2:*157, 1978.
108. Nuesch-Bachmann, I. H., and Hedinger, C. Atypische spermatogonien als präkanzerose. Schweiz. *Med. Wochenschr. 107:*795, 1977.
109. Skakkebaek, N. E. Atypical germ cells in the adjacent "normal" tissue of testicular tumours. *Acta Pathol. Microbiol. Scand. [A] 83:*127, 1975.
110. Gilbert, J. B., and Hamilton, J. B. Studies in malignant testis tumors. III-Incidence and nature of tumors in ectopic testes. *Surg. Gynecol. Obstet. 71:*731, 1940.
111. Skakkebaek, N. E., and Berthelsen, J. G. Carcinoma *in situ* of testis and orchiectomy. *Lancet 2:*204, 1978.
112. Testicular biopsy for early detection of testicular tumour. Editorial *Br. Med. J. 280:*426, 1980.
113. Batata, M. A., Whitmore, W. F., Jr., and Hilaris, B. S. Cancer of the undescended or maldescended testis. *AJR 126:*302, 1976.
114. Dow, J. A., and Mostofi, F. K. Testicular tumors following orchiopexy. *South. Med. J. 60:*193, 1967.
115. Krabbe, S., Skakkebaek, N. E., Berthelsen, J. G., Eyben, F. V., Volsted, P. Mauritzen, K., *et al.* High incidence of undetected neoplasia in maldescended testes. *Lancet 1:*999, 1979.
116. Whitaker, R. H. Management of the undescended testis. *Br. J. Hosp. Med. 4:*25, 1970.
117. Wangensteen, O. H. The undescended testicle. An experimental and clinical study. Doctoral dissertation, University of Minnesota, 1925.
118. DeCenzo, J. M., Leadbetter, G. W., Jr. Early orchiopexy and testis tumors. *Urology 5:*365, 1975.
119. Martin, D. C. Germinal cell tumors of the testis after orchiopexy. *J. Urol. 121:*422, 1979.
120. Gill, W. B., Schumacher, G. F. B., Bibbo, M., Strauss, F. H., II, and Schoenberg, H. W. Association of diethylstilbestrol exposure *in utero* with cryptorchidism, testicular hypoplasia, and semen abnormalities. *J. Urol. 122:*36, 1979.

3

Two Research Topics

Part A

Experimental Pathology

John F. Harris, Ph.D.
Michael A. S. Jewett, M.D., F.R.C.S.(C).

Most of the basic investigation of germinal testis tumors has been confined to the nonseminomas. Although approximately 50% of all germinal tumors are seminomas, there are no reliable experimental models and tumor tissue has yet to be maintained in the laboratory. This review will therefore focus on current experimental pathology of the nonseminomas and describe efforts to characterize the putative stem cell of both murine teratocarcinoma and human testicular tumor cell lines.

Germ cell tumors frequently consist of mixed cell types, some of which are malignant. In the murine teratocarcinoma model the identification and characterization of the stem cell of the tumor has greatly aided the understanding of the system. The different cell phenotypes are thought to be related by the normal pathways of differentiation, although the probabilities of transition to various stages may be altered. Several reviews have described the analogies observed with normal development using the mouse model of germ cell tumors.[1-11]

CHARACTERIZATION OF MURINE EMBRYONAL CARCINOMA CELLS

The spontaneous frequency of strain 129 mouse teratocarcinoma is small, but it may be enhanced by genetic factors.[12] The generation of independent embryonal carcinoma (EC) retransplantable tumors by the transplantation of primordial germ cells and presomatic embryos to ectopic sites is well documented.[13-16] The process of induction of teratocarcinoma is not only dependent primarily on the timing[13-16] of transplantation but also on genetic factors. The generation of independent teratocarcinomas has been mainly confined to 129 and C3H highly inbred laboratory mice. It appears that the process is not altered in that the one basic EC stem cell is generated by all these experiments; however, in the various methods of generation the frequency of teratocarcinoma may vary considerably. Thus, the available EC model is generated from a relatively restricted set of murine genes. A similar model system is not generated from embryo transplants performed in the rat. The yolk sac tumor (derived from extraembryonic cells) is only event observed in the rat.[17] Thus, the properties of the murine teratocarcinoma may be a unique occurrence in mammals.

The stem cell of teratocarcinoma is called the embryonal carcinoma (EC) cell. The properties of this cell most compare with the embryonal ectoderm cells of a 4-day embryo.[18, 19] The general properties described here are mainly derived from the cell lines *in vitro*.[20–35] The characterization encompasses the disciplines of histology, biochemistry, virology and immunology.

Stability

The use of tissue culture lines for genetic analysis *in vitro* has greatly increased the quantitative data on the rates of change of particular phenotypes. In addition, rigorous cloning and recloning procedures may be used to characterize presumptive variants occurring at random in cell populations to verify the stability of altered phenotypes. EC lines may exhibit different phenotypes but these differences are thought to be mutational rather than multiple classes of EC stem cells.

The tendency for tumor formation involving a mixture of malignant phenotypes occurs with high frequency in human disease. Is there anything to be learned from the murine EC model? On occasion, EC cells may form a malignant yolk sac tumor[14] but other differentiation derivatives may be benign.[1–11, 27, 36] It is not understood whether the malignant phenotype is transferred to yolk sac elements or whether there is a high probability *de novo* of malignancy in these differentiated cells. Why the malignant phenotype affects only a subset of murine developmental stages is not understood.

Morphology

They have a characteristic morphology as discussed in several reviews.[1–11] *In vitro* EC cell lines are small, epithelioid-like, with large nuclei, several prominent nucleoli and a small rim of cytoplasm.

Differentiation

The phenotype of independent clones of cultured lines may be quite variable with respect to the ability to differentiate. The observed variation is similar to individual clones of *in vivo* retransplantable lines[37] and differences observed may reflect the probability of differentiation (in that particular environment) rather than a qualitative change in the pathway. Multipotential EC tissue culture lines have been established with both 129/Sv and C3H genetic backgrounds.[20–22, 24–35] So called nullipotent cells of which the cell line F9 is the best known[23, 33] were thought not to differentiate; however, F9 may be induced to differentiate to parietal endoderm (discussed in a later section). Thus, the genetic and environmental factors that regulate EC cell differentiation are just beginning to be explored.

Chromosomes

The karyotype of many multipotent murine EC tissue culture lines is near diploid and stable. However, the G-banded karyotype is abnormal.[30] Similar chromosome abnormalities may appear in independent lines.[30] In the section under cell-cell hybridization a number of genetic experiments are discussed that deal with the relation between chromosome constitution and differentiation phenotype.

Biochemical Markers

There are several well-characterized enzyme activities which change upon transition of EC cells to a differentiation pathway. EC cells have high levels of alkaline phosphatase[24] and characteristic isozyme patterns of lactate dehydrogenase,[38] and creatine kinase.[39] EC cells do not produce plasminogen activator[40, 41] or α-fetoprotein,[39] and do not secrete fibronectin.[42, 43] They have a characteristic cytoskeleton[44] and type of collagen synthesized.[45]

Interaction of EC Cells with Virus

There is considerable evidence to suggest that EC cells differ from somatic tissues in their ability to support the growth and replication of certain murine exogenous viruses (reviewed in Ref. 8). EC cells are refractory to infection with minute virus of mice[46] ectopic C type viruses,[47, 48] polyoma,[49-51] simian virus 40 (SV-40).[49-51] Upon differentiation, the EC are sensitive to infection from these viruses.[52] In addition, murine EC cells, that are challenged with SV-40, do not express an early viral function called the T antigen.[49, 51, 52]

EC cells appear to have some features of RNA synthesis that differ from differentiated cells. EC multipotent cells express a 6-fold-greater level of endogenous xenotropic type C virus-related RNA than differentiated EC-derived tissue culture lines.[53] The EC cells do not contain viral particles or viral proteins.

With the ever-increasing development of cloned DNA probes, RNA markers may become more extensively characterized. These studies may lead to a better understanding of how cells control integrated viral genes, and also their own genetic material during differentiation.

Antigenic Markers

The technology used to define different cell surface markers is undergoing a high degree of refinement. A hybridoma is a (myeloma X spleen) cell hybrid that may be cloned and screened for specific antibody production.[54] The production of monoclonal antibodies to cell surface and organelle antigenic markers is being actively pursued in many laboratories. A well-characterized panel of such monoclonal antibodies may be used to define the molecular state of marker expression at a series of points in a particular differentiation pathway. Differentiation antigens defined thus far with monoclonal antibodies may have two extremes of expression. "Jumping" antigens may appear at several and apparently not functionally or ontogenetically related points in development.[55] "Lineage" antigens expression correlates with observable specialization during differentiation.[55] A general finding with regard to "jumping" determinants is species variation in the tissue distribution patterns.[55] The existence of two mapping classes of differentiation antigens suggests that care is required in the interpretation of relatedness of cells. The data from conventional sera and monoclonal antibody clearly show that EC cells share determinants with early embryo cells,[23, 32, 33, 56–61] and that these determinants are not expressed on most differentiated somatic tissues. EC cells lack the cell surface antigens of the major histocompatibility complex (H-2 complex).[62, 63] The kind of differentiation antigens detected thus far on murine EC cells with monoclonal antibodies behave like "jumping" antigens. The Forssman antigen has been identified on murine EC cells.[60] Another glycolipid determinant distinct from the Forssman specificity is detected by the Anti-SSEA-1 monoclonal antibody.[58, 59] This reagent is described here because it has been used in several studies to mark the transition of EC cells to differentiated cells and to characterize the human germ line tumor cell lines to be described.

SSEA-1 was identified using an allogeneic immunization of mice with EC cell lines. SSEA-1 is present on several multipotent and nullipotent EC cell lines, on preimplantation embryos at the 8-cell stage, on brain, kidney and sperm cells. It is not found on all differentiated murine cell lines examined. It reacts weakly with human germ cell tumor lines. Although the molecular nature of the glycolipid antigen has not been defined, SSEA-1 is a useful marker which possesses a "jumping" mapping distribution.

Cell-Cell Hybridization Experiments

The formation and analysis of cell-cell hybrids is a recent approach to understanding the role of chromosomes and differentiation.[64–68] In these experiments, cells with appropriate drug resistant markers are combined and fused. The hybrid cloned cells are compared with the phenotype of the two parent cells. If one parent is differentiated and the other is not, the fate of specific differentiation markers may be established. In addition, a process of chromosome loss occurs in such hybrid cells. After the loss of specific chromosomes, differentiation markers which were originally not expressed in the hybrid cell are reactivated.[69] Mapping of function may be performed by the analysis of karyotype.

The first type of cell-cell hybrid to be discussed is between two EC cell parents. Although the karyotype of such cells is much less stable, these (EC × EC) hybrids retain the ability to differentiate.[30] Another combination of interest is between two EC cells with different differentiation potentials. Hybrids formed between a multipotential × nullipotent EC cells retain the ability to differentiate.[70] The nullipotent × nullipotent hybrid remains unable to differentiate. Thus, the loss of ability of EC to differentiate does not appear to result from dominant factors that suppress differentiation.

The analysis of hybrids formed between an EC cell and a differentiated cell is much more complicated. There do not appear to be general rules to determine the phenotype of the hybrid in relation to the parents. The phenotype of (EC × fibroblast) hybrid clones is fibroblastoid.[71-74] The H-2 loci of both parents are expressed. This type of hybrid has been reported many times, using either 3T3, or L-cell parent. In this type of hybrid the EC properties are not expressed.

The phenotype of hybrid cells formed between EC and lymphocyte-derived differentiated cells are more variable. When the differentiated parent is derived from Friend leukemia, thymona, normal spleen or thymus, the hybrid resembled the EC parent in the majority of cases.[75-83] The multipotent EC phenotype was expressed in some of these hybrids. When the differentiated parent is derived from neuroblastoma, myeloma or hepatoma hybrid does not resemble either parent.[84-86]

In the reports reviewed, the EC phenotype was coordinately expressed or not expressed. Another study by Gmur *et al.*[82] suggests that EC properties are under coordinate control. In their studies of the regulation of phenotype in somatic cell hybrids, dramatic shifts of phenotype occurred in long-term cultures. In both (EC × normal spleen) and (EC × thymona) cell hybrids, transitions of phenotype occurred. Transitions of EC to fibroblastoid phenotype and fibroblastoid to EC phenotype appeared to occur at random and at a low frequency. The morphological changes in phenotype were checked using H-2 and monoclonal SSEA-1 reagent. The morphology of the tumors formed correlated with the phenotype of the hybrid cells in culture. No "mixed" cells were detected using immunofluorescent techniques. However, specific changes in karyotype were not associated unequivocally with the EC or fibroblastoid expression in the hybrid cells, although some of the fibroblastoid cell hybrids had a large number of chromosome rearrangements. This approach gives some suggestive evidence that the EC phenotype is coordinately controlled as a unit set of properties. The same set of hybrids was used to show that the regulation of H-2K and H-2D gene expression was independent.[79] Integrated regulation of numerous genes which are coordinately expressed or suppressed is suggested also by the analysis of somatic cell hybrids between mouse melanoma and rat hepatoma cells.[87]

The use of cell-cell hybrid techniques have limited applicability in the study of regulation. The high resolution techniques of DNA and chromosome transfer into EC cells may assist the effective application of this system in probing the control of gene expression. Cotransfer of genes for viral thymidine kinase and human β-globin into a multipotent EC appears to occur at workable frequencies.[88]

Environmental Factors that Alter the Probability of EC Differentiation

The ability to promote large populations of murine EC lines with the inducing agents, retinoids and substituted dioxins, is an important experimental finding. It has applications for studying biochemical processes of committment and differentiation, and for controlling the growth of the stem cell through differentiation into benign tissue.

It was documented more than 50 years ago that the pattern of epithelial cell differentiation is strongly influenced by retinoids.[89] Under vitamin-A deficient conditions in the rat, stratified and keratinizing layers have substituted for the normal and mucous-secreting epithelium. This abberant alteration of phenotype may be reversed with retinoic acid.

Vitamin A (retinoic acid) and related compounds greatly increase the probability of differentiation of EC cells *in vitro*.[90–93] The biochemical and antigenic markers expressed by F9 cells treated with retinoic acid were characteristic of parietal endoderm.[92] The effect of retinoic acid on EC cells is irreversible and dependent on the time of exposure. Detailed kinetic analyses have not been performed. Structure and activity relationships indicate that synthetic analogues may be effective since several portions of the retinoid molecule may be altered without losing the biological effect.[93]

Retinoic acid also increases the survival time of mice following challenge by a threshold number of tumorigenic F9 cells.[93] The differentiation of F9 tumor cells was suggested by an analysis of SSEA-1 and H-2 antigen expression. This might provide an alternate form of tumor therapy based not on cell killing but on inducing stem cell differentiation, but it would only be successful if the differentiated progeny of the stem cells were benign. This condition is true for murine tumors; however, it needs to be examined with human tumors. Another necessary requirement for success with the above approach is that there is a small mutation rate of the stem cell to a phenotype that is not responsive to the inducer.

One study indicates that there is a considerable range to the quantitative effects of retinoic acid induction on several independent embryonal carcinoma cell lines.[91] Mutant EC lines resistant to retinoic acid have been isolated.[94] Further analysis of this effect is necessary to determine the rate of occurrence.

Another example of chemical induction of differentiation of EC cells occurs with the XB teratocarcinoma cell line. This cell line under low density culture conditions will spontaneously differentiate to produce stratification and keratin layers.[29] Under high density culture conditions, however, differentiation occurs at a low rate.

Toxic agents such as 2,3,7,8-tetrachloro-dibenzo-*p*-dioxin will also increase the rate of differentiation in a dose-dependent fashion.[95] This class of toxic compounds affects the differentiation of epithelial cells by apparently inducing severe skin reactions. The binding affinity of the toxic compounds for a cytosol receptor was measured in these studies. These results suggest that a cytoplasmic receptor may mediate the pleiomorphic alterations of phenotype. Thus, the induction of differentiation in EC cells may serve as a sensitive method to detect very small concentrations of certain classes of toxic agents.

The Environmental Influence of the Blastocyst on the Development of EC Cells

The growth of retransplantable and tissue culture multipotential EC lines is a disorganized caricature of normal development in most sites in the mouse. In 1974 Brinster[96] reported the formation of chimeric mice from blastocysts that were injected with one EC cell. Several labs have duplicated this basic observation.[97–102] Thus, the EC cell may participate in normal development when directed by the field of the blastocyst. It is possible to envision introducing mutant genes carried by tissue culture EC cells into mouse stocks *via* the germ line of chimeric mice.

The general properties of this system noted to date are as follows. Four independent *in vitro* EC cell lines[99, 101] and three *in vivo* EC retransplantable tumors[96–98, 100] may all participate in normal development. However, the frequency of chimerism detected was low (less than 24%). In one report, germ line chimerism was detected in one male mouse.[98] Since the tissue culture lines employed provide either XO or XX they would be expected only to be able to form oocytes. A range of 8–80% of chimeric mice developed tumors when the tissue culture lines were the source of EC cells.[99] In contrast, the *in vivo* retransplantable tumor studies reported only one tumor.[100] The number and location of EC cells in the blastocyst also plays a role in tumor formation.[102] The histological examination of tumors from chimeric mice shows that EC cells are not always present, and fibrosarcomas were most detected. Thus, the blastocyst appears to be able to control a small number of EC cells.

It is not clear whether these tumors developed from injected cells which remained quiescent for several months or developed *de novo* from their differentiated progeny. The formation of fibrosarcomas has also been observed to segregate as a property of growth from (EC × normal spleen) cell hybrids.[82] It may be possible that the EC malignant phenotype may be transferred in some instances to other cells in a differentiated pathway.

The growth of EC cells in blastocysts provides a dramatic demonstration of the control of a malignant phenotype. This system raises several questions concerning the components of the blastocyst which influence the development of EC cells. How this effect is mediated may provide some fascinating clues on both normal development and neoplasia.

CHARACTERIZATION OF HUMAN GERM CELL LINES

Human cell lines are derived from a much more heterogeneous gene pool than the murine model. In the murine model, genetic components identified appear to affect the rate of occurrence of a stem cell with the properties of an EC cell. Genetic factors may also play a role in human tumors since there is reported association of HLA major histocompatibility and tumor incidence.[103] The much greater genetic heterogeneity may affect both the quantitative and qualitative properties of human germ cell tumors. Thus, there is no *a priori* reason to expect that an EC like cell will be characterized in the human model since different human tumors may be arrested at different points in development.

In human germ cell tumors there are various types of malignant cells recognized.[104–106] Yolk sac, choriocarcinoma, embryonal carcinoma are often mixed. The interrelationships of these malignant forms are not understood. Embryonal carcinoma is regarded by some as multipotential.[104–106] It may differentiate along extraembryonic or trophoblastic routes to form yolk sac carcinoma and choriocarcinoma. It may differentiate along the embryonic route to form a benign teratoma. Mostofi[107, 108] has suggested that the primordial germ cell may progress directly to yolk sac without an embryonal carcinoma compartment. An *in vitro* cell culture line would be desirable to study the transitions of these malignant forms.

Growth and Stability

Human germ cell tumors have been retransplanted as xenografts in immunosuppressed animals[109] and in congenital athymic or immunosuppressed mice.[110–112] Recloning experiments on human teratocarcinomas have not been reported *in vivo.* The success rate in establishing new retransplantable tumor is lower than 20%.[112]

Human testicular teratocarcinoma cell lines are being established in tissue culture for characterization.[113–117] To date, the growth of this tumor type has been difficult and there are now cell lines from approximately a dozen patients. One is therefore concerned that the cell type under selection for tissue culture growth may not be representative of the original malignancy. Does it represent the properties of the *in vivo* stem cell or does the cell line result from an *in vitro* transformation of differentiated cells of the *in vivo* stem cell? The answer to this question still depends on accumulating more well-characterized cell lines.

There have been no rigorous cloning experiments reported for cell lines derived from testicular patients. Without this kind of experiment it is difficult to interpret data concerning the observation of heterogeneity of cells. It remains to be seen if the technical conditions can be improved so that rigorous cloning can be performed for human testicular cell lines.

Morphology

Lines characterized resemble some aspects of the morphology of murine EC cells.[113–119] However, there is considerable variation in the lines themselves and between the same line under different growth conditions.

Differentiation

Differentiation of human EC lines has not been observed *in vitro* using similar conditions to promote differentiation of murine EC cells.[119] Although there is often some reference made to heterogeneous cell population in human teratocarcinoma cell lines[113–119] these changes are not under any known systematic control.

Chromosomes

The variance of the chromosome number distribution of the human lines is comparable to that of murine cell-cell hybrids and not of near-diploid murine EC cells.[118] Thus, the kind of genetic changes associated with numerical variations in the number of chromosomes may play a role in the human germ cell populations. The effect, if any, has not been reported systematically.

An analysis of chromosome 1 abnormalities by trypsin G-banding was performed on 14 cell lines derived from primary tumors or metastases of 11 patients with testicular cancer.[118] Nonrandom abnormalities in chromosome 1 were detected consistently. In addition, independent cell lines from the same patient had identical marker chromosomes. Wang *et al.*[118] have suggested that the consistent involvement of chromosome 1 rearrangements may be associated with the highly malignant nature of testicular cancers. Atkin and Pickthall[120] have suggested that the presence of chromosome 1 rearrangements may be a relatively late marker of malignant transformation and thus be associated with a poor prognosis and high degrees of metastatic disease.[120]

Biochemical Markers

With one exception, human testicular cell lines have high levels of alkaline phosphate as compared to diploid human fibroblasts.[113, 114, 117, 119] Although most of the activity was associated with the liver/bone isoenzyme, a significant but variable activity (0.3–30%) was found in the placental type. The presence of placental alkaline phosphatase is a shared feature with many other human tumor cell lines, and is restricted in expression to the placental trophectoderm during normal development. However, it is not known whether this isoenzyme is expressed at other times in the early embryo. This isoenzyme cannot be compared with the murine EC model because placental alkaline phosphatase is a relatively recent evolutionary event.[121–123] The hybridomas developed to alkaline phosphatase thus far are summarized by Slaughter *et al.*[124]

Andrews *et al.*[119] have compared the biochemical markers chorionic gonadotropin, α-fetoprotein, alkaline phosphatase and plasminogen activator expressed by eight independent human germ cell lines. Although markers characteristic of choriocarcinoma or yolk sac cells were detected, the eight lines more closely resembled murine EC cells. These results may suggest that limited differentiation of the human stem cells into trophectoderm and yolk cells occurs in culture. None of these enzyme markers are elusive or specific markers for the stem cell of testicular tumors. Plasminogen activator production was expressed by the human lines; whereas, murine EC cells do not express this marker. Thus, although murine and human germ cell tumors have many similar biochemical markers, there are exceptions.

Interaction with Virus

Type-A viral particles were detected at low frequency in Tera 1 cells.[125] Some cells in human germ cell lines express early virus antigen markers after an infection with SV-40 virus,[119] unlike the murine EC model. The population heterogeneity observed for the human cell lines may be a reflection of a mixture of virus-resistant stem cells and virus-sensitive differentiated cells. More analyses of clones of human lines may resolve these issues.

Antigenic Markers

All reports of human testicular tumor lines detected low levels of major histocompatibility complex markers; β-2-microglobulin and/or HLA markers.[113, 114, 117, 119] Since the levels of these marker expressions are low by quantitative binding, quantitative absorption and immunofluorescent techniques, conclusions about subpopulations were not drawn.[119] These cell lines were very weakly positive for SSEA-1, discussed earlier in the murine EC cell characterization. A human choriocarcinoma cell line and murine trophectoderm were much more reactive to SSEA-1. Although there are several parallels in the human and murine models for the expression SSEA-1, markers which have a higher binding activity for human testicular tumor stem cells are required to better characterize the heterogeneous cell cultures.

CONCLUSION

The analysis of the murine system has provided a model of teratocarcinoma based on the recognition of the EC cell as the malignant stem cell. There is considerable experience with this system that suggests that the probability of transfer of the malignant state to differentiated progeny is small. It is not known why most differentiated cells derived from EC are benign.

Chromosomal changes in hybrid cells that contain EC as one parent may express malignant phenotypes in differentiated cells. Malignant properties associated with differentiated cells may also arise from EC cells involved in the formation of a chimeric mouse. Thus, the probability of transfer of the malignant state in the murine system is low except under special conditions. In this respect, it is a very different model from human germ cell tumors.

In the analyses of the cell lines from testicular tumor cells characterized to date, there is heterogeneity within many cell types. These include biochemical and antigenic markers as well as resistance to virus. The observed heterogeneity of marker phenotypes such as HLA or SSEA-1 may reflect subpopulations of distinct phenotypes or a variation that is caused by other variables such as the position in the cell cycle. As Andrews *et al.*[119] point out, these uncertainties need to be resolved by the analysis of markers from small populations of cells that arose from a single cell. Such cloning experiments are necessary to ensure that the putative differentiated cells arose from the stem cell. The variable human cell lines do not appear to differentiate and do not form large numbers of choriocarcinoma and endodermal sinus (yolk sac) cells *in vitro.* Thus, the relationship between the heterogeneous cell phenotypes in germ-cell tumors awaits the isolation of a cell line appropriate for this characterization.

Andrews *et al.*[119] have suggested that the stem cell resembles a preblastocyst stage of development with low levels of HLA and SSEA-1. The stem cell may differentiate to a state that is SSEA-1 positive and secrete AFP or HCG. The markers in this context are suggestive of differentiation into the trophoblastic elements and along extraembryonic pathways.[119]

The analysis of this system requires more markers to characterize the differentiated cells that appear to arise in testicular tumor populations. In the human, we are uncertain about the number and properties of the putative stem cell phenotypes. Are these stem cells related by normal differentiation pathways or by transitions in phenotype more related to chromosome constitution changes? There are examples in the murine EC hybrid cells of transitions in phenotype that may also be the result of chromosome constitution changes. At this moment we are unable to answer these questions. Further analysis of the human germ cell lines *in vitro* may clarify some of these issues.

REFERENCES

1. Pierce, G. B., Jr. Teratocarcinoma: model for a developmental concept of cancer. *Curr. Top. Develop. Biol. 2:*223–246, 1967.
2. Pierce, G. B. The benign cells of malignant tumors. In *Developmental Aspects of Carcinogenesis and Immunity*, pp. 3–22, edited by T. J. King. Academic Press, New York, 1975.
3. Stevens, L. C. The biology of teratomas. *Adv. Morphogenesis 6:*1–31, 1967.
4. Damjanov, I., and Solter, D. Experimental teratoma. *Curr. Top. Pathol. 59:*69–130, 1974.
5. Martin, G. R. Teratocarcinomas as a model system for the study of embryogenesis and neoplasia. *Cell 5:*229–243, 1975.
6. Pierce, G. B. Teratocarcinoma: introduction and perspective. In *Teratomas and Differentiation*, pp 3–12, edited by M. I. Sherman and D. Solter. Academic Press. New York, 1975.
7. Graham, C. F. In: *Concepts in Mammalian Embryogenesis*, pp. 315–394, edited by M. Sherman. MIT press, Cambridge, Mass. 1977.
8. Hogan, B. L. M. Teratocarcinoma cells as a model for mammalian development. *Int. Rev. Biochem. 15:*333–376, 1977.
9. Jewett, M. A. S. Biology of testicular tumors. *Urol. Clin. North Am. 4:*495–507, 1977.
10. Pierce, G. B., Shikes, R., and Fink, L. M. *Cancer: A Problem of Developmental Biology*. Prentice-Hall, Engelwood Cliffs, N. J., 1978.
11. Solter, D. and Damjanov, I. Teratocarcinoma and the expression of oncodevelopmental genes. In *Methods in Cancer Research*, Vol 18, pp 277–332, edited by V. T. DaVita and H. Busch. Academic Press, New York, 1979.
12. Stevens, L. C. The biology of teratomas including evidence indicating their origin from primordial germ cell. *Ann. Biol. 1:*585–610, 1962.
13. Stevens, L. C. The development of teratomas from intratesticular grafts of tubal mouse eggs. *J. Embryol. Exp. Morphol. 20:*329–341, 1968.
14. Stevens, L. C. The development of transplantable teratocarcinomas from intratesticular grafts of pre- and postimplantation mouse embryos. *Develop. Biol. 21:*364–382, 1970.
15. Damjanov, I., Solter, D., Belicza, M., and Skreb, N. Teratomas obtained through extrauterine growth of seven-day-old mouse embryos. *J. Natl. Cancer. Inst. 46:*471–480, 1971.
16. Solter, D., Dominis, M., and Damjanov, I. Embryo-derived teratocarcinoma. II Teratocarcinogenesis depends on the type of embryonic graft. *Int. J. Cancer 25:*341–343, 1980.
17. Damjanov, I., Skreb, N., and Sell, S. Origin of embryo-derived yolk sac carcinomas. *Int. J. Cancer 19:*526–530, 1977.
18. Diwan, S. B., and Stevens, L. C. Development of teratomas from the ectoderm of mouse egg cylinders. *JNCI 57:*937–942, 1976.
19. Mintz, B., Cronmiller, C., and Custer, R. P. Somatic cell origin of teratocarcinomas. *Proc. Natl. Acad. Sci. 75:*2834–2838, 1978.
20. Kahan, B. W., and Ephrussi, B. Developmental potentialities of clonal *in vitro* cultures of mouse testicular teratoma. *JNCI 44:*1015–1036, 1970.
21. Rosenthal, M. D., Wishnow, R. M., and Sato, G. H. *In vitro* growth and differentiation of clonal populations of multipotential mouse cells from a transplantable testicular teratoma. *JNCI 44:*1001–1014, 1970.
22. Evans, M. J. The isolation of properties of a clonal tissue culture strain of pluripotent mouse teratoma cells. *J. Embryol. Exp. Morphol. 28:*163–176, 1972.
23. Artz, K., Dubois, P., Bennett, D., Condamine, H., Babinet, C., and Jacob, F. Surface antigens common to mouse cleavage embryos and primitive teratocarcinoma cells in culture. *Proc. Natl. Acad. Sci. 70:*2988–2992, 1973.
24. Bernstine, E. G., Hooper, M. L., Grandchamp, S., and Ephrussi, B. Alkaline phosphatase activity in mouse teratoma. *Proc. Natl. Acad. Sci. 70:*3899–3903, 1973.
25. Jakob, H., Bone, T., Gaillard, J., Nicolas, J. F., and Jacob, F. Teratocarcinome de la souris: isolment, culture et proprietes de cellules a potentialites multiples. *Ann. Microbiol. 124B:*269–282, 1973.
26. Gooding, L. R., and Edidin, M. Cell surface antigens of a mouse testicular teratoma. Identification of an antigen physically associated with H-2 antigens on tumor cells. *J.*

*Exp. Med. 140:*61–78, 1974.
27. Martin, G. R., and Evans, M. J. The morphology and growth of a pluripotent teratocarcinoma cell line and its derivatives in tissue culture. *Cell 2:*163–172, 1974.
28. Martin, G. R., and Evans, M. J. Differentiation of clonal lines of teratocarcinoma cells: formation of embryoid bodies *in vitro. Proc. Natl. Acad. Sci. 72:*1441–1445, 1975.
29. Rheinwald, J. G., and Green, H. Formation of a keratinizing epithelium in culture by a cloned cell line derived from a teratoma. *Cell 6:*317–330, 1975.
30. McBurney, M. W. Clonal lines of teratocarcinoma cells *in vitro*: differentiation and cytogenetic characteristics. *J. Cell Physiol. 89:*441–455, 1976.
31. Nicolas, J. F., Avner, P., Gaillard, J., Guenet, J. L., Jakob, H., and Jacob, F. Cell lines derived from teratocarcinoma. *Can. Res. 36:*4224, 4231, 1976.
32. Gachelin, G., Kemler, R., Kelly, F., and Jacob, F. PCC4, a new cell surface antigen common to multipotential embryonal carcinoma cells, spermatozoa, and mouse early embryos. *Dev. Biol. 57:*199–205, 1977.
33. Jacob F. Mouse teratocarcinoma and embryonic antigens. *Immunol. Rev. 33:*3–32, 1977.
34. Watanabe, T., Dewey, M. J., and Mintz, B. Teratocarcinoma cells as vehicles for introducing specific mutant mitochrondrial genes into mice. *Proc. Natl. Acad. Sci. 75:*5113–5117, 1978.
35. Reuser, A. J. J., and Mintz, B. Mouse teratocarcinoma mutant clones deficient in adenine phosphoribosyltransferase and developmentally pluripotent. *Somatic Cell Genet. 5:*781–792, 1979.
36. Pierce, G. B., Dixon, F. J., and Verney, E. L. Teratocarcinogenic and tissue-forming potentialities of the cell types comprising neoplastic embryoid bodies. *Lab. Invest. 9:*583–602, 1960.
37. Kleinsmith, L. J., and Pierce, G. B. Multipotentiality of a single embryonal carcinoma cell. *Cancer Res. 24:*1544–1552, 1964.
38. Lo, C. W., and Gilula, N. B. PC4 aza 1 teratocarcinoma stem cell differentiation in culture I biochemical studies. *Dev. Biol. 75:*78–92, 1980.
39. Adamson, E. D., Evans, M. J., and Magrane, G. G. Biochemical markers of the progress of differentiation in cloned teratocarcinoma cell lines. *Eur. J. Biochem. 79:*607–615, 1977.
40. Hall, J. D., Marsden, M., Rifkin, D., Teresky, A. K., and Levine, A. J. In *Teratomas and Differentiation*, pp 251–270, edited by M. I. Sherman and D. Solter. Academic Press, New York, 1975.
41. Linney, E., and Levinson, B. B. Teratocarcinoma differentiation: Plasminogen activator activity associated with embryoid body formation. *Cell 10:*297–304, 1977.
42. Wolfe, J., Mautner, V., Hogan, B. and Tilly, R. Synthesis and retention of fibronectin (LETS protein) by mouse teratocarcinoma cells. Exp. Cell Res. *118:*63–71, 1979.
43. Zetter, B. R., and Martin, G. R. Expression of a high molecular weight cell surface glycoprotein (LETS protein) by preimplantation mouse embryos and teratocarcinoma stem cells. *Proc. Natl. Acad. Sci. 75:*2324–2328, 1978.
44. Paulin, D., Forest, N., and Perreau, J. Cytoskeletal proteins used as markers of differentiation in mouse teratocarcinoma cells. *J. Mol. Biol. 144:*95–101, 1980.
45. Adamson, E. D., Gaunt, S. J., and Graham, C. F. The differentiation of teratocarcinoma stem cells is marked by the types of collagen which are synthesized. *Cell 17:*469–476, 1979.
46. Miller, R. A., Ward, D. C., and Ruddle, F. H. Embryonal carcinoma cells (and their somatic cell hybrids) are resistant to infection by the murine parvovirus MVM which does infect other teratocarcinoma-derived cell lines. *J. Cell. Physiol. 91:*393–402, 1977.
47. Peries, J., Alves-Cardoso, E., Canivet, M., Debons-Guillemin, M. C., and Lasneret, J. Lack of multiplication of ecotropic murine C-type viruses in mouse teratocarcinoma primitive cells: brief communication. *JNCI 59:*463–465, 1977.
48. Teich, N., Weiss, R. A., Martin, G. M., and Lowry, D. R. Virus infection of murine teratocarcinoma stem cell lines. *Cell 12:*973–982, 1977.
49. Boccara, M., and Kelly, F. Etude de la sensibilite au virus du polyome et e SV40 de plusieurs lignees cellulaires de teratocarcinoma. *Ann. Microbiol. (Paris) 129A:*227–238, 1978.
50. Swartzendruber, D. E., and, Lehman, J. M. Neoplastic differentiation: interaction of simian virus 40 and polyoma virus with murine teratocarcinoma cells *in vitro. J. Cell Physiol. 85:*179–187, 1975.

51. Speers, W. C., and Lehman, J. M. Increased susceptibility of murine teratocarcinoma cells to simian virus 40 and polyoma virus following treatment with 5-bromodeoxyuridine. *J. Cell. Physiol. 88:*297–306, 1976.
52. Segal, S., and Khoury, G. Differentiation as a requirement for simian virus 40 gene expression in F9 embryonal carcinoma cells. *Proc. Natl. Acad. Sci. 76:*5611–5615, 1979.
53. Emanoil-Ravicovitch, R., Hojman-Montes-De-Oca, F., Robert, J., Garcette, M., Callahan, R., Peries, J., and Boiron, M. Biochemical characterization of endogenous type C virus information in differentiated and undifferentiated murine teratocarcinoma-derived cell lines. *J. Virol. 34:*576–581, 1980.
54. Kohler, G., and Milstein, C. Derivation of specific antibody-producing tissue culture and tumour lines by cell fusion. *Eur. J. Immunol. 6:*511–519, 1976.
55. Springer, T. A. Cell-surface differentiation in the mouse characterization of "jumping" and "lineage" antigens using xenogenic rat monoclonal antibodies. In *Monoclonal Antibodies Hybridomas: A New Dimension in Biological Analyses*, edited by R. H. Kennett, T. J. McKearn, and K. B. Bechtol. Plenum, New York, 1980.
56. Stern, P. L., Martin, G. R., and Evans, M. J. Cell surface antigens of clonal teratocarcinoma cells at various stages of differentiation. *Cell 6:*455–465, 1975.
57. Dewey, M. J., Gearhart, J. D., and Mintz, B. Cell surface antigens of totipotent mouse teratocarcinoma cells grown *in vivo*: their relation to embryo adult and tumor antigens. *Dev. Biol. 55:*359–374, 1977.
58. Knowles, B. B., Aden, D. P., and Solter, D. Monoclonal antibody detecting a stage-specific embryonic antigen (SSEA-1) on preimplantation mouse embryos and teratocarcinoma cells. *Curr. Top. Microbiol. Immunol. 81:*51–53, 1978.
59. Solter, D., and Knowles, B. B., Monoclonal antibody defining a stage-specific mouse embryonic antigen (SSEA-1). *Proc. Natl. Acad. Sci. 75:*5565–5569, 1978.
60. Stern, P. L., Willison, K. R., Lennox, E., Galfre, G., Milstein, C., Secher, D., Ziegler, A., and Springer, T. Monoclonal antibodies as probes for differentiation and tumor-associated antigens: a Forssman specificity on teratocarcinoma stem cells. *Cell 14:*775–783, 1978.
61. Goodfellow, P. N., Levinson, J. R., Williams, V. E., II, and McDevitt, H. O. Monoclonal antibodies reacting with murine teratocarcinoma cells. *Proc. Natl. Acad. Sci. 76:*377–380, 1979.
62. Artz, K., and Jacob, F. Absence of serologically detectable H-2 on primitive teratocarcinoma cells in culture. *Transplantation 17:*632–634, 1974.
63. Morello, D., Gachelin, G., Dubois, P., Tanigaki, N., Pressman, D., and Jacob, F. Absence of reaction of a xenogenic anti-H-2 serum with mouse embryonal carcinoma cells. *Transplantation 26:*119–125, 1978.
64. Ephrussi, B. *Hybridization of Somatic Cells.* Princeton University Press, Princeton, N. J., 1972.
65. Davidson, R. L. Gene expression in somatic cell hybrids. *Annu. Rev. Genet. 8:*195–218, 1974.
66. Ringertz, N. R., and Savage, R. E. *Cell Hybrids.* Academic Press, New York, 1976.
67. Davis, F. M., and Adelberg, E. A. Use of somatic cell hybrids for analysis of the differentiated state. *Bacteriol. Rev. 37:*197–214, 1973.
68. Klebe, R. J., Chen, T. R., and Ruddle, F. H. Mapping of a human genetic regulator element by somatic cell genetic analysis. *Proc. Natl. Acad. Sci. 66:*1220–1227, 1970.
69. Weiss, M. C., and Chaplain, M. Expression of differentiation functions in hepatoma cell hybrids: reappearance of tyrosine aminotransferase inducibility after the loss of chromosomes. *Proc. Natl. Acad. Sci. 68:*3026–3030, 1971.
70. Rosenstraus, M. J., Balint, R. F., and Levine, A. J. Pluripotency of somatic cell hybrids between nullipotent and pluripotent embryonal carcinoma cells. *Somatic Cell Genet. 6:*555–565, 1980.
71. Finch, B. W., and Ephrussi, B. Retention of multiple developmental potentialities by cells of a mouse testicular teratocarcinoma during prolonged culture *in vitro* and their extinction upon hybridization with cells of permanent lines. *Proc. Natl. Acad. Sci. 57:*615–621, 1967.
72. Jami, J., Failly, C., and Ritz, E. Lack of expression of differentiation in mouse teratoma-fibroblast somatic cell hybrids. *Exp. Cell. Research. 76:*191–199, 1973.
73. McBurney, M. W., and Strutt, B. Fusion of embryonal carcinoma cells to fibroblast cells, cytoplasts, and karyoplasts. Developmental properties of viable fusion products. *Exp. Cell. Res. 124:*171–180, 1979.

74. Rousett, J. F., Dubois, P., Lasserre, C., Aviles, D., Fellous, M., and Jami, J. Phenotype and surface antigens of mouse teratocarcinoma × fibroblast cell hybrids. *Somatic Cell Genet. 5:*739–752, 1979.
75. Miller, R. A., and Ruddle, F. H. Pluripotent teratocarcinoma-thymus somatic cell hybrids. *Cell 9:*45–55, 1976.
76. McBurney, M. W. Hemoglobin synthesis in cell hybrids formed between teratocarcinoma and Friend erythroleukemia cells. *Cell 12:*653–662, 1977.
77. Miller, R. A., and Ruddle, F. H. Teratocarcinoma × Friend erythroleukemia cell hybrids resemble their pluripotent embryonal carcinoma parent. *Develop. Biol. 56:*157–173, 1977.
78. Miller, R. A., and Ruddle, F. H. Properties of teratocarcinomathymus somatic cell hybrids. *Somatic Cell Genet. 3:*247–261, 1977.
79. Andrews, P. W., and Goodfellow, P. N. Antigen expression by somatic cell hybrids of a murine embryonal carcinoma cell with thymocytes and L cells. *Somatic Cell Genet. 6:*271–284, 1980.
80. Gmur, R., Solter, D., and Knowles, B. B. Independent regulation of H-2K and H-2D gene expression in murine teratocarcinoma somatic cell hybrids. *J. Exp. Med. 151:*1349–1359, 1980.
81. Rousset, J. P., Jami, J., Dubois, P., Aviles, D., and Ritz, E. Developmental potentialities and surface antigens of mouse teratocarcinoma × lymphoid cell hybrids. *Somatic Cell Genet. 6:*419–433, 1980.
82. Gmur, R., Knowles, B. B., and Solter, D. Regulation of phenotype in somatic cell hybrids derived by fusion of teratocarcinoma cell lines with normal or tumor-derived mouse cells. *Dev. Biol. 81:*245–254, 1981.
83. McBurney, M. W., Featherstone, M. S., and Kaplan, H. Activation of teratocarcinoma-derived hemoglobin genes in teratocarcinoma Friend cell hybrids. *Cell 15:*1323–1330, 1978.
84. Bernstine, F. G., Koyama, H., and Ephrussi, B. Enhanced expression of alkaline phosphatase in hybrids between neuroblastoma and embryonal carcinoma. *Somatic Cell Genet. 3:*217–225, 1977.
85. Correani, A., and Croce, C. M. Expression of the teratocarcinoma phenotype in hybrids between totipotent mouse teratocarcinoma and myeloma cells. *J. Cell. Physiol. 105:*73–79, 1980.
86. Litwak, G. Somatic cell hybrids between totipotent mouse teratocarcinoma and rat hepatoma cells. *J. Cell. Physiol. 101:*1–8, 1979.
87. Fougere, C., and Weiss, M. C. Phenotype exclusion in mouse melanoma-rat hepatoma hybrid cells: pigment and albumin production are not reexpressed simultaneously. *Cell 15:*843–854, 1978.
88. Pellicer, A., Wagner, E. F., Kareh, A. E., Dewey, M. J., Reuser, A. J., Silverstein, S., Axel, R., and Mintz, B. Introduction of a viral thymidine kinase gene and the human β-globin gene into developmentally multipotential mouse teratocarcinoma cells. *Proc. Natl. Acad. Sci. 77:*2098–2102, 1980.
89. Wolbach, S., and Howe, P. Tissue changes following deprivation of fat-soluble A vitamin. *J. Exp. Med. 42:*753–777, 1925.
90. Strickland, S., and Mahdavi, V. The induction of differentiation in teratocarcinoma stem cells by retinoic acid. *Cell 15:*393–403, 1978.
91. Jetten, A. M., Jetten, M. E. R., and Sherman, M. I. Stimulation of differentiation of several murine embryonal carcinoma cell lines by retinoic acid. *Exp. Cell. Res. 124:*381–391, 1979.
92. Solter, D., Shevinsky, I., Knowles, B. B., and Strickland, S. The induction of antigenic changes in a teratocarcinoma stem cell line (F9) by retinoic acid. *Dev. Biol. 70:*176–182, 1979.
93. Strickland, S., and Sawey, M. J. Studies on the effect of retinoids on the differentiation of teratocarcinoma stem cells *in vitro* and *in vivo. Dev. Biol. 78:*76–85, 1980.
94. Schlindler, J., Matthai, K. I., and Sherman, M. I. Isolation and characterization of mouse mutant embryonal carcinoma cells which fail to differentiate in response to retinoic acid. *Proc. Natl. Acad. Sci. 78:*1077–1080, 1981.
95. Knutson, J. C., and Poland, A. Keratinization of mouse teratoma cell line XB produced by 2,3,7,8-tetrachlorodibenzo-*p*-dioxin: an *in vitro* model of toxicity. *Cell 22:*27–36, 1980.
96. Brinster, R. L. The effect of cells transferred into the mouse blastocyst on subsequent

development. *J. Exp. Med. 140:*1049–1056, 1974.
97. Ford, C. E., Evans, E. P., and Gardner, R. L. Marker chromosome analysis of two mouse chimeras. *J. Embryol. Exp. Morphol. 33:*447–457, 1975.
98. Mintz, B., and Illmensee, K. Normal genetically mosaic mice produced from malignant teratocarcinoma cells. *Proc. Natl. Acad. Sci. 72:*3585–3589, 1975.
99. Papaioannou, V. E., McBurney, M. W., Gardner, R. L., and Evans, M. J. Fate of teratocarcinoma cells injected into early mouse embryos. *Nature 258:*70–73, 1975.
100. Illmensee, K., and Mintz, B. Totipotency and normal differentiation of single teratocarcinoma cells cloned by injection into blastocysts. *Proc. Natl. Acad. Sci. 73:*549–553, 1976.
101. Papaioannou, V. E., Gardner, R. L., McBurney, M. W., Babinet, C., and Evans, M. J. Participation of cultured teratocarcinoma cells in mouse embryogenesis. *J. Embryol. Exp. Morphol. 44:*93–104, 1978.
102. Pierce, G. B. Tumorigenicity of embryonal carcinoma as an assay to study control of malignancy by the murine blastocyst. *Proc. Natl. Acad. Sci. 76:*6649–6651, 1979.
103. DeWolf, W. C., Lange, P. H., Einrson, M. E., Yunis, E. J. HLA and testicular cancer. *Nature 277:*216–217, 1979.
104. Friedman, N. B., and Moore, R. A. Tumors of the testis. A report of 922 cases. *Milit. Med. 99:*573–593, 1943.
105. Dixon, F. J., and Moore, R. A. Tumors of the male sex organs. In *Atlas of Tumor Pathology, Fascicle 316 and 32*, Armed Forces Institute of Pathology, Washington DC: 1952.
106. Pierce, G. B., Jr., and Abell, M. A. Embryonal carcinoma of the testis. In *Pathology Annual*, pp 27–60, edited by S. C. Sommers. Appleton-Century-Crofts, New York 1970.
107. Mostofi, F. K. Testicular tumors; epidemiologic, etiologic, and pathologic features. *Cancer 32:*1186–1201, 1973.
108. Mostofi, F. K. Pathology of germ cell tumor of testis: a progress report. *Cancer 45:*1735–1754, 1980.
109. Pierce, G. B., Jr., Verney, E. L., and Dixon, F. J. The biology of testicular cancer. I. Behavior after transplantation. *Cancer Res 17:*134–138, 1957.
110. Giovanella, B. C., Stehlin, J. S., and Williams, L. J. Jr. Heterotransplantation of human malignant tumors in "nude" thymusless mice. II. Malignant tumors induced by injection of cell cultures derived from human solid tumors. *JNCI 52:*921–930, 1974.
111. Selby, P. J., Heyderman, E., Gibbs, J., and Peckham, M. J. A human testicular teratoma serially transplanted in immune-deprived mice. *Br. J. Cancer. 39:*578–583, 1979.
112. Raghavan, D., Gibbs, J., Neville, A. M., and Peckham, M. J. Experimental germ cell tumors. *N. Engl. J. Med. 302:*811–813, 1980.
113. Holden, S., Bernard, O., Artzt, K., Whitmore, W. F., Jr., and Bennet, D. Human and mouse embryonal carcinoma cells in culture share an embryonic antigen (F9). *Nature 270:*518–520, 1977.
114. Hogan, B., Fellous, M., Avner, P., and Jacob, F. Isolation of a human teratoma cell line which expressed F9 antigen. *Nature 270:*515–518, 1977.
115. Fogh, J., Cultivation, characterization, and identification of human tumor cells with emphasis on kidney, testis and bladder tumors. *Natl. Cancer Inst. Monogr. 49:*5–9, 1978.
116. Yamamoto, T., Komatsubara, S., Suzuki, T., and Oboshi, S. *In vitro* cultivation of human testicular embryonal carcinoma and establishment of a new cell line. *Gan 70:*677–680, 1979.
117. Bronson, D. L., Andrews, P. W., Solter, D., Cervenka, J., Lange, P. H., and Fraley, E. E. Cell line derived from a metastasis of a human testicular germ cell tumor. *Cancer Res. 40:*2500–2506, 1980.
118. Wang, N., Trend, B., Bronson, D. L., and Fraley, E. E. Nonrandom abnormalities in chromosome 1 in human testicular cancers. *Cancer Res. 40:*796–802, 1980.
119. Andrews, P. W., Bronson, D. L., Benham, F., Strickland, S., and Knowles, B. B. A comparative study of eight cell lines derived from human testicular teratocarcinoma. *Int. J. Cancer 26:*269–280, 1980.
120. Atkin, N. B., and Pickthall, V. J. Chromosome 1 in 14 ovarian cancers. *Hum. Genet. 38:*35–33, 1977.
121. Goldstein, D. J., Rogers, C. E., and Harris, H. Expression of alkaline phosphatase loci

in mammalian tissues. *Proc. Natl. Acad. Sci. 77:*2857–2860, 1980.
122. Goldstein, D. J., and Harris, H. Human placental alkaline phosphatase differs from that of other species. *Nature 280:*602–605, 1979.
123. Hass, P. E., Wada, H. G., Herman, M. M., and Susman, H. H. Alkaline phosphatase of mouse teratoma stem cells: immunochemical and structural evidence for its identity as a somatic gene product. *Proc. Natl. Acad. Sci. 76:*1164–1168, 1979.
124. Slaughter, C. A., Coseo, M. C., Abrams, C., Cancro, M. P., and Harris, H. The use of hybridomas in enzyme genetics. In *Monoclonal Antibodies*, edited by R. H. Kennett, T. J. McKearn, and K. B. Bechtol, pp. 103–120. Plenum Press, New York, 1980.
125. Bronson, D. L., Fraley, E. E., Fogh, J., and Kalter, S. S. Induction of retrovirus particles in human testicular tumor (Tera 1) cell cultures: an electron microscopic study. *JNCI 63:*337–339, 1979.

Part B

Prevention of Intravascular Metastases of B16 Murine Melanoma: Adjuvant Chemotherapy with Actinomycin D*

Jerome P. Richie, M.D.

Actinomycin D was tested in an experimental preparation to determine its efficacy in the prevention of intravenous metastases. B16 melanoma cells were injected intravenously in syngeneic C57/BL6 mice. Two cell lines of the tumor, designated F1 and F10, with widely different metastatic potentials, were maintained in tissue culture and utilized for evaluation of pulmonary metastases.

When actinomycin D was given intraperitoneally at doses of 0.05 and 0.075 mg/kg for 5 days, the number of pulmonary metastases was significantly decreased ($p < 0.001$) in both the F1 and F10 cell lines. Although reduction did occur with a single dose, maximum reduction of pulmonary metastases was effected with a dose schedule administered over 5 days. Evaluation of a group of mice 2 and 3 weeks after injection of tumor cells revealed that the effects of actinomycin D were not secondary to delay in tumor growth but did represent highly significant differences in numbers of metastatic lesions.

It is concluded that in this experimental preparation actinomycin D, given in an adjuvant setting, can significantly reduce the number of pulmonary metastases. This study may have bearing on the design of adjuvant intraoperative and perioperative chemotherapy in order to destroy circulating tumor cells.

Radical exenterative surgical procedures may eradicate the primary tumor only to fail subsequently from distant metastases. This failure may be attributable either to intravascular spread of tumor from surgical

* Supported in part by BRSG #507–RR05489 and the Brigham Surgical Group, Inc.

manipulation, unrecognized small foci of tumor already present at distant sites, or both. Viable tumor cells, remote from the primary tumor, are invulnerable to surgical removal or radiation therapy. Thus, the need for effective systemic therapy in an adjuvant setting is apparent.

The complexity of cancer dissemination and the interaction of tumor cells with the host immune system contribute to the difficulty in understanding the process of metastasis. Successful prevention of metastases requires dissection of the metastatic cascade into its component parts. One aspect of the metastatic cascade is the entrapment of tumor cells in a distant capillary bed and establishment of new metastatic colonies.

An experimental preparation has been formulated to simulate escape of tumor cells into the circulation, presumably at the time of surgical manipulation and excision, and to evaluate the efficacy of adjuvant chemotherapy in this setting. The B16 melanoma and its sublines provide a well-documented tumor system in which to study metastases. Intravenous (I.V.) injection of tumor cells into the tail vein of C57/BL6 mice results in pulmonary metastases that can be counted under the dissecting microscope after necropsy. Fidler[1] has injected B16 melanoma cells into the C57/Bl6 mouse by the I.V. route, aseptically cultured the pulmonary metastases, and reinjected the cells into the circulation. By this process of selection, he has produced sublines of B16 melanoma with widely disparate potentials to metastasize. The B16 cell line (F1), produced by one injection, the harvesting of pulmonary metastases, and the reestablishment in tissue culture, has a low propensity to metastasize to the lungs. The B16-F10 cell line (F10), representing 10 such selection passages, has a high propensity to metastasize to the lungs.

The chemotherapeutic agent chosen for study is a well-tolerated antitumor antibiotic, actinomycin D. This agent has been shown to be an effective agent against B16 melanoma *in vitro* and *in vivo*. The minimal side effects of actinomycin D make it acceptable for consideration as an adjuvant treatment in the postoperative period.

MATERIALS AND METHODS

Two cell lines of the B16 melanoma, F1 and F10 (generously supplied by Dr. Isaiah Fidler, Frederick, Md.), were maintained in tissue culture on plastic plates in Weymouth's medium supplemented with 10% heat-inactivated fetal calf serum. Periodic passage *in vivo* assured viability and constant growth characteristics of the tumor cell lines.

For *in vivo* studies, C57/BL6J mice, 8–10 weeks old, were maintained on a standard laboratory diet. Tumor cell lines in the exponential growth phase were harvested by overlaying the cells with a thin layer of 0.25% trypsin-0.02% EDTA solution for 1 min. The flask was tapped to enhance removal of cells from the plastic, and media was added. Cells were then washed and resuspended in cold 0.9% NaCl solution. The cells were evaluated for viability by the trypan blue exclusion test and the cell suspension diluted to desired concentration. Viability of 98% + was obtained routinely.

The 5.0×10^4 cells were suspended in 0.2 ml of 0.9% NaCl and injected I.V. into the tail vein in unanesthetized C57BL6 mice. Groups of 10 mice each were allocated at random into either control or treated groups.

Treated mice received actinomycin D 0.05 or 0.075 mg/kg intraperitoneally (I.P.) 2 h prior to injection and once daily for the subsequent 4 days (days 0–4). At 2 weeks, all mice were killed and examined for gross evidence of pulmonary or other metastases. Nodules in the lungs (colonies) were counted under the dissecting microscope at 12.5 power magnification.

RESULTS

A dose response curve was generated for each cell line of tumor cells from *in vitro* sources injected I.V. into the tail vein (Table 3B.1). Either cell line of 5.0×10^4 cells reliably produced a readily countable but not overwhelming number (50–150) of pulmonary metastases at 2 weeks, and this dose inoculum was selected for the majority of experiments. Actinomycin D, administered I.P., was evaluated for toxicity with dose response curves. Given on a day 0–4 schedule, doses of 0.05 and 0.075 mg/kg could be tolerated with a weight loss of 15–20% and no mortality.

In experiment I, actinomycin D was tested for its effect on pulmonary metastases. A dose inoculum of 5.0×10^4 cells was injected I.V., and control or treated mice were sacrificed at 2 weeks. In the treated group, actinomycin D was given at doses of 0.05 mg/kg or 0.075 mg/kg I.P. on days 0–4. Actinomycin D significantly ($p < 0.001$) decreased the number of pulmonary metastases in both the F1 and F10 cell lines (Table 3.2). The effect was more pronounced with the F10 cell line and with the higher dose schedule.

In experiment II, the effect of single *versus* daily cumulative doses of actinomycin D, 0.075 mg/kg, was evaluated. Groups of 10 mice were injected I.V. with 5.0×10^4 cells (F1 or F10) and treated with a standard dose of actinomycin D given on day 0 only (2 h prior to injection of metastases), days 0–1, days 0–2, days 0–3, or days 0–4. In addition to standard control, an additional group of mice was injected I.V. with F1 or F10 melanoma cells premixed for 15 min with actinomycin D, 0.075 mg/kg, and the cells and actinomycin D then were injected I.V. together. This test established the most effective dose as 5 days, although significant reduction in pulmonary metastases ($p < 0.001$) was noted even with a single injection 2 h prior to the I.V. inoculation (Table 3.3). Admixture of actinomycin D with the cells for 15 min prior to injection produced the equivalent reduction of 3–4 days of therapy with actinomycin D I.P.

Table 3B.1.
Incidence of pulmonary metastases in C57B1/6 mice after I.V. injection of B16 melanoma cell lines.[a]

Cell Line	No. of Cells	No. of Pulmonary Metastases[b]
F1	2.5×10^4	22.6 ± 10.5
	5.0×10^4	88.2 ± 21.8
	1.0×10^5	273.0 ± 15.6 (3 deaths)
F10	2.5×10^4	74.4 ± 18.0
	5.0×10^4	130.6 ± 16.9
	1.0×10^5	243.2 ± 11.0

[a] Ten mice/group.
[b] Mean ± S.E.

Experiment III was formulated to verify if the difference in pulmonary metastases was secondary to mere delay in growth of colonies. A lower inoculum of F1 or F10 cells, 2.5×10^4 cells, was injected I.V. into groups of 20 mice. Ten mice served as controls and 10 received actinomycin D in a dose of 0.05 mg/kg I.P. on days 0–4. Five mice from each group were killed at 2 weeks postinjection and the remainder were killed at 3 weeks postinjection. The control group showed continued increase in both the number and size of pulmonary metastases in the intervening week; the treated groups failed to show any increase in number or size of metastases (Table 3.4). Furthermore, the difference in pulmonary metastases in the

Table 3B.2.
Effect of actinomycin D on pulmonary metastases in C57B1/6 mice after I.V. injection of B16 melanoma cell lines.[a]

Cell Line	No. of Cells	Treatment[b]	No. of Pulmonary Metastases[c]	p[d]
F1	5.0×10^4	Control	31.0 ± 2.8	
		ACT D 0.05 mg/kg	12.2 ± 1.6	<0.001
		ACT D 0.075 mg/kg	5.4 ± 0.7	<0.001
F10	5.0×10^4	Control	135.0 ± 14.0	
		ACT D 0.05 mg/kg	51.1 ± 6.9	<0.001
		ACT D 0.075 mg/kg	25.8 ± 3.8	<0.001

[a] Ten mice/group.
[b] ACT D = actinomycin D in mg/kg I.P. on days 0–4.
[c] Mean ± S.E.
[d] Probability of no difference from appropriate control group (Student's *t*-test).

Table 3B.3.
Incidence of pulmonary metastases with sequential doses of actinomycin D in C57B1/6 mice after I.V. injection of B16 melanoma cell lines.[a]

Cell Line	No. of Cells	Treatment[b]	Duration of Treatment	No. of Pulmonary Metastases[c]	p[d]
			Day		
F1	5.0×10^4	Control		34.0 ± 11.2	
		ACT D 0.075 mg/kg	0	13.7 ± 3.4	<0.05
			0–1	2.9 ± 0.7	<0.01
			0–2	4.3 ± 1.1	<0.05
			0–3	0.4 ± 0.1	<0.01
			0–4		<0.001
		Premixed		5.9 ± 1.7	<0.05
F10	5.0×10^4	Control		113.0 ± 19.3	
		ACT D 0.075 mg/kg	0	37.9 ± 6.2	<0.001
			0–1	40.5 ± 7.6	<0.001
			0–2	31.8 ± 8.2	<0.001
			0–3	25.5 ± 2.1	<0.001
			0–4	13.7 ± 1.6	<0.001
		Premixed		14.4 ± 4.5	<0.001

[a] Ten mice/group.
[b] ACT D = actinomycin D 0.075 mg/kg I.P. beginning 2 h prior to tumor inoculation. Premixed = tumor cells + actinomycin D 0.075 mg/kg mixed for 15 min and injected I.V. together.
[c] Mean ± S.E.
[d] Probability of no difference from appropriate control group (Student's *t*-test).

Table 3B.4.
Effect of longer observation period on development of pulmonary metastases in C57BL6 mice after I.V. injection of B16 melanoma cell lines.[a]

Cell Line	No. of Cells	Treatment[b]	Time to Death	No. of Pulmonary Metastases[c]	p^d
			Week		
F1	2.5×10^4	Control	2	8.0 ± 6.2	
		ACT D	2	2.8 ± 2.4	<0.05
		Control	3	28.8 ± 24.0	
		ACT D	3	3.1 ± 1.6	<0.001
F10	2.5×10^4	Control	2	23.3 ± 10.5	
		ACT D	2	5.3 ± 2.7	<0.001
		Control	3	50.6 ± 9.2	
		ACT D	3	6.0 ± 4.0	<0.001

[a] Twenty mice/group.
[b] ACT D = actinomycin D 0.05 mg/kg I.P. on days 0–4.
[c] Mean ±S.E.
[d] Probability of no difference from appropriate control group (Students' *t*-test).

control group at 2 weeks and the treated group at 3 weeks was highly significant ($p < 0.001$) for both the F1 and F10 cell lines.

DISCUSSION

More than 50% of the newly diagnosed cases of cancer each year will have metastatic disease at the time of diagnosis or a high risk of recurrence following the best available local therapy.[2] Circulating metastatic foci of tumor cells are the proper target of the medical oncologist, and chemotherapy and immunotherapy are the major potential mechanisms for tumor destruction on a systemic basis. Each of these two modalities of therapy has the ability to reach sanctuaries remote from the primary tumor site.

The theoretical considerations for adjuvant chemotherapy are based upon cell cycle kinetics and mechanical factors. Once the majority of tumor cells have been removed, the remaining microfoci have a higher tumor growth cell fraction,[3] less tumor in the resting or insensitive phase of chemotherapy, better vascularization,[4] and fewer competitive metabolites. Salmon[5] has shown that doubling time is proportional to the number of cells and is based on a Gompertzian curve. All the aforementioned factors, kinetic and anatomic, favor increased delivery of drug to the active tumor and increased susceptibility of tumor foci to chemotherapeutic agents in an adjuvant setting. Furthermore, patients with lower tumor burdens are less likely to be immunosuppressed. In animal systems, response to chemotherapy is inversely proportional to extent of disease.

The study of metastasis in an animal system has certain inherent limitations. Nonetheless, the ability to study metastasis from circulating tumor cells of different metastatic potentials in a syngeneic system should allow close scrutiny of the entire process. The lack of growing tumor burden at the time of I.V. inoculation provides a pure system in which to study metastatic phenomenon in an immunologically naive animal and allows quantification of circulating tumor cells without question of spontaneous metastases from active or excised tumor. Although immune modulation of the implantation of metastasis does occur,[6, 7] this preparation specifically precluded prior immune recognition of tumor.

Actinomycin D has been utilized as an adjuvant chemotherapeutic agent in other animal model systems. Blount and associates,[8] in a murine testicular tumor model system, have demonstrated the import of proper timing for effectiveness of an adjuvant chemotherapeutic agent. Using the embryonal ridge germ cell implantation technique for testicular tumor in the mouse, these authors have shown that actinomycin D, given on the day of grafting, is equally as effective as a four-drug combination (cyclophosphamide, vincristine (Oncovin), methotrexate, and fluorouracil) given 2 days subsequent to grafting of tumor. As predicted from a theoretical basis, lesser amounts of tumor burden should be more readily curable by adjuvant chemotherapeutic agents. In several other animal model systems, surgery followed by chemotherapy improved the cure rate of all metastatic animal cancers studied.[9]

Actinomycin D has proven effectiveness against the animal tumor model, B16 melanoma. The present study documents the ability of actinomycin D to significantly reduce the implantation and subsequent growth of pulmonary metastases secondary to circulating B16 melanoma cells. This has been demonstrated for two different sublines of the tumor, each with different metastatic potentials. A dose-response curve has been generated. Furthermore, the differences observed, both in number and in size of pulmonary metastasis, were not caused merely by a delay in growth of the tumor but represent actual diminution in the number of metastases.

There is demonstrated need for effective therapy in a surgical adjuvant setting. For an agent to be considered in an adjuvant setting, however, several factors must be considered. Toxicity that may be acceptable in a stable patient may be unacceptably high and fatal in a patient in the immediate postoperative period. The effects of chemotherapeutic agents on wound healing and general metabolic activity must be weighed carefully. The agent chosen should have demonstrated effectiveness against advanced states of the tumor, and the agent should not prejudice the ability of the patient to respond later to other effective chemotherapeutic agents.

Actinomycin D, an antitumor antibiotic, fulfills many of the requirements for an effective adjuvant chemotherapeutic agent. Its mode of action is binding deoxyribonucleic acid (DNA) and inhibiting DNA-dependent ribonucleic acid (RNA) synthesis.[10] It is a relatively noncycle-specific agent with demonstrated activity against lymphoma, childhood solid tumor, bone sarcoma, melanoma, ovarian and uterine tumors, and testicular germ cell tumors.[11] Its major toxicity, myelosuppression, may be effectively controlled by dose and schedule modifications. Because of its relatively mild toxicity and broad spectrum of antitumor activity, actinomycin D merits consideration in trials of surgical adjuvant chemotherapy. The ideal patient for adjuvant chemotherapy is the one with resected tumor but with a high likelihood of local or distant recurrence. Even though large numbers of patients may be required for statistical validity, an adequate randomized prospective trial of adjuvant chemotherapy in patients with minimal residual disease should provide the highest likelihood of demonstration of survival differences.

REFERENCES

1. Fidler, I. J. Selection of successive tumor lines for metastasis. *Nat. New Biol. 242:*148, 1973.
2. De Vita, V. T., Young, R. C., and Canellos, G. P. Combination *versus* single agent chemotherapy: Review of basis for selection of drug treatment of cancer. *Cancer 35:*98, 1975.
3. Skipper, H. E., and Schabel, F. M., Jr. Quantitative and cytokinetic studies in experimental tumor models. In *Cancer Medicine*, p. 629, edited by J. F. Holland and E. Frei. Lea & Febiger, Philadelphia, 1973.
4. Tannock, I. F. The relation between cell proliferation and the vascular system in a transplanted mouse mammary tumor. *Br. J. Cancer 22:*258, 1968.
5. Salmon, S. E. Kinetic rationale for adjuvant chemotherapy of cancer. In *Adjuvant Therapy of Cancer*, pp. 15–27, edited by S. E. Salmon and S. E. Jones. North-Holland, Amsterdam, 1977.
6. Fidler, I. J., Gersten, D. M. and Riggs, C. W. Relationship of host immune status to tumor cell arrest, distribution, and survival in experimental metastasis. *Cancer 40:*46, 1977.
7. Wexler, H., Chretien, P. B., Ketcham, A. S., and Sindelar, W. F. Induction of pulmonary metastases in both immune and nonimmune mice. *Cancer 36:*2042, 1975.
8. Blount, B. M., Stevens, L. C., and Whitmore, W. F., Jr. The effect of chemotherapy on germinal testicular tumors in mice. *Cancer 26:*570, 1970.
9. Griswold, D. P., Jr. The potential for murine tumor models in surgical adjuvant chemotherapy. *Cancer Chemother. Rep. 5:*187, 1975.
10. Kirk, J. M. The mode of action of actinomycin D. *Biochim. Biophys. Acta 42:*167, 1960.
11. Davis, H. L., Jr., von Hoff, D. D., Henney, J. E., and Rozencweig, M. The role of antitumor antibiotics in current oncologic practice. *Cancer Chemother. Pharmacol. 1:*83, 1978.

4

Germ Cell Tumors of Mice and Men: the Teratocarcinoma Models and Their Clinical Implications

David L. Bronson, Ph.D.
Judith Gunn Bronson, M.S.
Elwin E. Fraley, M.D.

"The choice of a suitable material is one of the major steps in biological research. It is not enough to ask the right questions—it is just as important to use the right material in order to get an answer."

François Jacob

Traditionally, cancer has been thought of as a rapid and uncontrolled growth of cells that arise by dedifferentiation resulting from spontaneous or chemically induced mutation or virus infection and which sometimes leads to the synthesis of abnormal (cancer-specific?) substances and to an unpredictable capacity to metastasize. Today, however, little is left of this traditional picture, and one of the chief contributors to its redrawing has been the mouse teratocarcinoma models that were developed by Leroy C. Stevens and G. Barry Pierce in the 1950s and 1960s.[1, 2] This chapter reviews that work briefly and describes the more recent studies of human testicular cancer cells. It then shows how the results have helped to construct a new picture of the nature of cancer.

MOUSE TERATOCARCINOMAS

Mouse (and human) teratocarcinomas are curious tumors: they contain both primitive malignant cells, called (because of their resemblance to the cells of the early embryo) embryonal carcinoma (EC) cells, and various partially or fully differentiated tissues—neurectoderm, cartilage, bone, striated and smooth muscle, respiratory and transitional epithelium—rather as if someone had stirred the tissues of a fetus. Occasionally, the

EC cells disappear, apparently by differentiation, leaving only a mass of mature or immature teratoma that is nearly always benign. This is scarcely the behavior one expects of a cancer cell.

Murine EC cells became even more puzzling when it was demonstrated that, when they are placed in a mouse blastocyst, they may participate in the creation of a normal mouse. (Blastocysts and EC cells from different strains of mice are used in order to provide markers for EC-derived cells.) This finding made it appear that the EC cell had accomplished the seemingly impossible feat of being malignant and normal simultaneously, its choice between the two behaviors being determined by its environment. As subsequent studies have confirmed, this is indeed true: in the EC cell, neoplasia and embryogenesis come together. This discovery made the murine teratocarcinoma one of the most useful tools of biological research, and these tumors now are used to analyze the function of the cell surface in embryogenesis, as a model of tumor-host interactions, as models of the control of cellular differentiation, and in studying the molecular specificity of natural killer (NK) lymphocytes, which kill EC cells but not their differentiated derivatives.

Spontaneous Murine Tumors

Athough most strains of mice rarely or never have spontaneous teratomas and teratocaricnomas, careful inbreeding of strains with low frequencies of such tumors has yielded valuable sublines such as 129/terSv, in which 30% of the males have spontaneous congenital testicular teratocarcinomas. These tumors are first visible as clusters of embryonic cells within the seminiferous tubules as early as the 14th day of fetal development. Other mouse strains, notably LT, have high frequencies of ovarian teratomas, which apparently develop postnatally by parthenogenesis of the oocytes.

The high incidence of testicular tumors in 129/terSv mice appears to have resulted from a single mutation in the parent 129/Sv line, which has only a 3% incidence of spontaneous testicular tumors; and Mintz and Fleischman[3] (whose excellent review of the mouse teratocarcinoma work is highly recommended) offer the interesting suggestion that tumor-susceptible strains of mice carry a mutant gene that predisposes the primordial germ cells of the male and the oocytes to spontaneous parthenogenetic cleavage.

Despite the interest in these spontaneous murine testicular tumors occasioned by the evidence for a genetic influence on the incidence of human testicular tumors,[4] this murine model has been of limited value in research because the tumors can rarely be sustained by serial transplantation into new hosts.

Embryo-Derived Tumors

A more useful model has been created by transplanting embryos containing egg-cylinder ectoderm to extrauterine sites such as the testis or beneath the kidney capsule, where they may gow into teratocarcinomas or teratomas that are histologically indistinguishable from those that arise spontaneously. (Other parts of the embryo form other tissues but not teratocarcinomas and teratomas). The frequency of teratocarcinoma production increases with the age of the embryo between the two-cell stage and the 8th day, after which only teratomas are produced.

Transplantation of an embryo alters both its biochemical environment and its physical constraints and disrupts its cell-cell associations. Thus, several reasons for the age limit on the production of teratocarcinomas can be postulated. First, the embryo may not be sufficiently disturbed by the procedure to deflect its cells from their differentiation pathway after the 8th day. Second, the primitive cells may already be committed to differentiation by that time. The difficulty with this hypothesis is that primitive primodial germ cells appear in the embryo shortly after this stage of development, so some uncommitted cells obviously do remain. Perhaps the remaining uncommitted cells cannot form tumors after the 8th day or do so only rarely. Alternatively, the primitive cells may be particularly susceptible to lethal damage during transplantation, a view for which there is some experimental evidence.[3]

Mice bearing embryo-derived tumors have splenomegaly, which is believed to represent an immunological response to antigenic stimulation.[5] Splenic enlargement is more pronounced in animals with teratocarcinomas than in those with teratomas and in those in which the embryo has been placed somewhere other than the testis. These findings suggest two things: first, that the embryo (especially its primitive cells) bears antigens that are recognized as nonself by the adult syngeneic animal and, second, that the testis is immunologically privileged; *i.e.* that material there has some protection against immunological assault.

Embryo transplants do not work in all strains of mice, and in some strains, the proportion of teratocarcinomas among the tumors is higher than it is in other strains. For example, in Balb/c mice, 50–70% of the tumors formed are malignant teratocarcinomas, whereas in other strains, such as C57BL/6, only 10% are. Such strains are called TC-permissive and TC-nonpermissive, respectively. In at least one strain, permissiveness is determined by some maternally transmitted factor, which could have affected the embryo during its brief stay in the uterus but more likely was derived from the cytoplasm of the zygote. The field of cytoplasmic inheritance is largely unexplored, and if the latter explanation proves correct, mouse teratocarcinomas would have yet another research application.

Genital-Ridge Tumors

This model, also called the Stevens model, is created by transplanting the genital ridges of appropriate strains of fetal mice into the testes of syngeneic adults. All of the resulting teratomas and teratocarcinomas have XY karyotypes, whereas the embryo-derived tumors may have either XX or XY karyotypes.*

One of the notable features of the Stevens model is that genital ridges are effective in producing teratocarcinomas between the 12th and 16th

* Genital ridges from female fetuses produce ovaries, not teratocarcinomas; apparently by the time these XX germ cells reach the genital ridges, they are already committed to one line of development.

days of development, in contrast to the embryonic ectoderm of the embryo transplants, which ceases to be tumorigenic after the 8th day. This finding focuses attention on one of the vexing questions of these models: which cells are involved? Does embryonic ectoderm form teratocarcinomas because it is a source of primordial germ cells? The ability of transplanted embryos to form both XX and XY tumors suggests that this is not so, that the embryonic cells are the direct ancestors of the tumor. Also, some strains of mice that are susceptible to embryo-derived tumors do not form tumors when genital ridges are transplanted. Thus it appears that primitive embryonic cells and male primordial germ cells can form histologically identical tumors.

Maintenance of Teratocarcinomas

Once a teratocarcinoma has been created, it often is possible to maintain it in various ways. For example, one tumor has been kept growing in the laboratory for more than 22 years by serial transplantation. However, during transplantation, a restriction in the types of differentiated tissues is common, as are changes in karyotype. (The two changes may be related in that a change in the gene dosage secondary to loss or reduplication of chromosomes could affect the range of differentiation.) Serially transplanted tumors often have XO karyotypes, but none has been found without an X chromosome, which appears to be critical for cell multiplication and maintenance.

A special form of transplanted tumor is the embryoid body, which is maintained in the peritoneal cavity of the host. There are two forms, simple and cystic, both of which contain a core of EC cells. The simple embryoid bodies have a rind of primitive endoderm; the cystic embryoid bodies may include nerve, muscle, and yolk sac tissue.[6]

Finally, EC cells can be maintained *in vitro.* Many lines, sublines, and clones have been established, with various abilities to differentiate. Cells maintained in an undifferentiated state remain capable of causing tumors in syngeneic mice. Cultured tumor cells have been useful in studies of early development because the EC cells closely resemble normal early embryonic cells yet are easier to propagate *in vitro.*

USES OF THE TUMOR MODELS

Control of Differentiation

It bears pointing out that much of the work on gene expression and its control has dealt with end stage differentiation products such as immunoglobulins rather than with "bread-and-butter" genes involved in the everyday activities of cells or their maturation. The mouse teratocarcinoma system provides an opportunity to study how differentiation genes are turned on and off. These studies have been conducted in blastocysts, in transplantable tumors, and in cultured cells.[6]

When one or a few murine EC cells are microinjected into or aggregated with a blastocyst and implanted in the uterus of a pseudopregnant female, the malignant behavior of the tumor cells is stopped. As shown by many experiments in which the tumor cells and the blastocyst differed in detectable ways such as adult skin pigmentation or isoenzymes, the EC cells become incorporated into normal tissues. The extent to which this happens varies; sometimes only one organ is involved, whereas some chimeras have tumor contributions to virtually all of their tissues. In one of the most spectacular successes of this type of work, cells taken from a tumor that had been maintained for almost 200 transplant generations for 8 years gave rise to the germ cells in a few of the chimeras, which fathered normal progeny. As yet, no one has reported obtaining both a male and a female with tumor-derived germ cells and mating them, although this accomplishment seems only a matter of time. As Mintz and Fleischman[3] point out, the offspring of such a union could boast (if that is the word) of being descended from a long line of distinguished tumors.

When murine EC cells are implanted subcutaneously, they remain malignant. However, in many other sites such cells will differentiate. Formation of neural tissue is common, but liver, kidney, lung, and thymus tissue has never been found in these teratomas. This probably results from a lack of proper association with other types of cells, because EC cells placed in a blastocyst are capable of contributing to such tissues. The extensive biochemical studies of these teratomas produced *in vivo* by EC cells have been described by Graham.[7]

Differentiation also can be studied *in vitro* with EC cells. Numerous lines are available that have different abilities to differentiate and form different types of tissue; *e.g.* some form neural derivatives, others endoderm, still others ectoderm, etc.[8] Some of these studies have explored stimulators of differentiation, such as retinoic acid. These experiments have made it clear that the first step in differentiation is, in fact, a two-step process. Thus, when the F9 cell line (one of the most popular and which is capable only of limited differentiation into endoderm) is treated for 2 days with retinoic acid, it loses its receptors to peanut agglutinin (PNA), receptors that are one of the primary characteristics of EC cells (*vide infra*). If, after 2 days, the F9 cells are transferred to medium without retinoic acid, these receptors reappear. However, after 4 days of growth in retinoic acid-containing medium, the F9 cells begin synthesizing plasminogen activator and basement membrane proteins. Once acquired, these properties are constitutive, and the cells cannot revert to EC cells.[9, 10]

Cell-Surface Antigens

"One might consider that the cell surface of teratocarcinoma is a world where carbohydrates are predominant," commented Takashi Muramatsu after surveying the abundant data about the antigens of EC cells. To date, all of the molecules found to be expressed preferentially on EC are carbohydrates.

A few of these antigens are of special interest. One of them, known as F9 because it was discovered on that cell line, was originally thought to be related developmentally and chemically to H-2, which is the major histocompatibility complex in mice and thus analogous to the human leukocyte antigens (HLA). It has since been found that this is not true.[11] Gachelin's group has partially purified the F9 antigen(s) from EC cells and early embryos and obtained both glycoproteins and glycolipids. The antigenic sites appear to be polysaccharide. The F9 antigens disappear from EC during differentiation.

The two other cell-surface antigens considered characteristic of murine EC are lectin-binding sites for the fucose-binding protein of *Lotus* (FBP) and for PNA, mentioned earlier. These sites also disappear during differentiation. The PNA sites are of special interest, as they are found on cells of several human cancers and are released into the circulation. It was recently suggested that this could be used as a laboratory test for the presence of certain cancers.[12]

Also present on EC cells and cells of the early embryo is a glycolipid called SSEA (stage-specific embryonic antigen)-1, which is defined by a monoclonal antibody raised against F9 cells.[13] A later antigen, SSEA-3, which was prepared by immunization of a rat with 4- to 8-cell-stage mouse embryos, does not react with murine EC cells but does react with human EC.[14] More will be said about this antigen later.

New antigens continue to be found on EC cells. Calcium-dependent cell-cell adhesion sites immunologically identical to those found on cleavage-stage embryos were described recently,[15] as was a surface lectin that appears to be involved in cell-cell adhesion.[16] Biochemical studies of these cell-surface carbohydrates recently led to the proposal of a model in which alteration of surface molecules by branching and chain elongation produces a continuous change in the cell surface that guides cell differentiation and ontogenesis.[17] As this interesting subject is outside the scope of this chapter, we refer the interested reader to Hakomori *et al.*[17]

STUDIES OF HUMAN GERM CELL TUMORS *IN VITRO*

The studies in our laboratory of human testicular germ cell cancers *in vitro* began in 1976 with the explanting of a mixed but predominantly EC tumor that had killed a 20-year-old man.[18] The tumor tissue, which was to become cell line 833K, was placed in culture by the coverslip technique, in which opposite edges of a square coverslip are embedded in 2 drops of sterile silicone grease so that the coverslip will hold the finely minced tissue against the growth surface of the culture plate. This method prevents detachment and loss of the tissue during manipulations such as medium changes. The coverslips also trap blood cells, and therefore this culture method often yields lymphoblastoid cell (LC) lines as well as tumor cell lines. LC are lines of polyclonal B lymphocytes that express Epstein-Barr virus antigens and multiply indefinitely, providing cells that are valuable as controls in experiments with the autologous testis tumor lines.

Since the 833K line was established, 26 additional testicular cancer cell lines have been derived from 108 specimens with various culture methods. An explant is most likely to develop into a line if the tissue donor has not received radiotherapy or chemotherapy, although some of our lines, including 833K, are from patients who have. Also, the tissue should be placed in physiological saline or culture medium immediately after it is excised and processed for culture within 1–2 h. It is imperative that the specimen and the resulting cell growth be handled gently, as the tumor cells are very fragile—a point that may surprise those whose clinical experience has shown how difficult they can be to kill *in vivo*. A few other cell lines have been established from human testicular cancers by other investigators.[19–23] Most of our lines, as well as most of those established elsewhere, appear to be EC; but a few lines appear to be malignant teratoma, two of our lines are a combination of EC and yolk sac carcinoma, and two are EC with choriocarcinoma. As one would expect, the yolk sac-EC lines are copious producers of α-fetoprotein (AFP), and the choriocarcinoma-EC lines readily produce human chorionic gonadotropin (HCG).

Virus Production

The first indication that there was something of special interest about the briskly growing 833K cells came from our electron microscopist, Donna Ritzi. During a routine examination of the cells for ultrastructural characteristics, she spotted two particles that closely resembled the retroviruses found in human placental tisues.[24–27] Retroviruses have an RNA genome and the ability to direct the encoding of their genetic material into DNA, which then becomes integrated with the genome of the host cell. Many retroviruses of subhuman species cause malignant transformation of cells *in vitro*, and some produce malignancies in animals.[28]

Further examination of the 833K cells revealed a few similar particles either outside of cells or budding from the outer membrane or microvilli, which is the way retroviruses mature (Fig. 4.1). These particles were

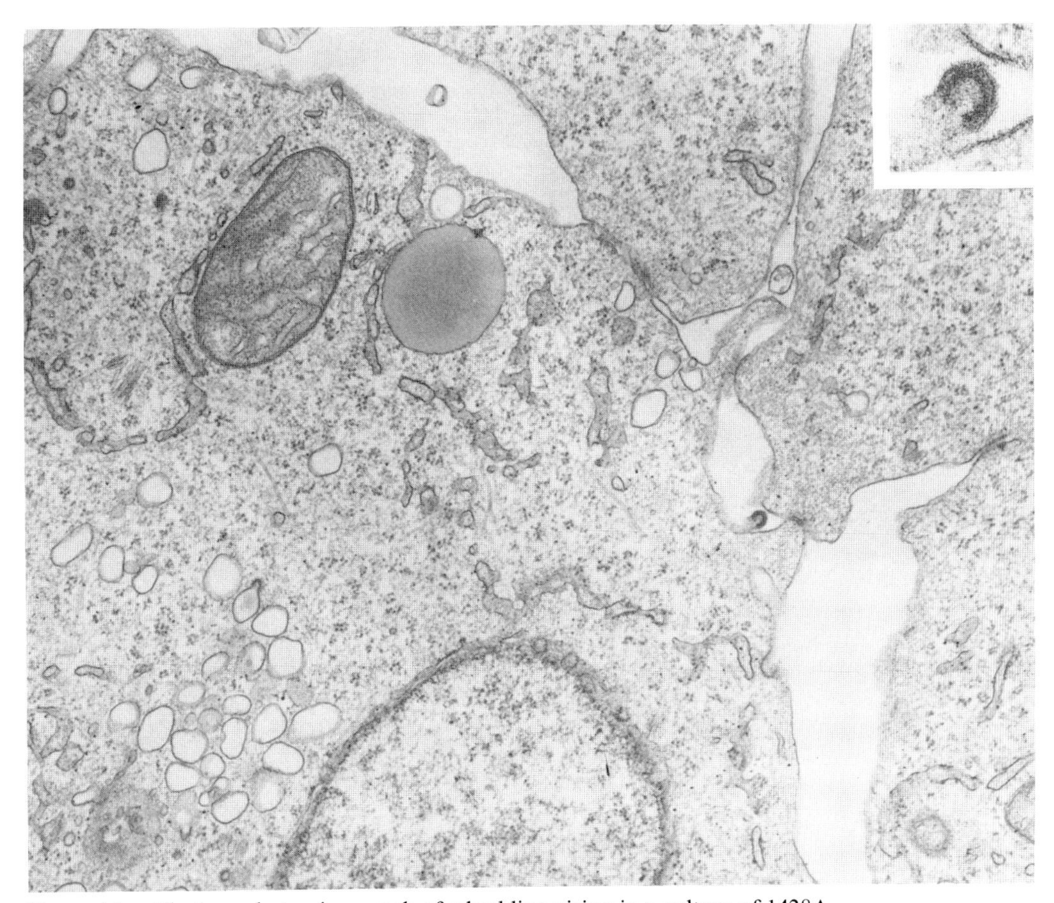

Figure 4.1. Electron photomicrograph of a budding virion in a culture of 1428A embryonal carcinoma cells (× 25,000 (*inset* × 90,000)).

produced by one of every 150–200 cells. Treatment of cultures with iododeoxyuridine (IUDR) and dexamethasone increased the number of particles per productive cell but did not appear to increase the proportion of cells producing the virus (Fig. 4.2). We sent electron micrographs to Dr. Albert J. Dalton, Scientist Emeritus of the National Cancer Institute (NCI) and a preeminent authority on the morphology of retroviruses, and he agreed that the particles look identical to the retrovirus, tentatively identified as a type C retrovirus, that is found in human placental tissues.[29]

To summarize the subsequent data, we have found that all 17 of our human EC lines produce these retroviruses, as does an EC line called Tera-1 established by Dr. Jørgen Fogh of Sloane-Kettering.[30] Further, our two lines from patient 2102E and the Tera-1 cells also produce a few spiked virions that have the morphological characteristics of type B retroviruses. On the other hand, the cell lines that do not have EC characteristics, such as our 577M lines and Dr. Fogh's Tera-2 (all of which are believed to be malignant teratoma and thus to be differentiated EC derivatives), do not produce either type of virion when stimulated with IUDR and dexamethasone. In addition, when the EC cells begin to differentiate, they stop producing virions. Collaborative studies with several other laboratories have established to the satisfaction of all the

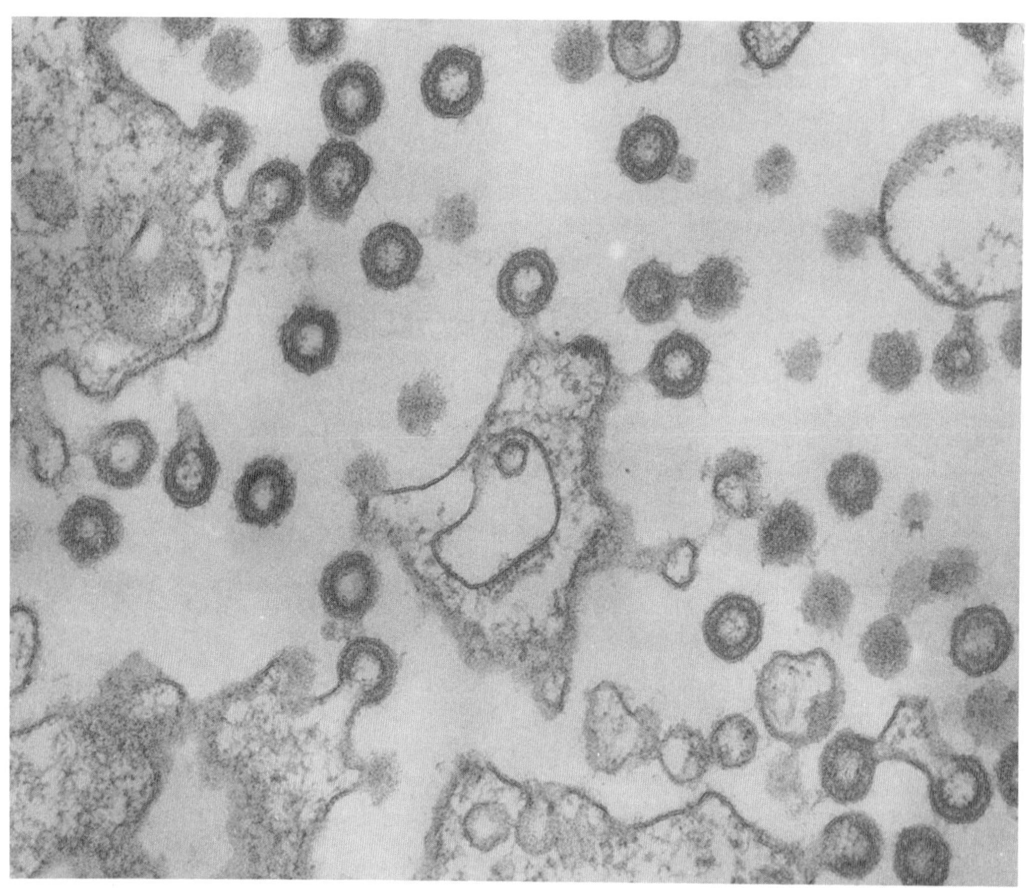

Figure 4.2. Budding and extracellular virions in a culture of 1075L-HEp (EC and choriocarcinoma grown on feeder cells) on day 4 after incubation with IUDR and dexamethasone (× 87,500).

investigators involved that, unlike so many earlier "human retroviruses," these are not laboratory contaminants but rather are indigenous to the EC cells.

Of course, in the world of retroviruses, more than morphology is required to prove membership in the group. A primary requirement is biochemical evidence of RNA-dependent DNA polymerase (reverse transcriptase) activity, as this is the enzyme that makes it possible to convert the virus's RNA genome into a DNA copy suitable for integration into the genome of the host. In the classical retrovirus laboratory models, such as the murine, avian (*e.g.* Rous sarcoma), and subhuman primate retroviruses, demonstration of viral-borne reverse transcriptase activity in culture fluids is generally not difficult, because titers of 10^9–10^{11} virions/ml can be achieved. It has been impossible to obtain such high titers of the virus produced by the human EC cells, even with high-producer sublines, and the first attempts to demonstrate reverse transcriptase activity failed. However, Dr. Robert Gallo's laboratory at the NCI recently used concentrates of 10 liters of supernatant fluids from EC cultures in reverse transcriptase assays and found low levels of activity.[31] This finding increases the probability that these particles are truly retroviruses.

What does the production of retroviruses by undifferentiated EC cells mean? Data available from other retrovirus systems permit some educated guessing. First, it must be emphasized that we do not know if the virus causes any kind of malignancy. The fact that it is produced only by undifferentiated EC cells and by placental cells suggests that the cells are producing it "deliberately" for some biological reason unrelated to malignancy. It may well be, for example, that the retroviruses of primitive and reproductive tissues are a messenger service, shuttling bits of information among cells to increase the shuffling of genetic information that nature encourages during the earliest stages of development. (Chromosome breakage and reunion during meiosis and mitosis is another example of such genetic revising.) This process, termed transduction, has long been known to occur in procaryotic systems such as bacteria, in which it is mediated by bacteriophage. Retroviruses are now believed capable of the same function. To a great extent, this conclusion is based on the recent demonstration that cells of vertebrates have a genetic sequence closely related to the retroviral transforming sequence, which is presumed to have originated in cellular genes. The normal function of the cellular gene is unknown, but it might be expressed during embryogenesis, a period of rapid cell growth. In nonmalignant cells, later expression of the sequence would then be tightly controlled whereas, in rare instances, it might be appropriated by a retrovirus and transduced to a susceptible cell. If this cellular gene were then integrated into the genome of the new host cell in the "wrong" position, so that it would not be subject to the usual regulator genes, or if it were integrated so that its expression was controlled by the retrovirus, the host cell would be unable to control its expression. The result would be unregulated growth—malignancy.

We can only speculate whether such transduction occurs between germ cells with the retrovirus found in EC cultures. It would be enlightening to examine normal germ cells for retrovirus production and for their response to infection by virions produced by the EC cultures. Unfortuately, the difficulty in obtaining pure populations of normal human germ cells and their reluctance to grow *in vitro* have so far precluded such a study.

Whatever the role of these retroviruses produced by EC cells and placental cells, it is significant that they apparently are not produced by differentiating EC cells or teratoma cells. Knowledge of the mechanism by which these cells control virus production would help greatly in attempts to understand the way eucaryotic cells regulate gene expression, a topic of obvious relevance to any understanding of malignant transformation and embryogenesis.

Cytogenetics

A routine part of our studies of cell lines is karyotyping with banding techniques that permit identification of the numerical and structural changes in the chromosome complement. These studies were performed on the cell lines by Dr. Nancy Wang and her colleagues[32] in the Dcpartment of Laboratory Medicine and Pathology at the University of Minnesota. They showed that each cell line has its own distinctive karyotype with unique marker chromosomes. There were some striking similarities among the lines, however, particularly in the number and types of abnormalities of chromosome 1. These abnormalities, found in all of the lines studied, are nonrandom, with break points occurring preferentially on the p arm in regions 12, 22, and 36 and on the q arm in region 12.[32] Because these changes are nonrandom, they yield morphologically identical marker chromosomes in different lines, calling to mind the Ph^1 (Philadelphia) chromosome of chronic myelocytic leukemia, the partial deletion of the p arm of chromosome 11 in many cases of Wilms' tumor, and the 3 → 8 translocation seen in hereditary renal cell carcinoma. Chromosome 1 abnormalities are common in human cancers, but the consistent finding of such similar changes in several specimens from the same histologic type of cancer is unusual.

Until very recently, it was not at all clear what these consistent chromosomal abnormalities might mean. However, it now is known that many abnormal chromosomes found in cancers contain misplaced genes that might thereby be "turned on" or transcribed in altered form.[33] This fascinating work, which has brought together investigations in immunology, cytogenetics, and viral oncology, may eventually explain the chromosome 1 abnormalities found in these cell lines.

Significantly, the cytogenetic studies of the cell lines established from tumor deposits at different sites in the same patient have identical features, although cells of somewhat different karyotypes may also be primary tumors. These findings reinforce the concept that metastases from a primary tumor represent the selective survival of subpopulations of tumor cells, not random events.[34] In light of this concept, the presence of three identical markers, M1, M2, and M3, in all of the 577M lines is particularly interesting. The 577MR line was established from a teratocarcinoma obtained at retroperitoneal lymphadenectomy, and the 577MF and 577ML lines were established from forehead and lung metastases, respectively, removed at warm autopsy almost 3 years later after the patient had received chemotherapy and radiation. These lines have slightly different karyotypes, but all have the aforementioned markers as well as the same modal chromosome number. The presence of these identical markers also proves that such chromosomes are native to the tumor, not artifacts of *in vitro* cultivation.[32]

Another finding in the cytogenetic studies was the presence of X chromosomes, sometimes of more than one, in the cells of all 14 lines studied with trypsin G-banding techniques.[35] For these chromosomes to be present, malignant transformation must have occurred before meiosis. This finding was not surprising. What was surprising was the discovery of Barr bodies—inactivated X chromosomes—in three of the five lines tested for them. In normal female cells, one of the two X chromosomes in each somatic cell is inactivated early in development, but in the normal male cell, the single X chromosome is not inactivated. Thus, these Barr body-containing tumors have differentiated independently of their male host. This finding has made the human testicular cancer cell lines a valuable model for students of the arcane subject of X chromosome inactivation.

Cell-Surface Antigens

In light of the extensive work on the surface of the mouse EC (stem) cell, studies of cell-surface molecules of human germ cell tumors were of obvious interest. Indeed, one of the first reports of a human testicular cell line focused on its expression of the F9 antigen.[19]

The immunological studies of the cell surface of our lines were performed by Drs. Peter W. Andrews and Davor Solter and their coworkers at the Wistar Institute, whose work on the mouse teratocarcinomas is well known. They looked both for such early antigens as SSEA-1 and SSEA-3 and for what are, in the murine system, evidences of the differentiated state, namely major histocompatibility antigens and β_2-microglobulin.

In murine EC cells, SSEA-1 is expressed but SSEA-3 is not. The latter is expressed, however, by cleavage-stage embryos up to the blastocyst stage. In the human EC lines, the reverse is true, *i.e.* the cells express SSEA-3 but little SSEA-1.[12, 18, 36] SSEA-1 also can be detected on human spermatozoa and human gestational choriocarcinoma, but neither it nor SSEA-3 is detectable on more differentiated human cells such as teratoma or cultured fibroblasts.

There also is a difference in the expression of the major histocompatibility antigens. Mouse EC cells do not express them, and for a long time it was thought that the F9 antigen was the precursor of these antigens (called H-2). We know now that this is not true.[11] Human EC cells, in contrast, do express major histocompatibility (HLA) antigens, and it was possible to prove this in experiments in which LC lines from our specimens were used as controls to determine the HLA type of the patient.[37] These findings show that in the human germ cell system the long-standing practice of equating expression of major histocompatibility antigens with differentiation may be incorrect. They also open up the prospect of a model for the study of these clinically important transplantation antigens, and they indicate that the human EC is more primitive than its mouse analogue.

Differentiation and Marker Production *in Vitro*

Early in our studies, it became evident that some cultures were more difficult to maintain in a vigorously growing state than were others. This problem was especially noticeable in cultures of some EC lines as, under certain conditions, a variable proportion of the cells became pleomorphic, and the cell growth rate diminished. An example is the 2044L line, which is an EC line established soon after we began this research. The 2044L cells were initially subcultured by scraping, because the primary and early passage cultures consisted of a dense growth of stromal fibroblasts with a few foci of tumor cells, which did not spread and grow well in competition with the stromal cells. After approximately eight passages, the fibroblasts began to degenerate, and the EC cells eventually overgrew them. It was then necessary to subculture the EC cells at high density because at a lower density, cells at the periphery of isolated clusters grew slowly and displayed distinct changes in morphology. These observations, as well as the findings in the mouse teratocarcinoma system and the apparent maturation of some germ cell tumors clinically, suggested that the human EC cells might differentiate.

Mouse EC cells (stem cells) lose their ability to differentiate rapidly and extensively *in vitro* if they are not grown continuously on "feeder" cells.[38] Similar results were obtained with our 2044L and other EC lines, in that continued passage of the cells after the stromal fibroblasts (which served as feeder cells) were no longer present led to cell lines that had the properties of EC cells but with little tendency to change morphology, growth rate, or growth pattern. Therefore, we began explanting human testicular germ cell tumors onto feeder monolayers of human lung (HL) fibroblasts that had been treated for 4 hours with mitomycin C. This drug inhibits the growth of the fibroblasts, and virtually all are destroyed within 3–4 days. When EC cells are added 24 h after mitomycin treatment of the HL, the EC cells attach rapidly, spread out, and form confluent monolayers. Further, attachment of tumor tissue is more efficient, and outgrowth is more rapid, when the minced tissue specimens are seeded on these feeder layers.

Two of the lines that were established and maintained continuously on feeder cells are the 1777N-Pr and 1777N-RP met lines, which represent, respectively, a primary teratocarcinoma and an EC retroperitoneal lymph node metastasis from the same patient. Several clones have been established from these lines by selecting single tumor cells with a micropipette and transferring each to a feeder monolayer in a separate well of a microtiter plate. When suspensions of the parent or cloned cell lines are seeded at low density without feeder layers, distinct changes in morphology and growth pattern are seen. In addition to being a possible model of controlled differentiation, these cells may be of interest to clinicians for the light they shed on AFP and HCG production.

When 1777N cells of either line are subcultured by trypsinization (which yields suspensions of dispersed cells) and seeded at low density without feeder cells, HCG is produced within 18 days, rises to a maximum level (often exceeding 3000 ng/ml) within 30–40 days, and then declines as the cells become crowded. Low levels of AFP are detected also. These cultures consist predominantly of syncytia, multinucleated giant cells, and clusters of typical EC cells, with lesser proportions of other cell types also being observed. The presence of numerous syncytia and the secretion of HCG suggest that the syncytial formations are trophoblastic elements.

However, when these same cell lines are subcultured by scraping (which yields cell clusters instead of dispersed cells) and seeded at low density without feeder cells, a longer time is required for a confluent monolayer to form. Therefore, differentiation is more extensive and diverse and yields, in addition to the cell types already described, fibroblastoid, spindle-shaped, stellate, and various other cells. These cultures produce both AFP and HCG, usually at maximum levels of 200–500 ng/ml of culture fluid. After one or two additional passages of scraped cells under these conditions, the cultures consist predominantly of fibroblasts and larger, elongated cells, and the growth rate of both types diminishes. Low levels of AFP, but not HCG, are detectable in the supernatant fluids of these cultures.

Continued passage of trypsinized or scraped cells without feeder layers generally results in one of two events. When seeded at a higher density (*e.g.* 5×10^6 cells/25-cm^2 flask), the EC cells begin to dominate and eventually are the only type that can be seen. These cells exhibit little tendency to differentiate under any of the conditions tested and secrete little or no AFP and HCG. Conversely, continued passsage of trypsinized cells at low density (*e.g.* 5×10^5 cells/25-cm^2 flask) yields cultures of enlarged, flat cells that show little or no growth, do not produce AFP or HCG, and eventually die. Similar events occur in cultures of scraped cells, except that the cells have a fibroblastoid morphology. These latter results suggest that these cells may represent different types of cells in a terminal, benign stage of differentiation. Some of our other EC lines that are maintained on feeder layers give similar responses when subcultured by these methods.

Thus, several of our cell lines exhibit properties of multipotential EC lines, require feeder layers to retain their differentiation potential, and produce AFP and HCG only while differentiating. The pattern of differentiation (*i.e.* the types of cells produced) and the levels of AFP and HCG secreted by the differentiating cells depend on the density at which the cells are seeded initially, the method of subculture, and the number of times the cells are subcultured by a particular method without feeder cells.

It appears, then, that marker production by EC cells *in vitro* is a concomitant of differentiation rather than a function of the most primitive cells. This finding provides another possible explanation for what has been called the "marker release phenomenon."[39] When a patient with a testicular germ cell tumor is given antitumor chemotherapy, his serum AFP and HCG levels often rise precipitously. This has been interpreted as the release of these markers from dying and lysing cells. However, on the basis of the results just described, it is also possible that some of this increase comes from increased marker production by primitive tumor cells nudged toward differentiation by the drugs.

CONCLUSION

To return to the question with which we started, what is cancer? The most satisfactory explanation, based in part on studies of germ cell tumors, is that it is a disease of malregulation of ordinary but developmentally significant genes. As a result, the stem cells of tissue fail to differentiate fully but, rather, stop at some point in the normal pathway. At that point, they produce the surface antigens and other products characteristic of that stage. This is particularly clear in the case of the many human tumors that produce HCG, which is one of the first differentiation products to appear in human cells. The critical abnormality may be genetic, such as in the hereditary tumors or those resulting from chemically induced mutations, or it may be epigenetic, as in the viral tumors. These viral tumors, in turn, may arise as the result of misplacement of normal cellular genes by transduction, leading to malregulation of gene expression.

The germ cell tumors thus have contributed significantly to our understanding of the seemingly disparate diseases known collectively as cancer. They also have brightened the clinical prospects, for they have shown us that at least some types of stem cells will, if placed in the proper environment, differentiate into the benign cells they were intended to become.

REFERENCES

1. Illmensee, K., and Stevens, L. C. Teratomas and chimeras. *Sci. Am. 240*(4)*:*120–132, 1979.
2. Pierce, G. B. Teratocarcinoma: model for a developmental concept of cancer. *Curr. Top. Dev. Biol. 2:*223–246, 1967.
3. Mintz, B., and Fleischman, R. A. Teratocarcinomas and other neoplasms as developmental defects in gene expression. *Adv. Cancer Res. 34:*211–278, 1981.
4. Fraley, E. E. Tumors of the human testis. In *Basic Reproductive Medicine*, Vol. 2, pp. 194–222, edited by F. Naftolin and D. W. Hamilton. MIT Press, Cambridge, 1982.
5. Damjanov, I., and Solter D. Embryo-derived teratocarcinomas elicit splenomegaly in syngeneic host. *Nature 249:*569–571, 1974.
6. Martin, G. R. Teratocarcinomas and embryogenesis. *Science 209:*768–776, 1980.
7. Graham, C. F. Teratocarcinoma cells and normal mouse embryogenesis. In *Concepts in Mammalian Embryogenesis*, pp. 315–394, edited by M. I. Sherman. MIT Press, Cambridge, 1977.
8. Nicolas, J. F., Avner, P., Gaillard, J., *et al.* Cell lines derived from teratocarcinomas. *Cancer Res. 36:*4224–4231, 1976.
9. Nishimune, Y., Ogiso, Y., Kume, A., *et al.* Identification of reversible and irreversible stages during the differentiation of pluripotential teratocarcinoma cell line. In *Teratocarcinoma and Embryonic Interactions*, pp. 229–236, edited by T. Muramatsu, G. Gachelin, and A. A. Moscona. Japan Scientific Societies Press, Tokyo, 1982.
10. Strickland, S. Mouse teratocarcinoma cells: prospects for the study of embryogenesis and neoplasia. *Cell 24:*277–278, 1981.
11. Gachelin, G., DeLarbre, C., Coulon-Morelec, C-J, *et al.* F9 antigens: a reevaluation. In *Teratocarcinoma and Embryonic Interactions*, pp. 121–138, edited by T. Muramatsu, G. Gachelin, and A. A. Moscona. Japan Scientific Societies Press, Tokyo, 1982.
12. Imagawa, K., Funatsu, A., Inui K., *et al.* A novel diagnostic method for cancer: quantitation of differentiation-dependent glycoconjugates. In *Teratocarcinoma and Embryonic Interactions*, pp. 239–248, edited by T. Muramatsu, G. Gachelin, and A. A. Moscona. Japan Scientific Societies Press, Tokyo, 1982.
13. Solter, D., and Knowles, B. B. Monoclonal antibody defining a stage-specific mouse embryonic antigen (SSEA-1). *Proc. Natl. Acad. Sci. USA 75:*5565–5569, 1978.
14. Shevinsky, L. H., Knowles, B. B., Damjanov, I., *et al.* Monoclonal antibody to murine embryos defines a stage-specific embryonic antigen expressed on mouse embryos and human teratocarcinoma cells. *Cell 30:*697–705, 1982.
15. Takeichi, M., Atsumi, T., Yoshida, C., *et al.* Molecular approaches to cell-cell recognition mechanisms in mammalian embryos. In *Teratocarcinoma and Embryonic Interactions*, pp. 283–293, edited by T. Muramatsu, G. Gachelin, and A. A. Moscona. Japan Scientific

Societies Press, Tokyo, 1982.
16. Martin, G. R., Rosen, S. D., and Grabel, L. B. Specificity and proposed role in intercellular adhesion of a teratocarcinoma stem cell lectin. In *Teratocarcinoma and Embryonic Interactions*, pp. 295–307, edited by T. Muramatsu, G. Gachelin, and A. A. Moscona. Japan Scientific Societies Press, Tokyo, 1982.
17. Hakomori, S-I, Fukuda, M., and Nudelman. E. Role of cell surface carbohydrates in differentiation: behavior of lactosaminoglycan in glycolipids and glycoproteins. In *Teratocarcinoma and Embryonic Interactions*, pp. 179–199, edited by T. Muramatsu, G. Gachelin, and A. A. Moscona. Japan Scientific Societies Press, Tokyo, 1982.
18. Bronson, D. L., Andrews, P. W., Solter, D., *et al.* Cell line derived from metastasis of a human testicular germ cell tumor. *Cancer Res. 40:*2500–2506, 1980.
19. Hogan, B., Fellous, M., Avner, P., *et al.* Isolation of a human teratoma cell line which expresses F9 antigen. *Nature 270:*515–518, 1977.
20. Fogh, J. Cultivation, characterization, and identification of human tumor cells with emphasis on kidney, testis, and bladder tumors. *Natl. Cancer Inst. Monogr. 49:*509, 1978.
21. Cotte, C. A., Easty, G. C., and Neville, A. M. Establishment and properties of human germ cell tumors in tissue culture. *Cancer Res. 41:*1422–1427, 1981.
22. Cotte, C., Raghavan, D., McIlhinney, R. A. J., *et al.* Characterization of a new human cell line derived from a xenografted embryonal carcinoma. *In Vitro 18:*739–749, 1982.
23. Yamamoto, T., Komatsubara, S., Suzuki, T., *et al. In vitro* cultivation of human testicular embryonal carcinoma and establishment of a new cell line. *Gann 70:*677–680, 1979.
24. Kalter, S. S., Helmke, R. J., Heberling, R. L., *et al.* C-type particles in normal human placentas. *JNCI 50:*1081–1084, 1973.
25. Vernon, M. L., McMahon, J. M., and Hackett, J. J. Additional evidence of type-C particles in human placentas. *JNCI 52:*987–989, 1974.
26. Dalton, A. J., Hellman, A., Kalter, S. S., *et al.* Ultrastructural comparison of placental virus with several type-C oncogenic viruses. *JNCI 52:*1379–1381, 1974.
27. Chandra, S., Liszczak, T., Korol, W., *et al.* Type-C particles in human tissues. I. Electron microscopic study of embryonic tissues *in vivo* and *in vitro. Int. J. Cancer 6:*40–45, 1970.
28. Robinson, H. L. Retroviruses and cancer. *Rev. Infect. Dis. 4:*1015–1025, 1982.
29. Bronson, D. L., Ritzi, D. M., Fraley, E. E., *et al.* Morphologic evidence for retrovirus production by epithelial cells derived from a human testicular metastasis. *JNCI 60:*1305–1308, 1978.
30. Bronson, D. L., Fraley, E. E. Fogh, J., *et al.* Induction of retrovirus particles in human testicular tumor (Tera-1) cell cultures: an electron microscopic study. *JNCI 63:*337–339, 1979.
31. Bronson, D. L., Saxinger, W. C., Ritzi, D. M., *et al.* Viruses produced by human embryonal carcinoma cells *in vitro* (Submitted for publication).
32. Wang, N., Trend, B., Bronson, D. L., *et al.* Nonrandom abnormalities in chromosome 1 in human testicular cancers. *Cancer Res 40:*796–802, 1980.
33. Marx, J. L. The case of the misplaced gene. *Science 218:*983–985, 1982.
34. Poste, G., and Fidler, I. J. The pathogenesis of cancer metastasis. *Nature 283:*139–146, 1980.
35. Wang, N., Perkins, K. L., Bronson, D. L., *et al.* Cytogenetic evidence for premeiotic transformation of human testicular cancers. *Cancer Res. 41:*2135–2140, 1981.
36. Andrews, P. W., Bronson, D. L., Benham, F., *et al.* A comparative study of eight cell lines derived from human testicular teratocarcinoma. *Int. J. Cancer 26:*269–280, 1980.
37. Andrews, P. W., Bronson, D. L., Wiles, M. V., *et al.* The expression of MHC antigens by human teratocarcinoma derived cell lines. *Tissue Antigens 17:*493–500, 1981.
38. Martin, G. R., and Evans, M. J. Differentiation of clonal lines of teratocarcinoma cells: formation of embryoid bodies *in vitro. Proc. Natl. Acad. Sci. USA 72:*1441–1445, 1976.
39. Vogelzang, N. J., Lange, P. H., Goldman, A., *et al.* Acute changes of α-fetoprotein and human chorionic gonadotropin during induction chemotherapy of germ cell tumors. *Cancer Res. 42:*4855–4861, 1982.

5

Immunocytochemistry of Testicular Cancer

Robert J. Kurman, M.D.

INTRODUCTION

The histopathologic classification of testicular cancer in current usage in the United States stems from the histologic observations of Friedman and Moore[1] and has been confirmed and broadened by ultrastructural,[2-4] animal transplantation[5-7] and comparative pathologic studies.[8-10] Despite the apparent precision of this classification, the histologic diagnosis of a particular tumor is at times uncertain, due in part to the conceptual difficulties regarding the nature and origin of the neoplastic cells and also to a failure to employ alternative methods of cellular identification to confirm the morphologic interpretations. These areas of uncertainty reflect fundamental deficiencies in a classification based solely upon morphological features. The shortcomings of this approach were revealed by the discovery that approximately 70% of patients with nonseminomatous germ cell tumors had elevated serum levels of α-fetoprotein (AFP) and/or human chorionic gonadotropin (HCG).[11-14] These findings were inconsistent with the fact that endodermal sinus tumor (yolk sac tumor or infantile embryonal carcinoma) and choriocarcinoma, the tumor elements thought to be responsible for the production of these markers, had been identified relatively rarely in testicular cancer in adults.[15-17] The adaptation of immunocytochemical techniques to the histologic analysis of these tumors now permits the identification of cells by their biochemical characteristics, independent of morphologic criteria. In this way a more holistic concept of the morphologic and functional nature of these neoplasms can be developed.

Although a number of placental, embryonic, and tumor-associated antigens have been studied in this group of tumors using immunocytochemical techniques, emphasis will be placed on the role of AFP and HCG since these are the only tumor markers that have been systematically correlated with clinical and immunohistologic studies. The purpose of this review is: (1) to correlate the results of tissue localization of AFP and HCG by immunoperoxidase techniques with the serum levels of these markers and with the morphologic features of germ cell tumors, (2) to reexamine our concepts of the histogenesis of these tumors based on the immunoperoxidase localization of AFP and HCG, and (3) to explore the role of immunocytochemical methods in developing new classifications based on functional as well as morphologic characteristics of these neoplasms.

IMMUNOPEROXIDASE METHODOLOGY

For a detailed discussion of the various types of immunoperoxidase methods, the reader is directed to two recent reviews.[18, 19] In the past, we have employed the indirect method in which incubation with the primary rabbit antiserum against human AFP or HCG is followed by an incubation with goat antirabbit immunoglobulin conjugated to peroxidase. The reaction product is then visualized by the addition of diaminobenzidine and hydrogen peroxide. Although this technique is generally satisfactory, we presently prefer the peroxidase-antiperoxidase (PAP) technique. Both methods are applicable to tissue that is routinely fixed in formalin and embedded in paraffin. Briefly, the PAP method depends on the addition of an excess of goat antirabbit immunoglobulin which links the primary rabbit antiserum (against AFP or HCG) to the rabbit antibody in the peroxidase-antiperoxidase complex. As in the indirect method, the reaction product is visualized by the addition of diaminobenzidine and hydrogen peroxide. By using nonconjugated antisera and low antibody dilutions the nonspecific background is markedly reduced and the sensitivity of the assay increased. A schematic representation of both the indirect and PAP methods is shown in Figure 5.1.

A number of controls must be performed in order to insure the specificity of the procedure. These include the use of tissues known to be positive and negative for the presence of AFP and HCG, sections incubated with the antiserum, *i.e.* rabbit anti-AFP preabsorbed with the specific antigen with the intent of abolishing the activity of the antiserum, and substitution of the primary antiserum with normal serum from the same species, *i.e.* normal rabbit serum.

RESULTS OF IMMUNOPEROXIDASE LOCALIZATION OF AFP AND HCG

Seminoma

In its pure form, seminoma is generally not associated with elevated serum levels of AFP or HCG, nor has AFP or HCG been identified in the typical seminoma cell with immunoperoxidase methods.[20] Tumor giant cells containing multiple nuclei identical to those found in individual seminoma cells also fail to show a positive reaction for AFP and HCG. Foreign body giant cells, present in approximately 20% of seminomas as part of the lymphocytic and plasma cell infiltrate, are also negative for AFP and HCG. In contrast, the giant cells that closely resemble the syncytiotrophoblastic element of choriocarcinoma have been shown to be positive for HCG (Fig. 5.2 and 5.3) but negative for AFP.[20, 21] These cells can be found in what is otherwise a pure seminoma. The cells have hyperchromatic pleomorphic nuclei with abundant eosinophilic or am-

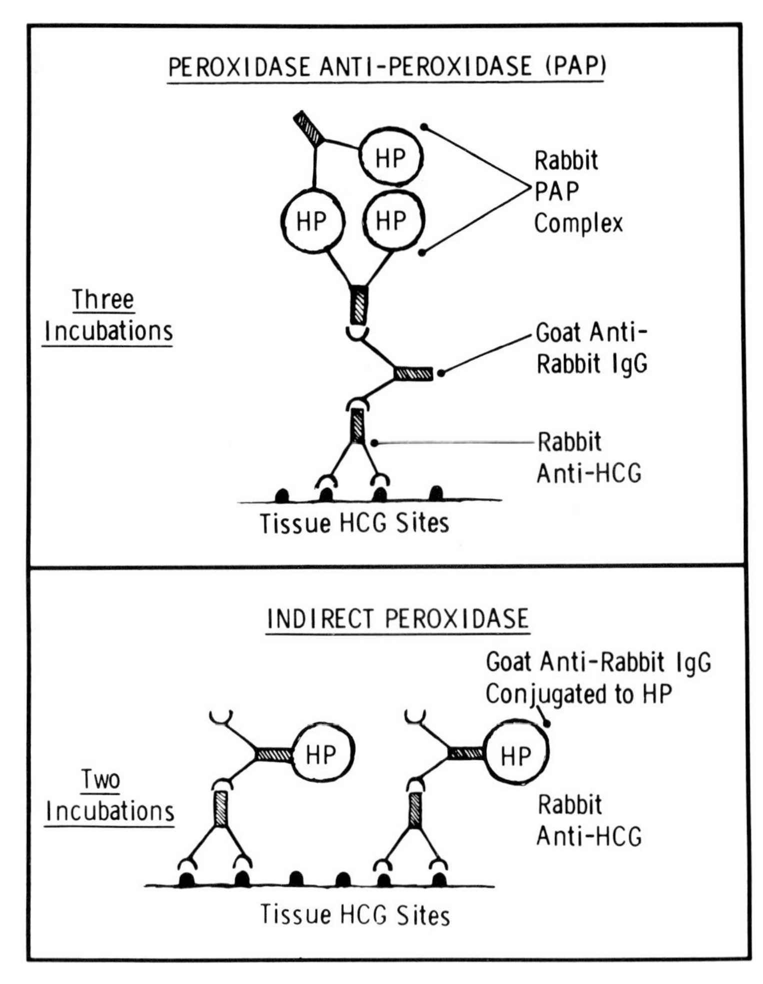

Figure 5.1. Schematic representation of the methodology of the indirect and peroxidase-antiperoxidase techniques. *HP*, horseradish peroxidase; *HCG*, human chorionic gonadotropin; IgG, immunoglobulin; PAP, peroxidase-antiperoxidase.

phophilic cytoplasm and are typically found near areas of hemorrhage (Fig. 5.2). Frequently, one or more large vacuoles are present within the cytoplasm (Fig. 5.3). In the past, the significance of these cells was not fully appreciated; in view of their cytologic and functional similarity to typical syncytiotrophoblast the term "syntiotrophoblasts" is appropriate. These cells should not be misconstrued as representing foci of choriocarcinoma, since the typical biphasic population of cytotrophoblast and syncytiotrophoblast is not present and the behavior of seminomas containing these cells may differ from seminoma containing foci of choriocarcinoma.[17]

Embryonal Carcinoma

Pure embryonal carcinoma is characterized by masses of large, primitive, somewhat pleomorphic cells containing amphophilic vacuolated cytoplasm and vesicular nuclei with coarse nuclear membranes and one

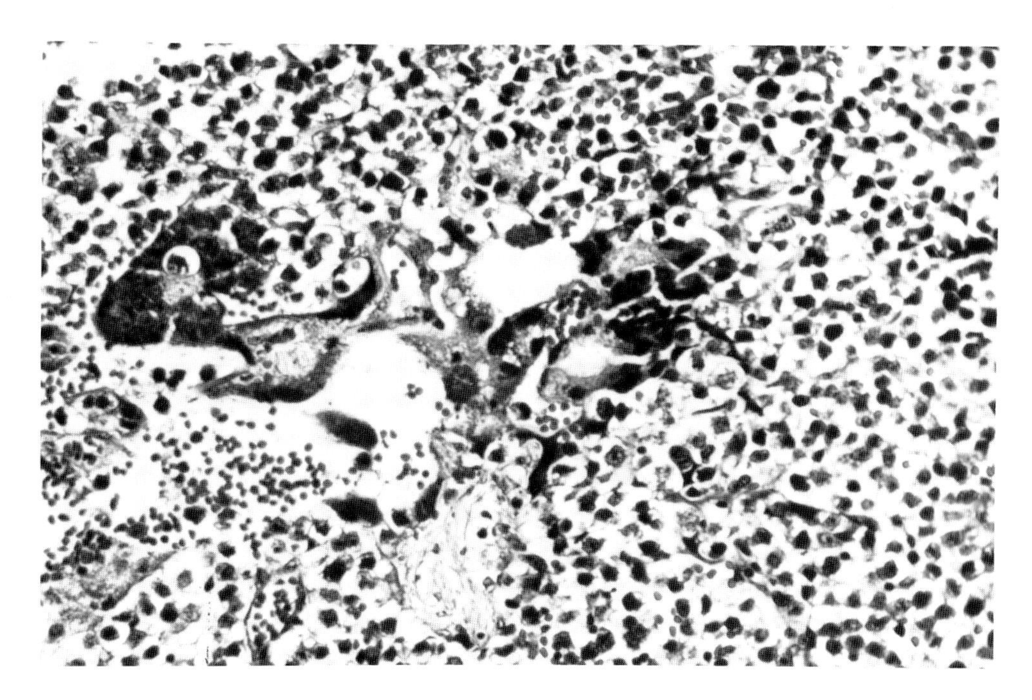

Figure 5.2. Seminoma with syncytiotrophoblasts adjacent to a hemorrhagic area (H & E).

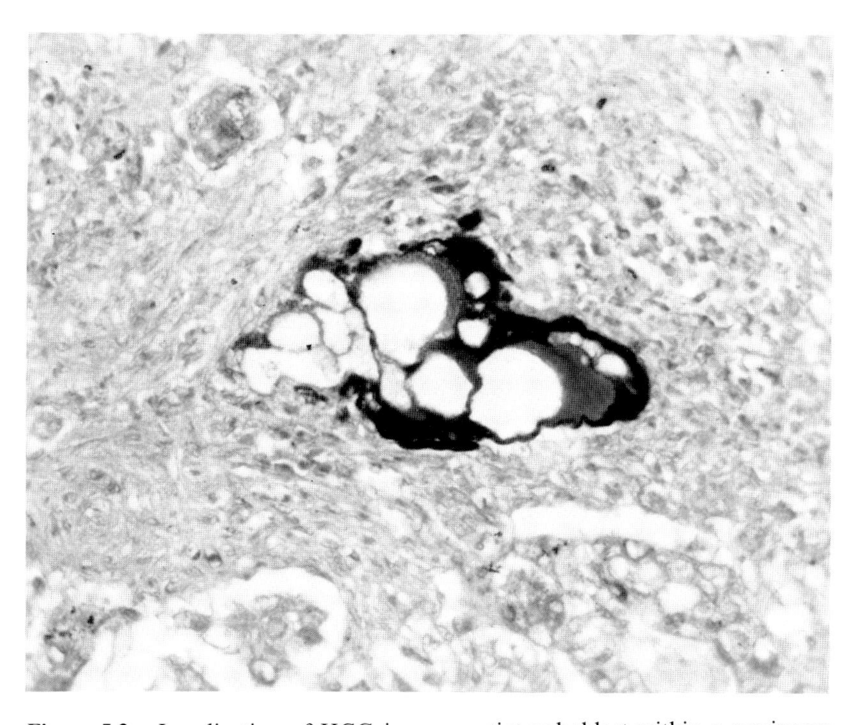

Figure 5.3. Localization of HCG in a syncytiotrophoblast within a seminoma (immunoperoxidase, anti-HCG).

or more prominent nucleoli. Occasionally, gland-like clefts and papillary processes are present within the masses of cells. The supporting stroma varies considerably, either being loose and edematous or cellular with spindle-shaped cells, resembling sarcoma. Syncytiotrophoblasts are frequently present, scattered randomly in the stroma, at the periphery, or within masses of embryonal carcinoma cells.

In their pure form, embryonal carcinoma and endodermal sinus tumor (yolk sac tumor) have distinctly different histologic patterns but in most instances considerable overlap exists. Embryonal carcinoma has a greater tendency to grow in solid masses composed of large primitive-appearing cells (Fig. 5.4) in contrast to endodermal sinus tumor which tends to form a loose meshwork of spaces and channels lined by flattened or cuboidal cells. (Fig. 5.5) AFP may be present within the primitive-appearing cells growing in masses of embryonal carcinoma but is more often found in flattened cells lining microcystic spaces. (Figs. 5.6*A* and 5.6*B*)[20–23] A positive reaction for AFP is frequently focal and is not present in all embryonal carcinoma cells; those that fail to react for AFP cannot be distinguished morphologically from those that do. On examination of slides stained with hematoxylin and eosin (H & E) the focal microcystic areas in embryonal carcinoma are easily overlooked (Fig. 5.7) but are unmasked with immunoperoxidase reactions for AFP. These microcystic areas may reflect one of the earliest morphologically recognizable patterns of yolk sac differentiation (Figs. 5.8 and 5.9) and appear to occur more commonly in embryonal carcinoma than was previously suspected.[24–26]

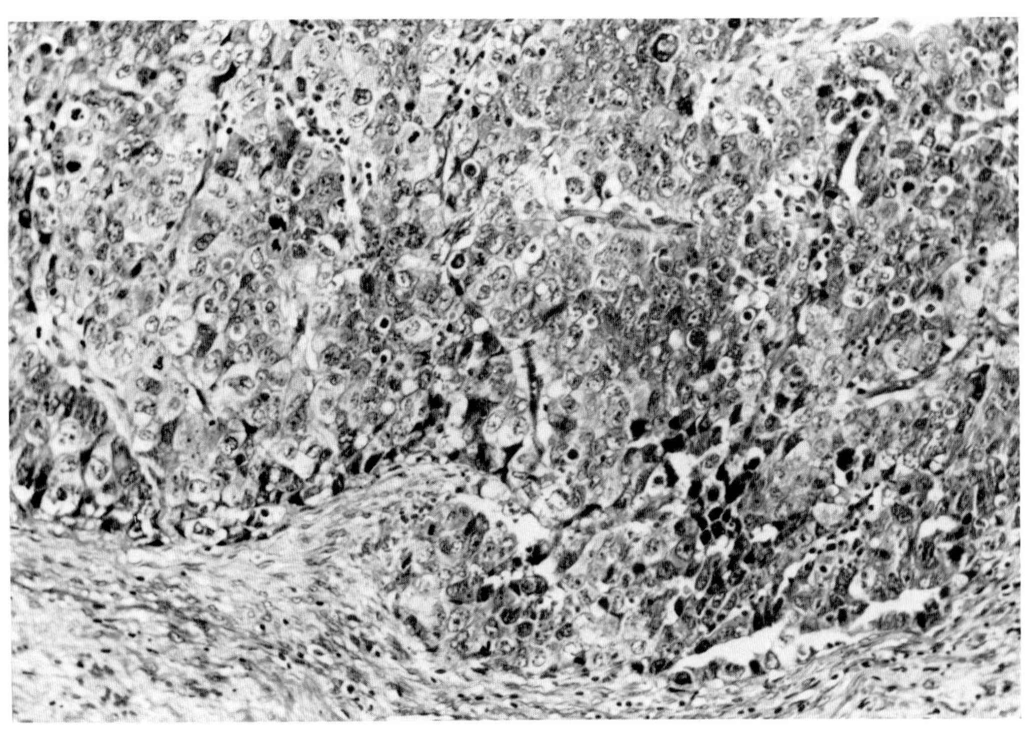

Figure 5.4. Embryonal carcinoma characterized by large primitive appearing cells growing in solid masses (H & E).

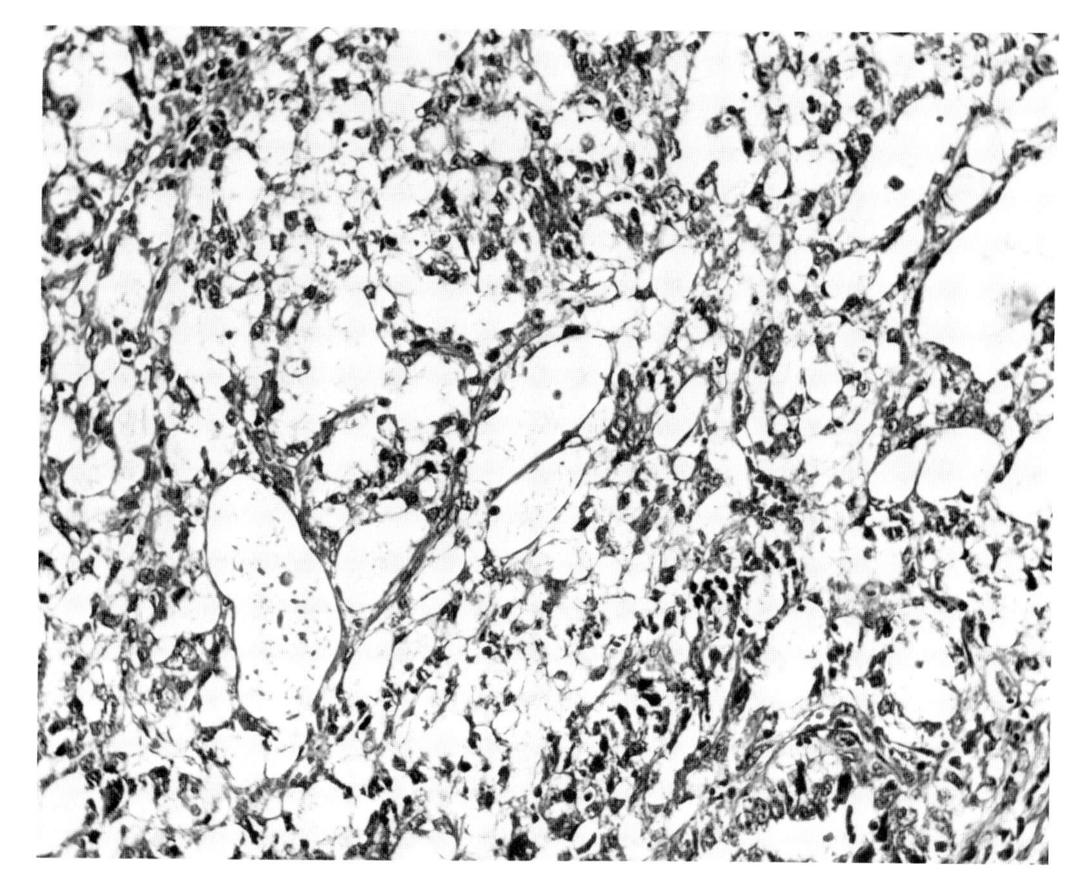

Figure 5.5. Endodermal sinus tumor showing a reticular pattern characterized by microcystic and macrocystic spaces lined by flattened cells (H & E).

In contrast to AFP, human chorionic gonadotropin is not localized in the embryonal carcinoma cells being confined to syncytiotrophoblasts only. Nonetheless, the frequent finding of syncytiotrophoblasts positive for HCG and embryonal carcinoma cells positive for AFP in embryonal carcinoma emphasize the close functional as well as morphologic relationship between choriocarcinoma, embryonal carcinoma and endodermal sinus tumor. A tendency of embryonal carcinoma to differentiate towards embryonal (teratoma) cell lines is manifested morphologically by the close association with cartilage, muscle and squamous epithelium.[27] Functional evidence of embryonic differentiation in embryonal carcinoma is based on the presence of "shared" markers such as AFP, α-1-antitrypsin and carcinoembryonic antigen which have recently been identified in components of teratoma.[22]

Endodermal Sinus Tumor (Yolk Sac Tumor)

Endodermal sinus tumor displays five interrelated histologic patterns which have been described in detail by Teilum.[8-10] These include: (1) a reticular pattern, the most common of all, (Fig. 5.5) which is composed of a loose meshwork of spaces and channels lined by flattened or cuboidal cells. Hyaline droplets, found in many endodermal sinus tumors, are

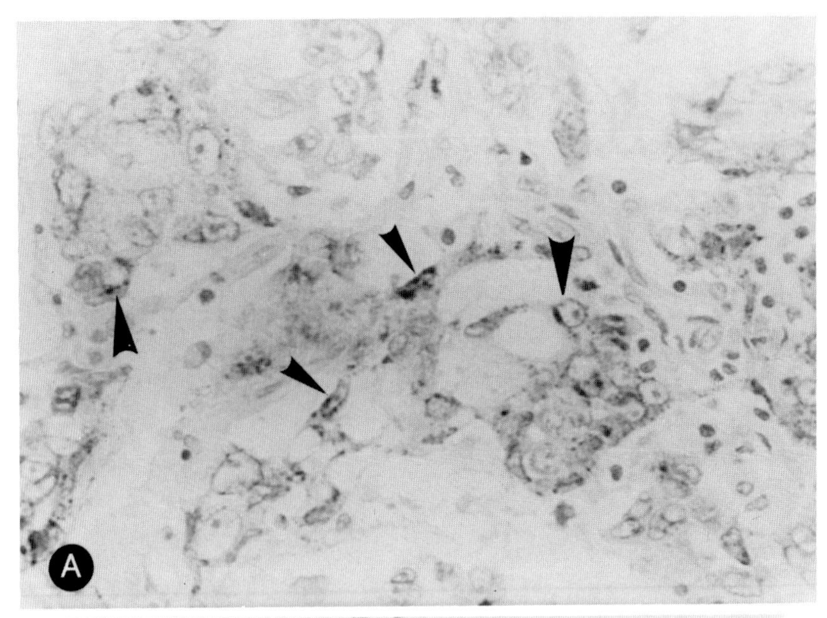

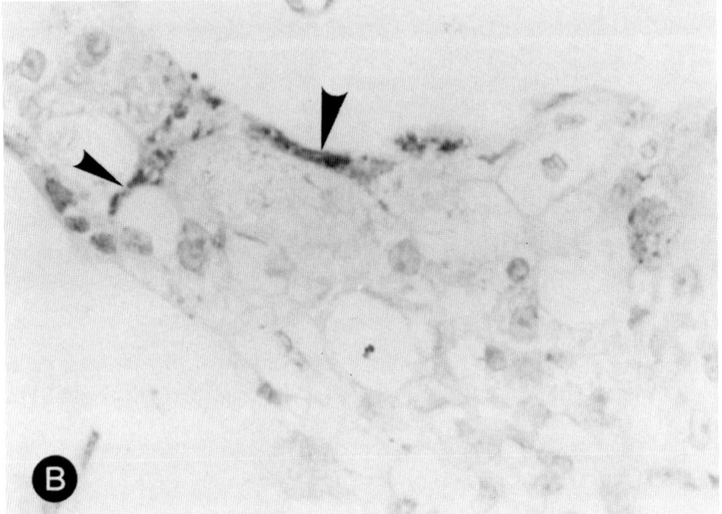

Figure 5.6 ***A*** **and** ***B*****.** *A*, localization of AFP (*dark black granules*) in primitive-appearing rounded cells (*large arrow*) and flattened cells (*small arrows*) within embryonal carcinoma (Immunoperoxidase, anti-AFP). *B*, localization of AFP in flattened cells lining microcystic (*small arrow*) and macrocystic spaces (*large arrow*) within embryonal carcinoma (immunoperoxidase, anti-AFP).

common in this pattern. (2) The endodermal sinus or festoon pattern, pathognomonic of the neoplasm, contains perivascular structures composed of a central capillary core surrounded by a mantle of primitive-appearing cells. (3) The polyvesicular vitelline pattern is characterized by multiple cystic vesicles with flat or columnar epithelium having clear cytoplasm and a dense fibroblastic stroma. (4) The alveolar glandular pattern is composed of cystic spaces lined by papillary processes with cuboidal epithelium. (5) The solid pattern is characterized by a relatively

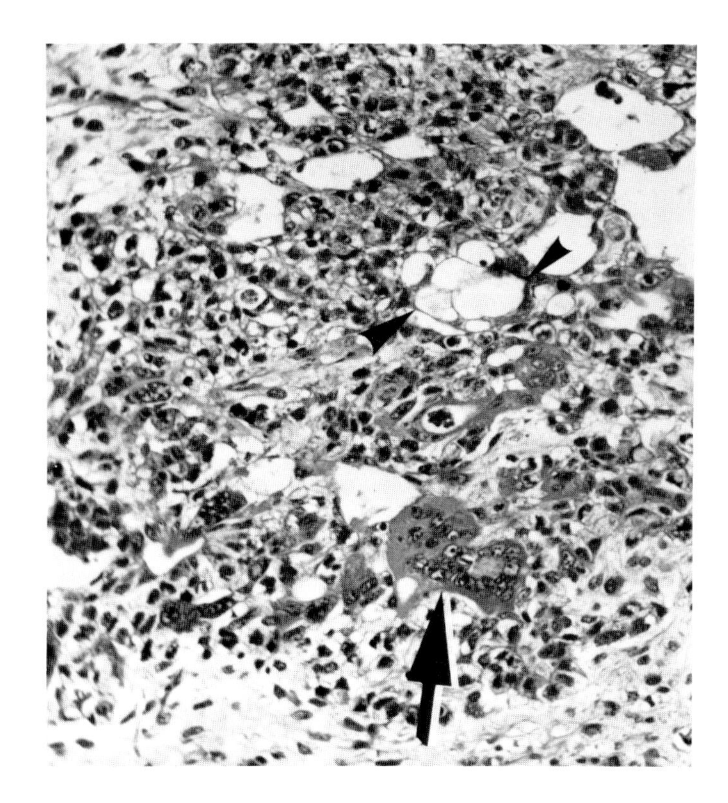

Figure 5.7. Embryonal carcinoma with several microcystic areas (*small arrows*) and a syncytiotrophoblast (*large arrow*) (H & E).

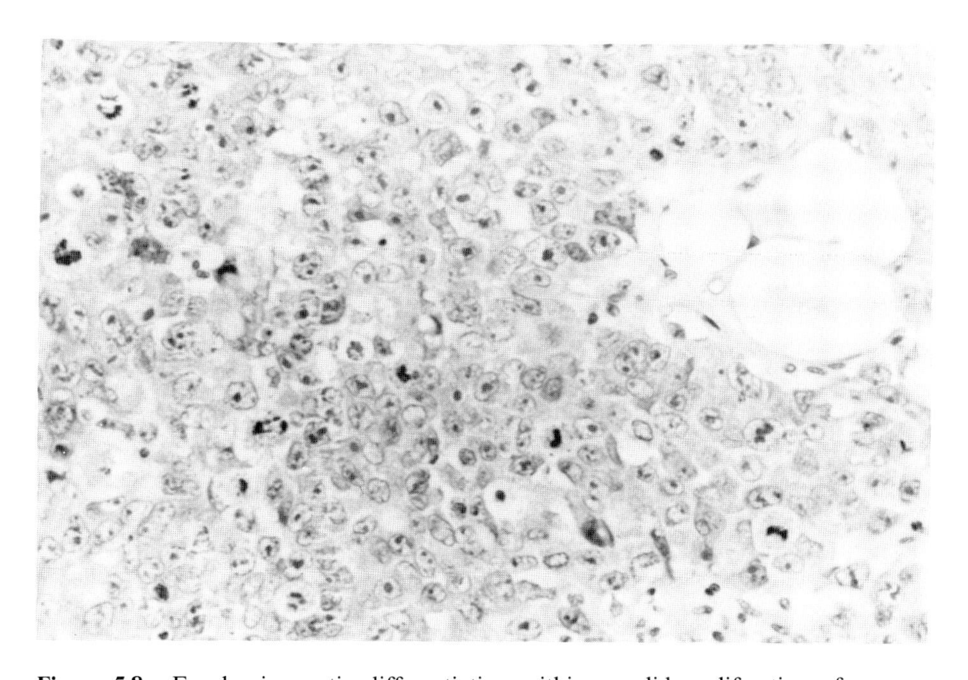

Figure 5.8. Focal microcystic differentiation within a solid proliferation of rounded cells in an embryonal carcinoma. Compare with Figure 5.9 (H & E).

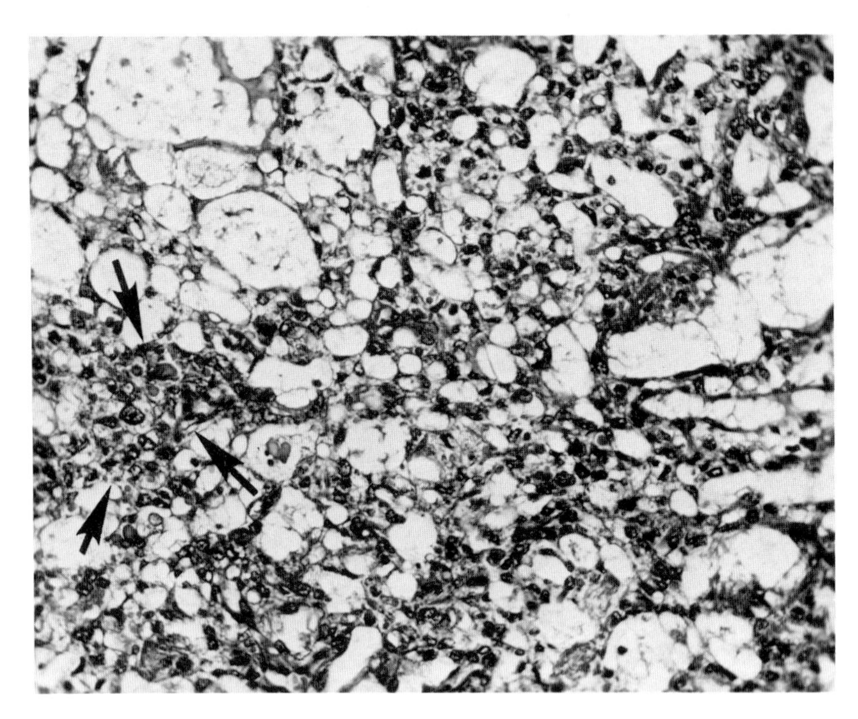

Figure 5.9. Focal solid area of rounded cells (*arrows*) amid profuse numbers of microcystic and macrocystic spaces in an endodermal sinus tumor (H & E).

solid growth of undifferentiated cells resembling embryonal carcinoma (Fig. 5.10).

Several reports have shown that this neoplasm produces AFP.[20, 22, 23, 28–38] Immunocytochemical studies have demonstrated that AFP is almost invariably present in this neoplasm although in many instances, as in embryonal carcinoma, its distribution may be quite focal. AFP is present within the cytoplasm of the cells arranged in all the various histologic patterns. The cells that contain AFP are cytologically indistinguishable from those that do not. The apparent heterogeneous population of positive and negative cells as well as the difference in staining intensity from one cell to the next also occurs in fetal liver and hepatocellular carcinoma, and may be a reflection of the synthesis and storage of AFP at different phases of the cell cycle.

Earlier studies using immunofluorescense and the indirect immunoperoxidase technique demonstrated the presence of AFP in the intracellular and extracellular hyaline droplets found in endodermal sinus tumor.[20, 28, 29, 31, 33, 37, 38] The intensity of the reaction product varied in these droplets, even in the same neoplasm, and only a minority of those present in a particular tumor were positive. Droplets that were negative for AFP were shown with immunofluorescence to be positive for other serum proteins such as albumin, prealbumin, α-1-antitrypsin and transferrin.[37] Since these proteins have also been shown to be synthesized by the fetal yolk sac[39, 40] this was interpreted as further support of the yolk sac origin of the tumors. More recently, using the PAP method, it has been found that these droplets are usually not positive for AFP.[41] Although the discrepancy between the earlier studies and the more recent PAP findings

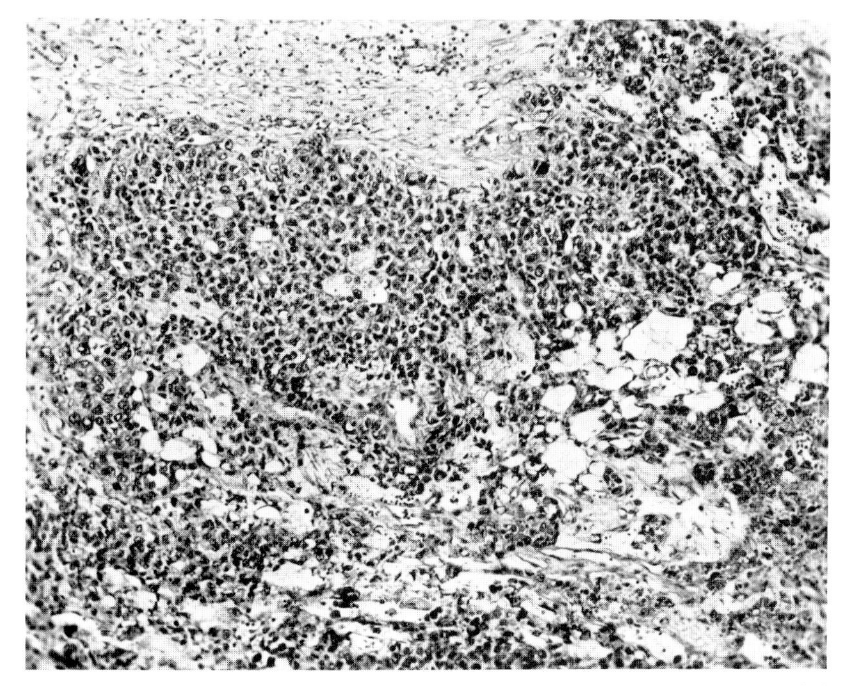

Figure 5.10. Endodermal sinus tumor showing a solid growth pattern on the *left* and a microcystic reticular pattern on the *right* (H & E).

has not been completely resolved, the difference may reflect the enhanced specificity of the PAP method. Both immunofluorescence and the indirect immunoperoxidase methods use dilutions of anti-AFP that are approximately five times more concentrated than what is presently used in the PAP technique. It is therefore conceivable that the positive reaction observed in the hyaline droplets may reflect nonspecific staining. Analysis of additional cases and further comparison of the PAP results with immunofluorescence and indirect immunoperoxidase will be necessary to shed further light on this issue.

Choriocarcinoma

Pure choriocarcinoma of the testis is exceedingly rare. There are only 18 cases among the first 6000 testis tumors accessioned at the Armed Forces Institute of Pathology.[15] Most choriocarcinoma occurs as a component within mixed germ cell tumors and is therefore best classified as such.[15, 42] Microscopically, choriocarcinoma is characterized by a biphasic population of syncytiotrophoblast and cytotrophoblast growing in a plexiform pattern. (Fig. 5.11*A*) The cytotrophoblast is comprised of sheets of primitive-appearing cells with single nuclei and clear cytoplasm with well-defined cell membranes closely resembling the embryonal carcinoma cell. Capping the masses of cytotrophoblast and often interdigitating with it, is the syncytiotrophoblast, containing multiple nuclei and abundant eosinophilic cytoplasm. Immunoperoxidase localization studies reveal that HCG but not AFP is present exclusively within the syncytiotrophoblast (Fig. 5.11*B*).[20] Neither HCG nor AFP has been thus far found in the cytotrophoblast.

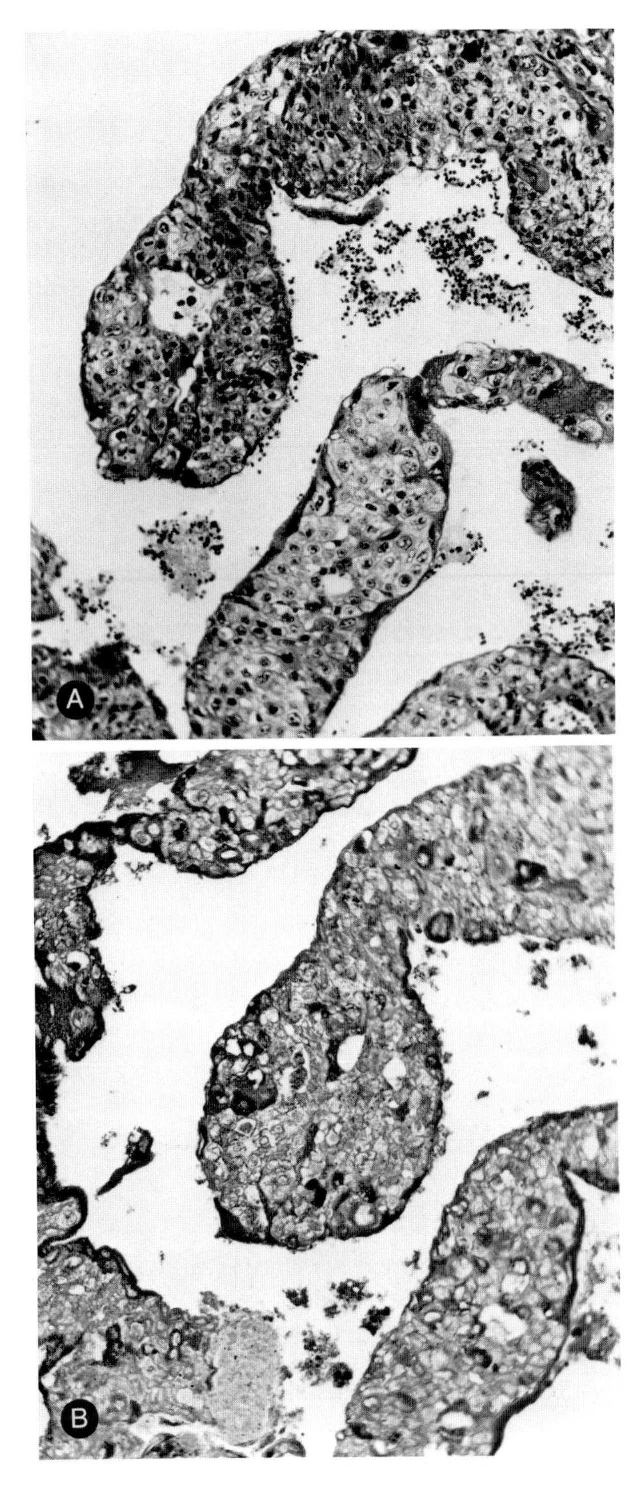

Figure 5.11 ***A*** **and** ***B*.** *A*, choriocarcinoma composed of syncytiotrophoblast and cytotrophoblast in a biphasic plexiform pattern (H & E). *B*, localization of HCG in syncytiotrophoblast exclusively (*dark black*). (Immunoperoxidase, anti-HCG).

Teratoma

Teratomas contain variable amount of tissue derived from two or more germ layers. The early immunohistologic analysis of a small number of teratomas containing mature and immature tissues failed to reveal AFP or HCG in the various cellular constituents[20] but more recent studies have demonstrated the presence of AFP-positive cells within epithelial-lined tubular structures.[22] Similar structures containing AFP-positive cells can be found in endodermal sinus tumor and embryonal carcinoma. Further study of a larger number of cases will be necessary before a definitive statement concerning the distribution of AFP and HCG in teratomas can be made.

Mixed Malignant Germ Cell Tumors (Including Teratocarcinoma)

This group of tumors is composed of mixtures of two or more of the previously described pure cell types. The capacity of these neoplasms to synthesize markers, is a function of their histologic composition. Tumors composed of endodermal sinus tumor or embryonal carcinoma generally synthesize AFP and those containing syncytiotrophoblast either as isolated syncytiotrophoblasts or as choriocarcinoma, synthesize HCG.

The term "teratocarcinoma" was used in the past to denote mixed germ cell tumors composed of embryonal carcinoma and teratoma, but has frequently been loosely applied often interchangeably with "malignant teratoma" and "teratoblastoma" to include a variety of histologic patterns. This terminology has obscured the precise assignment of AFP and HCG synthesis to particular cell types so it is therefore preferable to use the term "mixed germ cell tumor" and to enumerate the various cell types present. An estimation of the approximate proportion of each cell type present is also useful, since small foci of cells having the capacity to synthesize markers may produce enough of the marker to be detectable in the serum, a finding with important clinical significance in the management of these patients.

OTHER TUMOR MARKERS IN GERM CELL TUMORS

In addition to AFP and HCG, other placental and oncofetal proteins have been identified in this group of neoplasms. Carcinoembryonic antigen (CEA) has been localized with immunoperoxidase methods in areas of intestinal-like differentiation within teratomas[43] and occasionally in embryonal carcinoma.[22] Serum levels of CEA are elevated in 33% of patients with seminoma and 7% with nonseminomatous germ cell tumors, but CEA levels did not correlate with the course of disease.[44] The data, however, were not analyzed according to specific tumor types so it may be that CEA is of value in monitoring patients with teratomas but not in other types of germ cell tumors.

Human placental lactogen and pregnancy-specific β_1-glycoprotein have been localized in syncytiotrophoblasts.[22, 45] Usually these cells have also been positive for HCG but occasionally they have not been. Preliminary serum data have also shown that in an occasional patient these markers may be elevated when HCG levels are normal, so their measurement may be of value in monitoring patients in whom HCG levels are in the normal range.[45, 46] α-1-Antitrypsin has been localized in embryonal carcinoma, endodermal sinus tumor and teratomas.[22] Ferritin has also been identified using immunoperoxidase methods in the same tumors.[22] At this time, the value of markers other than AFP and HCG must be established by prospective studies in which these markers are measured in the serum and correlated with the course of the disease.

SOURCES OF CONFUSION IN THE INTERPRETATION OF SERUM AND TISSUE TUMOR MARKER DATA

Adequate sampling for routine histologic and immunohistochemical studies is of crucial importance. As a rule of thumb, two to three blocks of tissue for each centimeter of the greatest tumor diameter generally suffices, but additional samples may be necessary in certain situations. For example, we have had the experience of reviewing several different slides of a tumor showing only pure seminoma in a patient with an elevated serum HCG level without identifying choriocarcinoma or syncytiotrophoblasts. Processing of additional tissue revealed the presence of focal clusters of syncytiotrophoblasts within the seminoma which were positive for HCG with immunoperoxidase techniques.[20] Adequate sampling may be even more important for immunoperoxidase localization of AFP in view of the focal distribution of this marker in tissue. We have studied multiple blocks having the same histologic appearance from a particular neoplasm and have found a positive reaction for AFP in one block and not in the others.[41] It is not clear whether this reflects the synthesis or storage of AFP by the neoplasm, an "artifact" of fixation or tissue processing, or the limits of the sensitivity of the immunoperoxidase method in detecting low tissue levels of the marker.

Reliable correlation of serum and tissue tumor markers is only possible when all tumor is resected and extensively sampled for microscopic study. For neoplasms confined to the testis this can be readily accomplished, but in patients with metastatic disease this is usually not possible. The cell types present in a primary tumor may differ from those present in the metastases. This could result in an apparent discrepancy between the serum level of the tumor markers and immunohistologic analysis, which reflects only the markers in the particular specimen of tissue examined.

Although the immunoperoxidase method has proven to be very useful in correlating the serologic marker data with the histologic findings, it is important to be aware of the limitations of specificity and sensitivity with this method. The single most important factor to insure specificity is the use of a monospecific antiserum from a reliable source. Specificity controls using tissues known to be positive and negative for each particular marker must be performed. The sensitivity of the immunoperoxidase technique for AFP and HCG varies considerably. An approximate determination of the sensitivity of the method was attempted by correlating serum levels of HCG and AFP with their presence in tissue as revealed by immunoperoxidase. In cases in which the actual serum determination was made several days after tissue acquisition, an estimated serum level was calculated by extrapolation. The major shortcoming of such an analysis is that if only a few cells secrete the hormone, the serum level may be low although the tissue concentration is high. Nevertheless, it was shown by this analysis that HCG could almost always be identified in tissue sections when the serum level was above 1–5 ng/ml (Table 5.1), but AFP was consistently localized in tissue sections only when serum levels were quite elevated, approximately 800 ng/ml or higher (Table 5.2). This data was

Table 5.1.
Correlation of human chorionic gonadotropin (HCG) in tissue with serum levels in patients with testicular germ cell tumors[a]

Histology	Serum HCG	Tissue HCG
	ng/ml	
Emb + ST	1	+
Emb + ST, Tera	1.6	+
Sem + ST	2.5	+
Emb + ST	3.2	+
Sem	3.6	−
Emb + ST	6.9	+
Emb + ST	7.0	+
Emb + ST	9.6	+
Emb + ST	33	+
Emb + ST, Chorio	35	+
Emb + ST	65	+
Emb + ST, EST + ST, Tera	169	+
Emb + ST, Chorio	2,619	+
Emb + ST	31,000	+

[a] The abbreviations used are: Emb, embryonal carcinoma; ST, syncytiotrophoblasts; Tera, teratoma; Sem, seminoma; Chorio, choriocarcinoma; EST, Endodermal Sinus Tumor.

Table 5.2.
Correlation of α-fetoprotein (AFP) in tissue with serum levels in patients with testicular germ cell tumors[a]

Histology	Estimated serum AFP[b]	Actual serum AFP	Tissue AFP
	ng/ml	*ng/ml*	
Emb + ST	22	22	+
Emb, EST, Tera, Sem	130	59	−
EST, Tera	170	50	−
Emb, Sem	380	260	−
Emb + ST	450	100	−
Emb + ST	?[c]	130	±
Emb + ST	?	88	−
Emb + ST	?	88	+
Emb + ST, EST + ST, Tera	820	330	+
Emb + ST	870	52	+
Emb, Chorio	900	330	+
EST, Tera	2,000	1,850	+
Emb, Sem	4,800	1,400	+
Emb + ST, Tera	40,000	13,000	+

[a] For abbreviations, see Table 5.1.
[b] Calculated for time of tissue acquisition.
[c] ?, insufficient data to make estimate.

based on the use of the indirect immunoperoxidase method. At the present time, we employ the PAP method and have found that it is more sensitive, but a similar correlation of tissue localization with serum levels has not yet been performed.[41]

THE ROLE OF IMMUNOCYTOCHEMISTRY IN ELUCIDATING THE HISTOGENESIS OF GERM CELL TUMORS OF THE TESTIS

The contribution of immunocytochemistry in elucidating the histogenesis of germ cell tumors of the testis depends on the correlation of the biochemical features of the tumor cell populations with their morphologic features using traditional histologic techniques. Since it is likely that the biochemical differentiation of a tumor precedes the morphologic differentiation, immunoperoxidase findings provide important clues to some of the earliest recognizable forms of morphologic differentiation which have not been previously appreciated using hematoxylin and eosin stains. Furthermore, by identifying cells according to biochemical parameters, the varying morphologic expression of a particular cell can be followed at different stages in the course of the disease process. Although the findings of immunoperoxidase studies must still be considered preliminary they have already prompted a reappraisal of views on the classification of these tumors based on morphologic criteria only.[47]

Trophoblastic Differentiation

Serologic studies have revealed that approximately 70% of nonseminomatous germ cell tumors are associated with elevated serum levels of HCG[11, 14] and immunocytochemical analysis has shown that HCG is localized in the syncytiotrophoblastic component of choriocarcinoma or in isolated syncytiotrophoblasts.[20] Current histologic classifications place great emphasis on the importance of recognizing and distinguishing foci of choriocarcinoma from syncytiotrophoblasts[16, 17] but the morphologic distinction may not always be clear.

Syncytiotrophoblasts are often present focally in embryonal carcinoma, so the diagnosis of choriocarcinoma depends on whether the cells adjacent to the syncytiotrophoblast are nontrophoblastic embryonal carcinoma cells or cytotrophoblast and therefore are choriocarcinoma. The distinction may be impossible on morphologic grounds because neither light nor electron microscopic analysis can consistently distinguish the cells of embryonal carcinoma from the cytotrophoblastic element of choriocarcinoma.[15] Immunocytochemical analysis has not revealed differences between the syncytiotrophoblast of choriocarcinoma and isolated syncytiotrophoblasts[20] but has shown that occasionally embryonal carcinoma cells contain AFP whereas cytotrophoblast does not. However, only a small number of such tumors have been studied.

The serum level of HCG can not be used as a criterion to distinguish a tumor-containing choriocarcinoma from one containing syncytiotrophoblasts only, since it has been shown that embryonal carcinoma with abundant syncytiotrophoblasts can produce higher levels of HCG than a tumor containing lesser amounts of choriocarcinoma.[20] It therefore appears likely that the serum level of HCG reflects the volume of functioning syncytiotrophoblast. Although data from the British Testicular Tumor Panel indicate that the presence of syncytiotrophoblasts does not alter prognosis whereas elements of choriocarcinoma do, this data has not been stratified according to the stage of the disease and the treatment. In the future, carefully designed prospective studies using modern forms of chemotherapy may show that there are no differences and, therefore, perhaps invalidate the distinction that is currently being made between these tumors.

Endodermal Sinus (Yolk Sac) Differentiation

Localization of AFP in germ cell tumors is playing an important role in delineating the histogenesis of neoplasms within the embryonal carcinoma-endodermal sinus tumor group. The finding that tumors with the pattern of endodermal sinus tumor synthesize AFP in conjunction with the demonstration that the fetal yolk sac is a potent source of AFP[39] confirmed Teilum's[8-10] claim that the endodermal sinus tumor is of yolk sac origin. The rarity of this tumor in its pure form in adults, contrasted with the serological data showing a 70% frequency of elevated serum AFP levels in patients with nonseminatomous germ cell tumors,[11-14] led to immunohistologic studies which revealed that tumor cells having the morphologic criteria of embryonal carcinoma contained AFP also.[20] More recent studies[22] have confirmed these findings and have substantiated observations that yolk sac differentiation occurs more frequently than previously suspected. Of additional interest has been the finding of solid areas within endodermal sinus tumor that are positive for AFP and bear a close resemblance to hepatocellular carcinoma.[48] In addition to yolk sac tumor, AFP may be produced by hepatocellular carcinoma, gastric carcinoma and pancreatic carcinoma.[11] Since the fetal gut, as well as the liver and yolk sac, produce AFP, synthesis of this protein may reflect endodermal differentiation rather than yolk sac differentiation specifically.

BIOCHEMICAL-MORPHOLOGIC CLASSIFICATION OF GERM CELL TUMORS

As a result of refinements in immunocytochemical methodology and the increased use of serologic assays for the measurement of tumor markers, attention is now being directed to the identification of the various heterogeneous populations of cells that comprise germ cell neoplasms using immunologic techniques. Following the course of these markers in the serum has played a paramount role in improving survival by detecting early recurrence and by recognizing that different cell populations may respond in a different manner to chemotherapeutic agents.[49-53] A comparable situation exists in the management of women with gestational trophoblastic disease where it has been shown that the serum level of HCG and its regression pattern in response to chemotherapy is even more important in management than the histologic grading system.[54-57] Presently, AFP and HCG are the primary tumor markers in the diagnosis and management of germ cell tumors of the testis but as greater clinical experience is gained with other markers such as pregnancy-specific β-1-glycoprotein, human placental lactogen, α-1-antitrypsin, CEA and ferritin, it may become evident that tumors may be additionally classified by qualitative and quantitative patterns of tumor markers. In the future, the pathologist may report that a tumor displays a particular pattern of tumor markers as determined by immunocytochemistry and thereby indicate to the clinican which markers may be used to help monitor the effect of therapy. This information will be complementary to and possibly even more relevant to the clinician than the precise morphologic diagnosis.

The immunocytochemistry of testicular cancer is still in its infancy. This review is an attempt to summarize the present status of this rapidly evolving field and to speculate on its potential impact in modifying histopathologic classifications for the future. As appropriate commercial antisera become more readily available and as pathologists gain wider experience in the application of immunocytochemical techniques in the surgical pathology laboratory, immunocytochemistry will take on a greater role in the diagnosis and classification of germ cell tumors. It is clear that we have advanced beyond the characterization of these tumors solely by morphologic methods and have entered into an era of combined morphologic and functional classification.

REFERENCES

1. Friedman, N. B., and Moore, R. A. Tumors of the testis: a report 922 cases. *Milit. Surg 99:*573, 1946.
2. Pierce, G. B., and Dixon, F. J. Testicular teratomas. I. Demonstration of teratogenesis by metamorphosis of multipotential cells. *Cancer 12:*573, 1959.
3. Pierce, G. J., Jr. Ultrastructure of human testicular tumors. *Cancer 19:*1963, 1966.
4. Pierce, G. B., Jr., Stevens, L. C., and Nakane, P. K. Ultrastructural analysis of the early development of teratocarcinomas. *J. Natl. Cancer Inst. 39:*755, 1967.
5. Stevens, L. C., and Hummel, K. P. A description of spontaneous congenital testicular teratomas in strain 129 mice. *J. Natl. Cancer Inst. 18:*719, 1957.
6. Stevens, L. C. The biology of teratomas including evidence indicating their origin from primordial germ cells. *Ann. Biol. 11:*585, 1962.
7. Stevens, L. C. Experimental production of testicular teratomas in mice. *Proc. Natl. Acad. Sci. U.S.A. 5:*661, 1964.
8. Teilum, G. Gonocytoma—homologous ovarian and testicular tumors. I. With discussion of "mesonephroma ovarii" (Schiller: *Am. J. Cancer,* 1939). *Acta Pathol. Microbiol. Scand. 27:*249, 1950.
9. Teilum, G. Endodermal sinus tumors of the ovary and testis. Comparative morphogenesis of the so-called mesonephroma ovarii (Schiller) and extraembryonic (yolk-sac-allantoic) structures of the rat's placenta. *Cancer 12:*1092, 1959.
10. Teilum, G. Classification of endodermal sinus tumor (mesoblastoma vitellinum) and so-called 'embryonal carcinoma' of the ovary. *Acta. Pathol. Microbiol. Scand. 64:*407, 1965.
11. Waldmann, T. A., and McIntire, K. R. The use of a radioimmunoassay for alpha-fetoprotein in the diagnosis of malignancy. *Cancer 34:*1510, 1974.
12. Kohn, J. Orr, A. H., Mcelwain, T. J., Bentall, M., and Peckham, M. J. Serum alpha-fetoprotein in patients with testicular tumors. *Lancet 2:*433–436, 1976.
13. Grigor, K. M., Detre, S. I., Kohn, J., and Neville, A. M. Serum alpha-fetoprotein levels in 153 male patients with germ cell tumors. *Br. J. Cancer 35:*J2–58, 1977.
14. Javadpour, N. McIntire, K. R., Waldmann, and T. A., Bergman. The role of alpha-fetoprotein and human chorionic gonadotropin in seminoma. *J. Urol 120:*687–690, 1978.

15. Mostofi, R. K., and Price, E. B. Tumors of the Male Genital System. *Atlas of Tumor Pathology, Second series, Fascicle 8.* Armed Forces Institute of Pathology, Washington, D.C. 1973.
16. Mostofi, F. K., and Sobin, L. H. Histological typing of testicular tumors. *International Histological Classification of Tumors.* World Health Organization, Geneva, 1977.
17. Pugh, R. C. B. (ed). *Pathology of the Testis.* Blackwell, Oxford, 1976.
18. Kurman, R. J., and Casey, C. Immunoperoxidase techniques in surgical pathology. Principles and practice. In *Manual of Clinical Immunology,* Ed. 2, pp. 60–69, edited by Noel and Friedman, American Society for Microbiology, Washington, D.C., 1980.
19. Taylor, C. R. Immunoperoxidase Techniques: practical and theoretical aspects. *Arch. Pathol. Lab. Med. 102:*113, 1978.
20. Kurman, R. J., Scardino, P. T., McIntire, K. R., Waldmann, T. A., and Javadpour, N. Cellular localization of alpha-fetoprotein and human chorionic gonadotropin in germ cell tumors of the testis using an indirect immunoperoxidase technique. A new approach to classification utilizing tumor markers. *Cancer 40:*2136, 1977.
21. Nochomovitz, L. E., Lange, P. H., Fraley, E. E., and Rosai, J. Testicular seminoma with human chorionic gonadotropin (HCG) production: a study of 16 cases with special reference to anaplastic seminoma. *Lab. Invest. 42:* 140, 1980.
22. Jacobsen, G. K., Jacobsen, M., and Clausen, P. P. The distribution of tumor-associated antigens in the various histologic components of germ cell tumors of the testis. *Am. J. Surg. Pathol. 5:*257, 1981.
23. Beilby, J. O. W., Horne, C. H. W., Milne, G. D., and Parkinson, C. Alpha-fetoprotein, alpha-1-antitrypsin, and transferrin in gonadal yolk-sac tumors. *J. Clin. Pathol. 32:*455, 1979.
24. Talerman, A. The incidence of yolk sac tumor (endodermal sinus tumor) elements in germ cell tumors of the testis in adults. *Cancer 36:*211, 1975.
25. Neville, A. M., Grigor, K., and Heyderman, E. Clinicopathologic role of tumor index substances in paediatric neoplasia. In *Recent Advances in Histopathology,* pp. 23–44, edited by P. P. Anthony and N. Woolf. Churchill Livingston, Edinburgh, 1978.
26. Parkinson, C., and Beilby, J. O. W. Features of prognostic significance in testicular germ cell tumors. *J. Clin. Pathol. 30:*113, 1977.
27. Kurman, R. J., and Norris, H. J. Embryonal carcinoma of the ovary. A clinicopathologic entity distinct from endodermal sinus tumor resembling embryonal carcinoma of the adult testis. *Cancer 38:*2420, 1976.
28. Kurman, R. J., and Norris, H. J. Endodermal sinus tumor of the ovary. A clinical and pathologic analysis of 71 cases. *Cancer 38:*2404, 1976.
29. Itoh, T., Shirai, T., and Matsumoto, S. Yolk sac tumor and alpha-fetoprotein. Clinico-pathological study of four cases, Gann *65:*215, 1974.
30. Norgaard-Pedersen, B., Albrechtsen, R., and Teilum, G. Serum alpha-fetoprotein as a marker for endodermal sinus tumor (yolk sac tumor) or a vitelline component of teratocarcinoma. *Acta. Pathol. Microbiol. Scand. (A), 83:*573, 1975.
31. Tsuchida, Y., Saito, S., Ishida, M., *et al.* Yolk sac tumor and alpha-fetoprotein. A report of three cases. *Cancer 32:*917, 1973.
32. Wilkinson, E. J., Friedrich, E. G., and Hosty, T. A. Alpha-fetoprotein and endodermal sinus tumor of ovary. *Am. J. Obstet. Gynecol. 116:*711, 1973.
33. Palmer, P. E., Safaii, H., and Wolfe, H. J. Alpha-1-antitrypsin and alpha-fetoprotein. Protein markers in endodermal sinus (yolk sac) tumors. *Am. J. Clin. Pathol. 65:*575, 1976.
34. Grigor, K. M., Detre, S. I., John, J., *et al.* Serum alpha-fetoprotein levels in 153 patients with germ cell tumours. *Br. J. Cancer 35:*52, 1977.
35. Rimbaut, C., Caillaud, J. M., Caillou, B., *et al.* Alpha-fetoprotein (AFP) and germ cell tumors: biological and histological correlation. *Scand. J. Immunol. (Suppl.) 8:*201, 1978.
36. Sell, A., Sogaard, H., and Norgaard-Pedersen, B. Serum alpha-fetoprotein as a marker for the effect of post-operative radiation and/or chemotherapy in eight cases of ovarian endodermal sinus tumor. *Int. J. Cancer 18:*574, 1976.
37. Endo, Y., Ruano, Y., Tsuchida Y., Asaka, T., Kaneko, Y., Kaneko, M., Sakashita, S., Tsukada, Y., Watabe, Y., Hirai, H., and Oda, T. Protein synthesis in yolk sac tumor: histochemical studies of human and rat yolk sac. *Scand. J. Immunol. (Suppl.) 8:*171, 1978.
38. Teilum, G., Albrechtsen, R., and Norgaard-Pedersen, B. Immunofluorescent localization

of alpha-fetoprotein synthesis in endodermal sinus tumor (yolk sac tumor). *Acta Pathol. Microbiol. Scand.* (*A*) *82:*586–588, 1974.
39. Gitlin, D., and Petricelli, A. Synthesis of serum albumin, prealbumin, alpha-fetoprotein, alpha-1-antitrypsin and transferrin by the human yolk sac. *Nature 228:*995, 1970.
40. Gitlin, D. Normal biology of alpha-fetoprotein. *Ann. N.Y. Acad. Sci. 259:*7, 1975.
41. Kurman, R. J., and McIntire, K. R. (Unpublished data).
42. Nochomovitz, L. E., and Rosai, J. Current concepts on the histogenesis, pathology, and immunocytochemistry of germ cell tumors of the testis. *Pathol. Annu. 13:*327, 1978.
43. Heyderman, E. Multiple tissue markers in human malignant testicular tumors. *Scand. J. Immunol.* (*Suppl.*) *8:*119, 1978.
44. Scardino, P. T., Cox, H. D., Waldmann, T. A., *et al.* The value of serum tumor markers in the staging and prognosis of germ cell tumors of the testis. *J. Urol. 118:*994, 1977.
45. Horne, C. H. W., and Towler, C. M. Pregnancy-specific beta-1-glycoprotein: a review. *Obstet. Gynecol. Surv. 33:*761, 1978.
46. Rosen, W. S., Javadpour, N., Calvert, I., *et al.* Pregnancy specific beta-1-glycoprotein (SP_1) is increased in certain nonseminomatous germ cell tumors. *J. Natl. Cancer Inst. 62:*1439, 1979.
47. Parkinson, C., Beilby, J. O. W. Testicular germ cell tumors: Should current classification be revised? *Invest. Cell. Pathol. 3:* 135, 1980.
48. Scully, R. E. Tumors of the Ovary and Maldeveloped Gonads. *Atlas of Tumor Pathology. Second series, Fascicle 16.* Armed Forces Institute of Pathology, Washington, D.C. 1979.
49. Perlin, E., Engeler, J. E., Jr., Edson, M., *et al.* The value of serial measurement of both human chorionic gonadotropin and alpha-fetoprotein for monitoring germinal cell tumors. *Cancer 37:*215, 1975.
50. Thompson, D. K., Haddow, J. E. Serial monitoring of serum alpha-fetoprotein and chorionic gonadotropin in males with germ cell tumors. *Cancer 43:* 1820, 1979.
51. Javadpour, N., McIntire, K. R., Waldmann, T. A., Bergman, S., and Anderson, T. The role of the radioimmunoassay of serum alpha-fetoprotein and human chorionic gonadotropin in the intensive chemotherapy and surgery of metastatic testicular tumors. *J. Urol. 119:*759, 1978.
52. Scardino, P. T., and Skinner, D. G. Germ-cell tumors of the testis: Improved results in a prospective study using combined modality therapy and biochemical tumor markers. *Surgery 86:*86, 1979.
53. Skinner, D. G., and Scardino, P. T. Relevance of biochemical tumor markers and lymphadenectomy in management of nonseminamatous testis tumors. Current perspective. *J. Urol. 123:*378, 1980.
54. Elston, C. W., Bagshawe, K. D. The value of histological grading in the management of hydatidiform mole. *J. Obstet. Gynaecol. Br. Comwlth. 79:*717, 1972.
55. Bagshawe, K. D. Risk and prognostic factors in trophoblastic neoplasia. *Cancer 38:* 1373, 1976.
56. Curry, S. L., Hammond, C. B., Tyrey, L., Creasman, W. T., Parker, R. T. Hydatidiform mole. Diagnosis, Management and long-term follow up of 347 patients. *Obstet. Gynecol. 45:* 1, 1975.
57. Morrow, C. P., Kletzky, O. A., DiSaia, P. J., Townsend, D. E., Mishell, D.R., Nakamura, R. M. Clinical and laboratory correlates of molar pregnancy and trophoblastic disease. *Am. J. Obstet. Gynecol. 128:*424, 1977.

6

Clinical Applications of Tumor Markers in Testicular Cancer

Paul H. Lange, M.D.
Derek Raghavan, M.B., B.S., F.R.A.C.P.

Although the technology of tumor imaging has become increasingly sophisticated with the introduction of radioisotope scans and computed axial tomography, these methods are unable at present to detect tumor masses smaller than 5–10 mm in diameter (10^8–10^9 cells)[1] and usually cannot show whether the malignant cells present are viable. These limitations have stimulated the search for more sensitive and specific methods of tumor detection, methods which are theoretically capable of detecting a mass of fewer than 10^5 cells.[2] One possible approach is the scrutiny of chemical or molecular probes: tumor markers.

The ideal tumor marker would be a substance produced only by one type of tumor cell; which could be reliably and reproducibly measured in minute amounts in the tissues, body fluids, or excreta; which would be excreted rapidly; and which would be present in amounts directly related to the mass of the tumor. In current practice, however, most tumor markers also are present in the normal state, and their utility depends more on quantitative than on qualitative differences. Furthermore, few marker substances are specific for only one tumor cell type, and they are thus most useful when considered in the context of a particular disease in a particular patient.

Most of the tumor markers in current use are proteins; several are enzymes (*e.g.* lactic acid dehydrogenase, placental alkaline phosphatase). Because of the marked immunogenicity of proteins in unrelated species, antisera can be raised against the marker in a variety of animals. These antisera, when suitably adsorbed and purified, can be highly specific for the tumor antigen and thus are suitable for use in a variety of very sensitive immunological assays including radioimmunoassay (RIA) and enzyme-linked immunosorbent assay (ELISA).[3-5] The enzymatic properties of some tumor markers permit a biochemical approach, in which the detection system is based on the ability of the marker to initiate a biochemical reaction, the product of which can be measured. Alternatively, simple biochemical or electrophoretic techniques can be used to detect or measure these proteins. In general, the sensitivity and specificity of the immunological methods render them more useful clinically than are the biochemical techniques.

In testicular cancer, most of the known tumor markers are "oncodevelopmental" or "oncofetal" antigens—substances that are associated both with tumor cells and with cells of the developing embryo. Because these antigens normally are found during development, their presence on tumor cells is probably not the result of mutation but rather of re-expression of genes that have been repressed at some stage during development. It has been suggested that this phenomenon reflects a close interrelationship between the processes of normal organ development (ontogenesis) and the mechanisms of malignant transformation (oncogenesis).[6, 7]

The application of sensitive assays for the oncodevelopmental antigens α-fetoprotein and human chorionic gonadotropin in the management of patients with testicular cancer represents one of the most useful clinical implementations of tumor markers.[4, 8–12] Nevertheless, these antigens fall far short of the requirements for an ideal tumor marker. In this article, we will review the uses and limitations of tumor markers in the management of patients with testicular cancer and will assess some of the innovations in this rapidly developing area of cancer research and treatment.

PATHOPHYSIOLOGY OF TUMOR MARKERS

α-Fetoprotein

α-Fetoprotein (AFP), a glycoprotein with a molecular weight of approximately 70,000, is a single-chain molecule produced by the fetal yolk sac, liver, and gastrointestinal tract in many species. In the human fetus, AFP is a major serum protein, which reaches peak levels at about the twelfth week of gestation and then declines. After 1 year of age, it usually is not detectable by the older, less sensitive assay procedures, although RIA has demonstrated "normal" levels as high as 16 μg/liter (16 ng/ml). The function of AFP is unknown, although it appears to act as an albumin-like serum protein in the fetus. An immunoregulatory function also has been proposed, but there is conflicting evidence.[13] In man, AFP can be detected in the serum, extracellular fluid, amniotic fluid, urine, and cerebrospinal fluid. It also can be detected in AFP-producing tumor tissue.

α-Fetoprotein was first detected about 20 years ago, in the sera of animals with chemically induced hepatomas. With the older immunodiffusion assays, it also was demonstrated in the sera of patients with hepatomas and occasionally in patients with germ cell tumors. Radioimmunoassays with lower limits of sensitivity of <5 μg/liter have shown this marker to be present in 70% of patients with hepatomas and as many as 70% of those with germ cell tumors. However, with the increased sensitivity of the newer assay procedures, there has been a decrease in specificity, AFP being found in a variety of other diseases also (Table 6.1).

The metabolic half-life of AFP in normal persons is approximately 5

Table 6.1.
Causes of elevated circulating levels of tumor markers

	AFP	Microhetero-geneity	HCG	Comments
Ataxia telangiectasia	+	?	−	
Hereditary tyrosinemia	+	?	−	
Nonmalignant liver disease	+	+[a]	−	Disease usually severe; AFP levels almost always <1000 ng/ml
Luteinizing hormone	−		+	May cause apparent HCG elevation in some cases; see text
Marijuana	−		+?	Ref. 32; see text
Hepatocellular carcinoma	+	+[a]	+	
Pancreatic carcinoma	+	+?	+	
Gastric carcinoma	+	+?	+	
Lung carcinoma	+	+?	+	
Breast carcinoma	−		+	
Renal carcinoma	−		+	Rare; levels usually low
Bladder carcinoma	−		+	Rare; levels usually low
Seminoma	−		+	
NSGCT	+	+[a]	+	
Benign genitourinary disease	−		−	

[a] May be means of distinguishing AFP from germ cell tumors from that from other sources; see text.

days.[14] The metabolic clearance rate in patients with cancer or in the postoperative period has not been measured directly, but observations in clinical practice are consistent with a value of 4–6 days (Lange, unpublished; Kohn and Orr, personal communication).

Biochemical and immunological characterization has shown that AFP, like many glycoproteins, exhibits intraspecies microheterogeneity; *i.e.* different molecular variants are present within each species. For example, two AFP variants have been demonstrated in man on the basis of binding properties with lectins such as concanavalin A (Con-A). AFP produced by the fetal liver has a Con-A unbound fraction of approximately 5%, whereas in AFP from the yolk sac it is approximately 50%.[15] Whether this property will be of clinical value remains to be determined; however, one potentially useful application is in distinguishing between AFP from active testicular tumor and AFP from a liver damaged by metastatic deposits, chemotherapy, or other hepatotoxins (Lange and Vessella, in preparation).

Human Chorionic Gonadotropin

Human chorionic gonadotropin (HCG) is a glycoprotein with a molecular weight of approximately 38,000, which is secreted normally by the trophoblastic tissue of the placenta. It is composed of two dissimilar polypeptide chains, designated alpha (α) and beta (β). The α-subunit closely resembles the α-subunits of the pituitary hormones luteinizing hormone (LH), follicle-stimulating hormone (FSH), and thyroid-stimulating hormone (TSH) and therefore is not antigenically distinct. However, the β-subunit is structurally different from the β-subunits of the pituitary hormones, a property that confers both biological and immunological specificity.[16, 17] Some antibodies raised against purified β-HCG subunits cross-react to a small extent with physiologic concentrations of LH,[16] although there has been controversy about the extent of this cross-reactivity.[16–18] Antisera also have been raised against the COOH-terminal fragment of HCG[19]; although they are more specific, they are less sensitive because of their lower affinity for native HCG.[17] One of the most important principles for the use of these assays clinically is that cross-reactivity with LH differs markedly among the various "standard" β-HCG immunoassays, depending on the particular antibody used, and caution must be exercised in interpreting the significance of borderline-abnormal values.

It has been known since 1930 that HCG is present in the sera of some patients with germ cell tumors.[20] With the development of more sensitive assay procedures, the prevalence of detectable HCG in the sera of patients with nonseminomatous germ cell tumors (NSGCT) has increased to 40–60%. However, HCG also has been detected in the sera of patients with other malignancies (including seminoma; *vide infra*) and with nonmalignant conditions (Table 6.1).[16, 17, 21–23] Also, bacterial proteases may mimic the effects of HCG in RIAs,[24] distorting low level-positive results, and it remains to be proved that the HCG-like activity detected in extracts of some normal tissues (*e.g.* testis, pituitary, liver[21–23]) is not also the result of proteases.

The metabolic half-life of the whole HCG molecule is between 24 and 36 hours.[16, 17] However, the subunits have much shorter half-lives: 20 min for the α-chain and less than 45 min for the β-chain.[8, 16] Neoplasms associated with HCG production do not always secrete the whole molecule, some tumors secreting free α- or β-chains exclusively and others producing abnormal forms of the whole molecule or its subunits. As a result, some caution is necessary in interpreting the rate of decline of circulating marker levels after treatment (*vide infra*). As with AFP, lectin-binding assays have demonstrated microheterogeneity in HCG.[23]

Other Tumor Markers

A detailed discussion of the biology of markers that might prove to be of use in the management of patients with testicular cancer is beyond the scope of this review. The physicochemical characteristics of some of these substances are summarized in Table 6.2 and have been reviewed extensively.[2, 4, 25, 26]

SENSITIVITY AND SPECIFICITY OF AFP AND HCG IN TESTICULAR CANCER

In discussing the applications of tumor markers to clinical practice, certain terms must be defined. "Sensitivity," which refers to the proportion of true-positive results found in patients known to have the tumor in question,[27] is a function both of the smallest number of tumor cells

Table 6.2.
Serum markers other than AFP/HCG evaluated for possible use in the management of testicular tumors[ab]

	Molecular Weight	Cross-Reactivity	Detectable in Tumor Tissue?	Probable Clinical Value?
CEA	180,000	NCA	Yes	No
LDH	134,000		No	Sometimes
PlAP	120,000	Other p'tases	Yes	Yes?
SP-1	90,000		Yes	Yes?
α_1-Antitrypsin	90,000		Yes	No
Ferritin	Aggregates[c]		Yes	No
Human placental lactogen	20,000	Growth hormone	Yes	No
Fibronectin	450,000		Yes	?

[a] Data from references 4, 9, 10, 13, 68–79, 81; Lange and Millan, unpublished.
[b] The abbreviations used are: AFP, α-fetoprotein; HCG, human chorionic gonadotropin; CEA, carcinoembryonic antigen; NCA, natural cross-reacting antigen; LDH, lactic acid dehydrogenase; PlAP, placental alkaline phosphatase; and SP-1, Schwangerschaftsproteine-1.
[c] Aggregates of subunits with molecular weights of 19,000–21,000.

required to produce detectable levels of the marker and of the number of those cells present in the patient, and also depends on such variables as the affinity of the antiserum for the tumor marker being assayed. "Specificity" is a measure of the uniqueness of the marker for the tumor and reflects the incidence of true-negative results in subjects known to be free of the disease.[27] The "false-negative" rate is the proportion of patients with the tumor in whom the marker is not detected; the "false-positive" rate is the proportion of subjects without the tumor in whom the marker is detected.

The necessary lower limits of sensitivity for the assays for AFP and HCG have not been finally determined, but, in general, 5–10 μg/liter (5–10 ng/ml; 5.15–10.3 mIU/ml) for AFP and 1–2 μg/liter (5–10 mIU/ml) for HCG appear to be satisfactory, depending on the assay used.[4] In addition, intramural and interlaboratory variations in the assay results should be considered when interpreting marker values, and rigorous quality control should be incorporated into all systems.[4]

To be of maximum clinical value, AFP and HCG both should be measured because of the large proportion of patients with increased circulating levels of only one marker. In more than 400 patients with metastatic NSGCT, 25% had increased levels of AFP only, and nearly 15% had HCG as the only detectable marker.[10] Furthermore, in the course of the disease, the fluctuations in the levels of AFP and HCG may not be parallel (discordance), and the level of one marker may fall in response to treatment while the other remains unchanged or rises.[28–30] Alternatively, the level of one marker may be within normal limits initially, only to rise later. It also should be noted that as many as 30% of patients with stage II NSGCT and approximately 10% of those with untreated stage III disease have neither marker present in increased amounts.[9, 10] Finally, a much higher proportion of patients with pure seminoma will not have detectable levels of these markers, as will be discussed. These phenomena probably reflect the cellular heterogeneity of germ cell tumors, the variable patterns of tumor-marker elevation being a function of the different "clones" of cells present.[10, 30]

Although either marker may be elevated occasionally in a variety of other malignant and nonmalignant conditions, our experience has shown that in patients with testicular cancer these markers are, for practical purposes, very specific (especially with respect to NSGCT). We know of no documented case in which a persistently elevated tumor-marker level in a patient with known testicular cancer was due solely to any of the conditions listed in Table 6.1. Furthermore, in the unlikely event that this should occur, other causes for elevated marker levels could be excluded by clinical and laboratory evaluation, perhaps augmented by lectin-binding assays, as mentioned earlier.

There are caveats to the statement that true false-positive results do not occur for AFP/HCG in testicular cancer. A marker level may be elevated in a tumor-free patient if the serum sample is obtained too soon after tumor removal for the substance to have been cleared metabolically. This applies particularly to AFP, which has a longer half-life than does HCG. Thus it is important to obtain serial samples; a single estimation may have little clinical value.[9, 10]

A second caveat is that persistent slight elevations of HCG occasionally are recorded in patients who actually have only elevated LH levels. This phenomenon, which usually occurs when one of the less-specific commercial HCG assays is used, is particularly relevant to the patient with testicular cancer who may have elevated LH levels because of hypogonadism induced by chemotherapy or orchiectomy. In distinguishing true HCG elevations from those resulting from cross-reactivity with LH, the following should be noted:

1. When reliable RIAs are used, these rare falsely elevated HCG levels are usually only borderline (1–3 μg/liter).
2. False elevations may fluctuate but do not rise steadily.
3. Equivocal elevations must be considered in the clinical context, and assays showing slight elevations and those in which the results do not fit the clinical picture should be repeated.
4. The simultaneous determination of testosterone and LH levels often will be helpful. As noted above, most LH assays cross-react greatly with HCG, whereas the β-HCG assays cross-react only slightly with LH. Thus an elevation of 2 μg/liter in a β-HCG assay when the LH level is 100 μg/liter is compatible with LH cross-reactivity. However, for an LH level of 100 μg/liter to be caused by an elevated HCG level, the circulating HCG level would have to be greater than 75 μg/liter.
5. Retesting for circulating LH and HCG levels after a short course of testosterone in order to suppress LH production often will resolve the issue.[31]

The significance of increased circulating levels of HCG in marijuana smokers has yet to be assessed.[32] This finding may assume considerable importance if verified, in view of the increasing use of the marijuana derivative tetrahydrocannabinol (THC) as an antiemetic for patients receiving combination chemotherapy.

CLINICAL INTERPRETATION

Diagnosis

Knowledge of the prevalence and significance of elevated marker levels in patients with undiagnosed scrotal masses has lagged behind that of other aspects of the use of tumor markers in testicular cancer. Until recently, these assays were performed primarily in referral centers, where patients usually are not seen until after orchiectomy. However, with the increasing awareness of the value of markers, the assays have become more widely available, and more primary care physicians are sending preorchiectomy blood specimens for analysis. Our current preorchiectomy marker data are shown in Table 6.3. These data and those from other medical centers permit the following conclusions. First, marker levels are not elevated in patients whose scrotal masses are found to be benign or composed of nongerm cell tissues (*e.g.* lymphomas, Leydig-cell tumors). Second, if the AFP level is elevated, the patient has a nonseminomatous germ cell tumor (with or without concurrent seminoma). However, an elevated HCG level may occur in pure seminoma, pure NSGCT, or "combined" tumors (seminoma plus NSGCT). Third, the prevalence of raised AFP or HCG levels before orchiectomy probably increases with increasing stage of disease (Table 6.3).

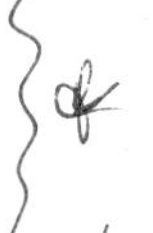
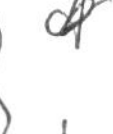
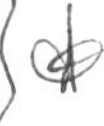

Marker assays performed on fluid aspirated percutaneously from hydroceles or other intrascrotal lesions are diagnostically useless and medically ill-advised. Transscrotal aspiration carries a high risk of contamination of the inguinal lymphatic chains, altering the pattern of spread of testicular tumors. Furthermore, it has been reported than an HCG-like substance, which does not appear to be LH, can be found in testicular fluid in benign conditions.[33]

Hence, on the basis of our present knowledge of markers in patients with scrotal masses, AFP and HCG can be considered useful in diagnosis only if the levels are elevated, in which case it is almost certain that the mass is a malignant germ cell tumor. However, the cornerstone of diagnosis remains the histologic examination, and no patient should be started on treatment for testicular cancer solely on the basis of a testicular mass and raised marker levels. Furthermore, the absence of detectable AFP or HCG before orchiectomy does not mean that a scrotal mass is not a germ cell tumor.

Table 6.3.
Preorchiectomy marker levels at the University of Minnesota

Diagnosis	Elevated AFP or HCG Levels (%)
Benign intrascrotal mass ($N = 43$)	0 (0)
Seminoma ($N = 70$)	16 (23)
NSGCT	
Stage I ($N = 32$)	22 (69)
Stage II–III ($N = 57$)	50 (88)

Staging

The inaccuracy of conventional staging techniques can be reduced drastically by incorporating tumor marker data.[8–11, 34] This requires a working knowledge of the metabolic clearance of these markers. For example, after orchiectomy, at least two values, obtained several days apart, often are needed to prove that the marker is originating in a metastatic deposit rather than from the excised testicle. Thus, if the marker-producing tumor tissue truly was confined to the testicle (stage I), the rate of decline of the marker(s) in the circulation should be in accordance with the physiological half-life of the substance in the blood, since the source of the marker has been removed.

With two or more values, one can calculate the expected marker level either by drawing an elimination curve or from the following equations[9]:

$$\text{For HCG: } X_F = X_0 e^{-0.023(t_h)}$$

$$\text{For AFP: } X_F = X_0 e^{-0.139(t_d)}$$

where X_0 is the initial concentration and X_F the concentration at time (t) in hours (h) or days (d).

The metabolic effects of operation on marker clearance remain to be clarified. However, in patients undergoing lymphadenectomy, the rates of decline often are affected by factors such as blood transfusions, and values determined immediately before and after such operations may be misleading.

When metabolic decay is taken into consideration, some patients who have pathologically proved retroperitoneal metastases have normal prelymphadenectomy marker levels (Table 6.4). In some of these cases, the marker levels were elevated before orchiectomy.[9, 10, 30] Thus, one cannot assume that the patient has no remaining disease if the marker levels return to normal after orchiectomy or lymphadenectomy.

Noninvasive diagnostic techniques (*e.g.* lymphography, echography, computed tomography) have well-documented false-negative and false-positive rates.[1, 35] However, tumor markers may be falsely negative in a significant number of patients with retroperitoneal metastases. Therefore, it appears that retroperitoneal lymphadenectomy, in addition to its efficacy as a therapeutic technique, remains the best single staging method for disease confined to the abdomen. However, we believe that to achieve the maximum staging accuracy, the operation must be augmented with other procedures, particularly tumor-marker assays. In this way, it is

Table 6.4.
Frequency of elevated prelymphadenectomy marker levels in patients with NSGCT

Reference	Stage of Disease			Total (%)
	II_A	II_B	II_C	
Scardino and Skinner[11]	6/12	12/22	5/5	23/39 (59)
Lange *et al.*[9]	7/15	11/15	8/10	26/40 (65)
Friedman *et al.*[42]	1/11	18/40	8/10	27/61 (44)
Total (%)	14/38 (37)	41/77 (53)	21/25 (84)	76/140 (54)

possible to detect micrometastatic disease beyond the retroperitoneum. Because combination chemotherapy for germ cell malignancy appears to be most effective against small amounts of disease,[36, 37] early diagnosis of residual tumor (within or beyond the abdomen) after lymphadenectomy probably materially affects the chances for cure.

In centers where retroperitoneal lymph-node dissection is not practiced routinely, tumor markers assume even greater importance in staging, particularly in apparent clinical stage I disease.[37–39] In this situation, a postorchiectomy treatment plan is formulated after rigorous noninvasive staging (conventional radiography, lymphography, intravenous pyelography, computed axial tomography, radioisotope scanning, echography, and tumor-marker determination). In most European medical centers, the results of this initial assessment determine whether radiotherapy or chemotherapy is given. With the recent initiation of a "no treatment" trial for some patients with clinical stage I disease,[37, 38] the greatest possible accuracy in noninvasive staging has become crucial.

Monitoring of Treatment

The principal value of AFP/HCG serum determinations in testicular cancer is in the monitoring of disease during and after initial therapy. In fact, these markers have become indispensible, because they usually reflect or predict progression or remission of disease, sometimes several months before other methods can.

Persistently elevated blood levels of one or more tumor markers in a patient who has completed a definitive course of treatment means that viable tumor is still present (providing, of course that metabolic decay rates and possible LH cross-reactivity have been excluded as causes). In this situation, the primary treatment has failed to produce a "cure," and a second-line treatment should be commenced. Similarly, if marker levels rise or fail to decline during a long course of treatment (*e.g.* radiotherapy), an alteration in the treatment usually is indicated (see also section on actual half-life determinations). However, we believe that a rapid decline of marker levels to "normal" during treatment does NOT justify early termination of therapy. With current assay methods, a "normal" tumor-marker level may mask as many as 10^4–10^5 marker-producing tumor cells.

The recent observation of raised levels of HCG-like activity in two marijuana smokers with germ cell tumors thought to be in remission presents a problem, because in both cases discontinuation of drug use resulted in normalization of the marker levels.[32] In the past, we have suggested that a rising marker level is, by itself, often sufficient evidence of disease recurrence to justify starting treatment, but in such cases it appears prudent to rule out drug use as a cause of marker elevations before deciding to start treating the patient for tumor. Clearly, this matter requires further study.

In patients with NSGCT who have completed chemotherapy but have persistent masses detected by noninvasive methods, 20–50% will have normal markers.[9, 11, 30] Some of these masses will prove to be differentiated teratoma, seminoma, treatment-induced fibrosis or necrosis, or benign lesions. Nevertheless, some will be viable NSGCT accompanied by falsely negative marker values.

Prognosis

One of the more controversial issues in tumor-marker use in germ cell malignancy has been whether raised marker levels are themselves a prognostic variable; *i.e.* is a marker elevation merely a reflection of tumor bulk or does production of markers by a tumor indicate inherent aggressiveness or resistance to treatment? When the data are not corrected for tumor bulk or histologic type, high marker levels appear to be an adverse prognostic sign.[37, 40–42] However, when the cases are separated into subgroups on the basis of histology and bulk, increased AFP and HCG levels have not seemed to be independent prognostic variables,[11, 37, 38] although we believe that further scrutiny of this issue is needed. Parenthetically, in a preliminary study of 59 patients with clinical stage I NSGCT, the presence of HCG-positive cells (demonstrated by immunocytochemical staining of tumor tissue) was of no prognostic significance.[38] We know of no comparable data for AFP, but such studies have been hampered by technical problems with histochemical staining for that marker.

Actual Half-Life (AHL)

It has been proposed that analysis of the rate of decline of AFP/HCG levels in the circulation in response to treatment may be a useful prognostic indicator.[43] According to this concept, patients with a rapid rate of decline of marker levels during induction chemotherapy or radiotherapy will become free of disease, whereas those with a rate of decline considerably slower than the physiological rate will have an unfavorable clinical course, even if the markers return to "normal." There is some evidence that this is true for AFP.[43–45]

In a detailed, although retrospective, study of both AFP and HCG levels during 35 clinical episodes, investigators at the University of Minnesota found that 87% of patients in whom disease was eradicated had favorable AHLs, whereas 89% of those who failed to become disease-free during chemotherapy had prolonged AHLs.[46] However, in view of the false-negative rate with the available tumor markers, further assessment, perhaps prospectively, is required before the AHL method can be recommended for routine clinical use.

Tissue Fluid Marker Levels

The utility of AFP/HCG assays is not restricted to the blood. Elevations may be detected in pleural fluid, ascites fluid, and cerebrospinal fluid (CSF)[47, 48] and may denote local metastatic deposits.

HCG has been of particular use in the management of central nervous system metastases in gestational choriocarcinoma.[2] The two causes of elevated CSF gonadotropin levels are local disease and passive diffusion resulting from greatly increased blood levels.[49] A blood:CSF ratio of less than 40 suggests the presence of disease in the central nervous system. However, a ratio greater than 40 does not preclude metastases in the nervous system, and it may be necessary to begin treatment and achieve normal blood levels of HCG before attempting to define the blood:CSF ratio further. One potential problem is the occasional lag phase, in which HCG diffuses out of the CSF more slowly than it declines in blood during treatment. These same principles may be applied to the management of testicular choriocarcinoma with possible cerebral or spinal metastases, although the results appear somewhat less reliable, probably because of the histologic heterogeneity of germ cell tumors.

The limited evidence available suggests that AFP is of less value in detecting or monitoring metastases in the central nervous system, because the correlation of increased CSF levels with the presence of tumor in the central nervous system is less reliable.[47, 48] Both false positives and false negatives occur.

TUMOR MARKERS AND SEMINOMA

Traditionally, it has been held that seminomas and NSGCT, despite a common germinal origin, follow distinct developmental paths. This view was based on the histologic differences between classical seminoma and the nonseminomatous tumors, the far greater radiosensitivity of pure seminoma, and the fact that in mixed seminomatous and nonseminomatous tumors the two histologic patterns often occur in separate regions.[50]

The histologic demonstration of "anaplastic" seminoma[50] and of patterns apparently intermediate between seminoma and NSGCT,[51, 52] the immunocytochemical demonstration of HCG-positive giant cells in seminoma,[53, 54] the clinical histories of some patients with seminoma and elevated HCG levels,[55] and the recent findings with a xenograft model of an AFP-producing "seminoma"[52] have suggested that there is a continuum between seminoma and NSGCT or, alternatively, that there is a form of solid yolk sac carcinoma that resembles seminoma at the light microscope level.[52, 56] This concept would explain the occurrence of nonseminomatous metastases from "pure" primary seminomas and the coexistence of seminomatous and nonseminomatous elements in extragonadal sites.[56] It may be possible to identify patients with "high-risk" seminomas at initial presentation on the basis of histologic study, tumor-marker measurements, immunocytochemical staining, and, perhaps, ultrastructural analysis and plan their treatment accordingly.[55, 57]

Although the accumulated clinical experience with tumor markers in seminoma is more limited than in NSGCT, certain features have emerged:

1. If the AFP level is elevated, NSGCT is present either in the primary tumor or in manifest or occult metastases (whatever the accuracy of our conception of the histogenesis of germ-cell tumors). Thus if the AFP level is elevated, a "seminoma" should be managed as NSGCT unless there is unquestionable evidence that the AFP originates from a nontumor source, such as the liver.[58] In this context, lectin-binding studies may be helpful.
2. The prevalence of raised circulating HCG levels in patients with pure seminoma is between 10 and 30%.[9, 10] At the University of Minnesota Hospitals, nearly 30% of patients with pure seminoma have elevated blood levels of HCG, although this may be influenced by patterns of patient referral (uncomplicated, low-stage, marker-negative cases may be referred less frequently).
3. If HCG alone is elevated, the patient may have either pure seminoma or a mixed tumor. Accordingly, the primary tumor should be examined thoroughly for nonseminomatous elements, and immunocytochemical staining should be performed to locate the source of HCG within the tumor (*vide infra*).

4. The prognostic implications of raised blood levels of tumor markers in patients with "seminoma" have not been fully defined. It is clear that if the AFP level is elevated, the prognosis is that of NSGCT. However, the significance of HCG remains controversial, and there is evidence to suggest both that it means a worse prognosis[59, 60] and that it does not affect the prognosis.[61] In a recent series of 31 patients, it appeared that HCG had no prognostic implications in low-stage disease but that it was associated with a poor outcome in more advanced disease when conventional treatment was used.[55]

Despite the extent of this debate, it is well to remember that the majority of patients with seminoma do not have elevated blood levels of either AFP or HCG. It is for these patients that new tumor markers are particularly needed, a point we will discuss later.

TUMOR LOCATION TECHNIQUES

In addition to the conventional assay techniques, which document increased circulating marker levels and hence the presence of viable tumor somewhere in the patient, two methods have been introduced that are designed to show where that tumor is.

Selective Catheterization

At the National Cancer Institute, selective percutaneous catheterization of the veins draining the groin and retroperitoneum has been used to obtain samples of the venous blood at several levels for assay for the α-subunit of HCG. Because of the short half-life of α-HCG (20 min), there is little accumulation in the peripheral circulation; and sharp local increases in α-HCG concentration can be detected. Such an increase is said to indicate a tumor deposit in the area drained by that vein. As the technique is somewhat cumbersome and is useful only for solitary deposits of HCG-producing tumors, its usefulness is probably limited.[8]

Radioimmunodetection

Radiolabeled anti-CEA antibodies can be used to locate deposits of CEA-producing tumors in animals and humans.[62] The technique involves conjugation of a specific antibody with a radionuclide such as ^{125}I and the use of ^{131}I-labeled albumin and subtraction imaging techniques to eliminate the blood-pool background from circulating CEA on the computer printout or screen.

As an extension of these studies, antibodies raised against HCG or AFP and conjugated with ^{125}I have been used to locate metastases of germ cell tumors that produce these markers. Although early successes have been reported, [63–66] it is not clear whether the sensitivity and resolution of this technique will be superior to those of conventional radiography and computed tomography (assuming that both are performed under optimal conditions). Also, interpretation of the scans is often a significant problem,[66, 67] and the occurrence of tumors that apparently do not produce AFP or HCG may limit the value of the method further. Nonetheless, the potential of radioimmunodetection represents an exciting new application of AFP/HCG and possibly other marker such as SSEA-1 and LICR-LON-HT13 (*vide infra*) to the management of patients with testicular tumors.

NEW MARKERS

Because of the false-negative rates associated with AFP and HCG, new tumor markers of germinal malignancy are being sought. Although several tumor-associated antigens have been demonstrated, the evidence to date suggests that at best they will be useful in only a few patients. For example, CEA is produced by teratomas with gut-like differentiation[68] but the levels do not correlate well with changes in tumor mass.[41, 69–71] Similarly, human placental lactogen, α_1-antitrypsin, and ferritin appear unlikely to be of clinical value because they are not prevalent, specific, or sensitive enough or because they add little to the information already available from AFP and HCG.[70]

It has been suggested that, despite its lack of specificity, serum lactic acid dehydrogenase (LDH) or one of its isoenzymes may be of use in monitoring the progress of treatment for NSGCT.[72–74] Occasionally, rising serum LDH levels are the only marker of persistent or recurrent tumor. As yet, however, false-positive and false-negative rates are undefined, and we believe that treatment should not be altered or initiated solely on the basis of this marker.

The pregnancy protein SP-1 (*Schwangerschaftsproteine*-1), produced by syncytiotrophoblastic cells of the placenta, is found during normal pregnancy and in patients with gestational choriocarcinoma. Elevated levels of this protein also have been detected in as many as half of patients with metastatic testicular cancer,[75, 76] usually in association with increased levels of HCG. Occasionally, SP-1 is of clinical value in patients without detectable AFP or HCG.[75] The discrepancies found in the prevalence of SP-1 are a significant problem, however, and are caused by differences in assay techniques and in the limits of normal defined in each laboratory.[75, 76] Further studies will be required to define the clinical value of SP-1 as a marker.

Placental alkaline phosphatase (PlAP), a fetal isoenzyme that can be distinguished biochemically from the adult alkaline phosphatase isoenzymes (from bone, liver), has been demonstrated in the sera of patients with a variety of malignancies. It has been suggested that PlAP is a marker for seminoma; but with both enzymatic assays and RIA, a large proportion of cases had false-positive or false-negative results.[77, 78] At the University of Minnesota Hospitals, raised serum PlAP levels were detected in 18% of patients when an enzymatic method was used, but this did not add anything useful to the information already available from the other markers. However, more recent experience with a more sensitive immunoassay suggests that PlAP may, in fact, become a useful marker for seminoma, correlating with the presence of disease in patients without detectable HCG.[79]

Fibronectin, a glycoprotein found in insoluble form at the cell surface and in the surrounding extracellular matrix, is produced by mouse teratocarcinoma cells *in vitro*[80] and by xenografted human germ cell tumors in immunosuppressed mice[81] and has been demonstrated in fixed specimens of human NSGCT (Raghavan and Ruoslahti, unpublished). It appears that the fibronectin isolated from the xenografted tumors resembles the form found in amniotic fluid but differs from other types found in human plasma.[81] Whether this substance will be of use as a tumor marker is uncertain. However, its presence in germ cell tumors and in normal amniotic fluid may have important implications for the understanding of growth, differentiation, and cell-cell interaction of these tumors.

Another group of potential markers of germ-cell tumors is the "F9-like" cell-surface antigens. Embryonal carcinoma cells from strain 129 mice share common cell-surface antigens with normal uncommitted embryonic cells.[82] The "prototype" of this group of antigens, F9, was originally found on the surface of a cell line (F9) derived from a teratocarcinoma from a strain 129 mouse, being detected by antiserum raised in normal adult 129 mice.[82] F9 antigenic activity is present on murine germ cells throughout life but disappears from all somatic cells after the second week of gestation. It also is present on human germ cell tumor lines *in vitro* and on normal human spermatozoa.[83-85] Other cell-surface antigens, characterized with monoclonal antibodies raised against germ cell tumors, have distributions similar to that of F9: SSEA-1[86, 87] and LICR-LON-HT13.[88, 89]

With the available assay methods, neither F9, SSEA-1, nor LICR-LON-HT13 reactivity has been found in circulating blood. However, these antigens may have applications in radioimmunodetection. Preliminary studies in mice bearing 129 strain teratocarcinoma[90] and in immunosuppressed mice with human germ cell tumor xenografts[91] show that small tumors can be located with radiolabeled antisera raised against SSEA-1 and LICR-LON-HT13, respectively. These antisera may be of use in patients with germ cell tumors.

DEMONSTRATION AND MEASUREMENT OF MARKERS IN TUMOR TISSUE

Several techniques have been used to demonstrate and measure markers within the tumors themselves: immunofluorescence (IF), immunocytochemistry (IC), radioimmunoelectrophoresis (RIE), and tissue-slurry RIA.[4, 12, 25, 26, 53, 54, 92-95] The advantages of studying tumor markers *in situ* include:

1. Increased sensitivity: direct demonstration of a marker in fresh or fixed tissue reduces the effect of "dilution" by the patient's serum.
2. Permanence: fixed tissues can be stored for a long time before use (particularly for IC), thus facilitating retrospective studies.
3. Cellular localization: both IF and IC allow marker production to be attributed to specific types of cells (*e.g.* HCG production to syncytial giant cells in seminoma) and hence yield data relating marker production to histology and prognosis.
4. Elimination of the effects of marker metabolism: in referral centers, where patients often are not seen until weeks after initial treatment, tumor markers may no longer be detectable in the circulation. In this situation, IF or IC

performed on tumor sections can define the most appropriate markers to monitor and provide information of the prevalence of each marker (and, indirectly, data relating marker positivity to prognosis).

However, there are technical problems with these techniques. Antigens may be denatured during fixation (causing false-negative results) and artifacts of staining may cause false-positive or false-negative results, particularly with antisera that have not been purified adequately. As with the assays for circulating markers, rigorous quality control procedures, with positive and negative controls, must be incorporated in each method.[4, 92]

Several markers have been demonstrated in the tissue of germ cell tumors: HCG in syncytial giant cells of seminoma and NSGCT[53, 54] and in trophoblastic tissue;[53, 54, 96] AFP in cells with the morphology of classic yolk sac carcinoma,[54, 96] undifferentiated cells,[54] and cells with features common to seminoma and yolk sac carcinoma;[52, 96] CEA in regions of intestine-like differentiation[68]; and human placental lactogen,[68] PlAP,[78] fibronectin,[81] and ferritin[68] in a variety of cell types.

Thus, with judicious combinations of assay techniques for markers in the circulation and in tumor tissues, it may be possible to define more accurately the prevalence of each potential tumor marker, its potential usefulness in a particular patient, and its prognostic significance. However, it should not be forgotten that false negatives may occur as a result of sampling error, inadequate antisera, or staining artifacts; hence, failure to demonstrate the common markers in tissue sections should not preclude their inclusion in the battery of markers to be assayed in that particular patient. In the future, however, with increasing sensitivity and specificity of these techniques, it may be possible to define which markers should be followed clinically on the basis of tissue-demonstration methods.

CONCLUSION

We have reviewed the uses and limitations of the available tumor markers and assay techniques in the management of patients with germ cell tumors. At present, AFP and HCG are firmly established in diagnosis, monitoring of treatment, and follow-up. However, as currently applied, these markers fall short of ideal, and it remains to develop new assays and markers that ultimately can result in marker sensitivities and specificities sufficient to detect nearly all occult metastases.

REFERENCES

1. Husband, J. Diagnostic techniques: their strengths and weaknesses. *Br. J. Cancer. 41 (Suppl 4) 41:*21–29, 1980.
2. Bagshawe, K.D., and Searle, F. Tumour markers. *In Essays in Medical Biochemistry.* Vol. 3. pp. 25–74, edited by V. Marks and C. N. Hales. Biochemical Society, London, 1977.
3. Masseyeff, R., Maiolini, R., and Ferrua, B. Assay methods for carcino-embryonic proteins. *In Carcino-Embryonic Proteins,* Vol. 1, pp. 495–503, edited by F. G. Lehmann. Elsevier/North Holland Biomedical Press, Amsterdam, 1979.
4. Nørgaard-Pedersen, B., and Raghavan, D. (eds). Germ cell tumours: a collective review. *Oncodev. Biol. Med. 1:*327–350, 1980).
5. Sell, S. Alpha-fetoprotein. *In Cancer Markers: Diagnostic and Developmental Significance,* pp. 249–294, edited by S. Sell. Humana Press, Clifton, N.J., 1979.

6. Abelev, G. I. Alpha-fetoprotein as a marker of embryo-specific differentiations in normal and tumor tissue. *Transplant. Rev. 20:*3–37, 1974.
7. Uriel, J. Retrodifferentiation and the fetal patterns of genetic expression in cancer. *Adv. Cancer. Res. 29:*127–174, 1979.
8. Javadpour, N. The role of biologic tumor markers in testicular cancer. *Cancer 45:*1755–1761, 1980.
9. Lange, P. H., McIntire, K. R., and Waldmann, T. A. Tumor markers in testicular tumor: current status and future prospects. *In: Testicular Tumors: Management and Treatment*, pp. 69–81, edited by L. E. Einhorn. Masson Publishing, New York, 1980.
10. Kohn, J., and Raghavan, D. Tumour markers in malignant germ cell tumours. *In The Management of Testicular Tumours*, edited by M. J. Peckham. Edward Arnold, London, (In press).
11. Scardino, P. T., and Skinner, D. G. Germ cell tumors of the testis: improved results in a prospective study using combined modality therapy and biochemical tumor markers. *Surgery 86:*86–94, 1979.
12. Nørgaard-Pedersen, B. Human alpha-fetoprotein: a review of recent methodological and clinical studies. *Scand. J. Immunol. (Suppl) 4:*7–45, 1976.
13. Ruoslahti, E., and Hirai, H. (eds). Alpha-fetoprotein. *Scand. J. Immunol. (Suppl) 8:*3–26, 1978.
14. Gitlin, D., and Boesman, M. Serum α-fetoprotein, albumin, and γ-G-globulin in the human conceptus. *J. Clin. Invest. 45:*1826–1838, 1966
15. Ruoslahti, E., Engvall, E., Pekkala, A., and Seppälä, M. Developmental changes in carbohydrate moiety of human alpha-fetoprotein. *Int. J. Cancer 22:*515–520, 1978.
16. Vaitukaitis, J. L. Human chorionic gonadotropin: a hormone secreted for many reasons. *N. Engl. J. Med. 301:*324–326, 1979.
17. Vaitukaitis, J. L. Secretion of human chorionic gonadotropin by tumors. *In Carcino-Embryonic Proteins*, Vol 1, pp. 447–456, edited by F-G Lehmann. Elsevier/North Holland Biomedical Press, Amsterdam, 1979.
18. Mann, K., Lamerz, R., Hellmann, T., Kumper, H. J., Staehler, G., and Karl, H. J. Use of human chorionic gonadotropin and alpha-fetoprotein radioimmunoassays: specificity and apparent half-life determination after delivery and in patients with germ cell tumors. *Oncodev. Biol. Med. 1:*301–306, 1981.
19. Ayala, A. R., Nisula, B. C., Chen, H-C, Hodgen, G. D., and Ross, G. T. Highly sensitive radioimmunoassay for chorionic gonadotropin in human urine. *J. Clin. Endocrinol. Metab. 47:*767–773, 1978.
20. Zondek, B. Versuch einer biologischen (hormonalen) Diagnostik beim malignen Hodentumor. *Chirurg 2:*1072–1073, 1930.
21. Braunstein, G. D., Rasor, J., and Wade, M. E. Presence in normal human testes of a chorionic-gonadotropin-like substance distinct from human luteinizing hormone. *N. Engl. J. Med. 293:*1339–1343, 1975.
22. Matsuura, S., Ohashk, M., Chen, H-C., *et al.* Physicochemical and immunological characterisation of an HCG-like substance from human pituitary glands. *Nature 286:*740–741, 1980.
23. Yoshimoto, Y., Wolfsen, A. R., and Odell, W. D. Human chorionic gonadotropin-like substance in nonendocrine tissues of normal subjects. *Science 197:*575–577, 1977.
24. Richert, N. D., Bramley, T. A., and Ryan, R. J. Hormone binding, proteases and the regulation of adenylate cyclase activity. *In Novel Aspects of Reproductive Physiology*, pp. 81–106, edited by C. H. Spilman and J. W. Wilks. Scientific Products Medical & Scientific Books, New York, 1978.
25. Nørgaard-Pedersen, B., and Axelsen, N. H. (eds). *Carcinoembryonic Proteins: Recent Progress. Scand J. Immunol. (Suppl) 8:*1–683, 1978.
26. Lehmann, F-G, (ed). Carcino-Embryonic Protein, Vol. 1, pp. 1–557. Elsevier/North Holland Biomedical Press, Amsterdam, 1979.
27. Ransohoff, D. F., and Einstein, A. R. Problems of spectrum and bias in evaluating the efficacy of diagnostic tests. *N. Engl. J. Med 299:*926–930, 1978.
28. Braunstein, G. C., McIntire, K. R., and Waldmann, T. A. Discordance of human chorionic gonadotropin and alpha-fetoprotein in testicular teratocarcinomas. *Cancer 31:*1065–1068, 1973.
29. Lange, P. H., McIntire, K. R., Waldmann, T. A., Hakala, T. R., and Fraley, E. E. Alpha-fetoprotein and human chorionic gonadotropin in the management of testicular tumors. *J. Urol 118:*593–596, 1977.

30. Raghavan, D., Gibbs, J., Costa, R. N., *et al.* The interpretation of marker protein assays: a critical appraisal in clinical studies and a xenograft model. *Br. J. Cancer (Suppl 4) 41:*191–194, 1980.
31. Catalona, W. J., Vaitukaitis, J. L., and Fair, W. R. Falsely positive specific human chorionic gonadotropin assays in patients with testicular tumors: conversion to negative with testosterone administration. *J. Urol. 122:*126–128, 1979.
32. Garnick, M. D. Spurious rise in human chorionic gonadotropin induced by marihuana in patients with testicular cancer. *N. Engl. J. Med. 303:*1177, 1980.
33. Scardino, P. T., Waldmann, T. A., and McIntire, K. R. Elevated local fluid levels of human chorionic gonadotropin in benign testicular conditions. Presented at the Annual Meeting, American Urological Association, San Francisco, 1980.
34. Bosl, G. J., Lange, P. H., Fraley, E. E., Goldman, A., Nochomovitz, L. E., Rosai, J., Waldmann, T. A., Johnson, K., and Kennedy, B. J. Human chorionic gonadotropin and alphafetoprotein in the staging of nonseminomatous testicular cancer. *Cancer 47:*328–332, 1981.
35. Fraley, E. E., Lange, P. H., and Kennedy, B. J.: Germ-cell testicular cancer in adults. *N. Engl. J. Med. 301:*1370–1377; 1420–1426, 1979.
36. Einhorn, L. H., and Donohue, J. *Cis*-diamminedichloroplatinum, vinblastine, and bleomycin combination chemotherapy in disseminated testicular cancer. *Ann. Intern. Med. 87:*293–298, 1977.
37. Peckham, M. J., Barrett, A., McElwain, T. J., Hendry, W. F., and Raghavan, D. Nonseminoma germ cell tumours (malignant teratoma) of the testis: results of treatment and an analysis of prognostic factors. *Br. J. Urol. 53:*162–172, 1981.
38. Raghavan, D., Peckham, M. J., Heyderman, E., and Tobias, J. S. Prognostic factors in clinical stage I nonseminomatous germ cell tumors of the testis managed by orchiectomy and lymph node irradiation. *Cancer* (In Press).
39. Raghavan, D., Heyderman, E., Peckham, M. J., McElwain, T. J., Kohn, J., and Orr, A. H. Tumour markers and the management of testicular malignancy. *In Tumour Markers: Impact and Prospects*, pp. 281–288, edited by E. Boelsma and Ph. Rumke. Elsevier/North Holland Biomedical Press, Amsterdam, 1979.
40. Newlands, E. S., Begent, R. H. J., Kaye, S. B., Rustin, G. J. S., and Bagshawe, K. D. Chemotherapy of advanced malignant teratomas. *Br. J. Cancer 42:*378–384, 1980.
41. Scardino, P. T., Cox, H. D., Waldmann, T. A., McIntire, K. R., Mittemeyer, B., and Javadpour, N. The value of serum tumor markers in the staging and prognosis of germ cell tumors of the testis. *J. Urol. 118:*994–999, 1977.
42. Friedman, A., Vugrin, D., and Golbey, R. B. Prognostic significance of serum tumor biomarkers (TM), alpha-fetoprotein (AFP), beta subunit of human chorionic gonadotropin (bHCG), and lactate dehydrogenase (LDH) in nonseminomatous germ cell tumors (NSGCT) (abstract). *Proc. Am. Soc. Clin. Oncol. 21:*323, 1980.
43. Kohn, J. The dynamics of serum alpha-fetoprotein in the course of testicular teratoma. *Scand. J. Immunol. (Suppl) 8:*103–107, 1978.
44. Kohn, J. The value of apparent half-life assay of alpha-1 fetoprotein in the management of testicular teratoma. *In Carcino-Embryonic Proteins*, Vol. 2, pp. 383–386, edited by F-G Lehmann. Elsevier/North Holland Biomedical Press, Amsterdam, 1979.
45. Thompson, D. K., and Haddow, J. E. Serial monitoring of serum alpha-fetoprotein and chorionic gonadotropin in males with germ cell tumors. *Cancer 43:*1820–1829, 1979.
46. Lange, P. H., Vogelzang, N. J., Goldman, A., Kennedy, B. J., and Fraley, E. E. Marker half-life analysis as a prognostic tool in testicular cancer. *J. Urol.* (In press).
47. Kaye, S. B., and Bagshawe, K. D. Chemical markers in spinal fluid for tumours of the central nervous system (CNS). *In CNS Complications of Malignant Disease*, pp. 306–323, edited by J. M. A. Whitehouse and H. E. M. Kay. Macmillan Press, London, 1979.
48. Schold, S. C., Vugrin, D., Golbey, R. B., and Posner, J. B. Central nervous system metastases from germ cell carcinoma of testis. *Semin Oncol. 6:*102–108, 1979.
49. Bagshawe, K. D., and Harland, S. Immunodiagnosis and monitoring of gonadotropin-producing metastases in the central nervous system. *Cancer 38:*112–118, 1976.
50. Mostofi, F. K. Tumors of the male genital system. *In Atlas of Tumor Pathology. Second Series*, pp. 1–84, edited by F. K. Mostofi and E. B. Price, Jr. Armed Forces Institute of Pathology, Washington, D.C., 1973.
51. Friedman, M., and Pearlman, A. W. "Seminoma with trophocarcinoma": a clinical variant of seminoma. *Cancer 26:*46–64, 1970.
52. Raghavan, D., Heyderman, E., Monaghan, P., *et al.* Hypothesis: When is a seminoma

not a seminoma? *J. Clin. Pathol. 34:*123–128, 1981.
53. Heyderman, E., and Neville, A. M. Syncytiotrophoblasts in malignant tumours. *Lancet 2:*103, 1976.
54. Kurman, R. J., Scardino, P. T., McIntire, K. R., Waldmann, T. A., and Javadpour, N. Cellular localization of alpha-fetoprotein and human chorionic gonadotropin in germ cell tumors of the testis using an indirect immunoperoxidase technique. *Cancer 40:*2136–2151, 1977.
55. Lange, P. H., Nochomovitz, L. E., Rosai, J., Fraley, E. E., et al. Serum alpha-fetoprotein and human chorionic gonadotropin in patients with seminoma. *J. Urol. 124:*472–478, 1980.
56. Raghavan, D., and Neville, A. M. The biology of testicular tumours. *In Scientific Foundations of Urology*, Ed. 2, edited by D. Innes-Williams and G. Chisholm. William Heinemann Medical Books, London, (In press).
57. Raghavan, D., Sullivan, A., Peckham, M. J., and Neville, A. M. Elevated serum alpha-fetoprotein and seminoma: clinical evidence for a histological continuum? *Cancer 50:*982–989, 1982.
58. Javadpour, N. Significance of elevated serum alpha-fetoprotein (AFP) in seminoma. *Cancer 45:*2166–2168, 1980.
59. Wilson, J. M., and Woodhead, D. M. Prognostic and therapeutic implications of urinary gonadotropin levels in the management of testicular neoplasia. *J. Urol. 108:*754–756, 1972.
60. Maier, J. G., and Sulak, M. H. Radiation therapy in malignant testis tumors: carcinoma. *Cancer 32:*1217–1226, 1973.
61. Mauch, P., Weichselbaum, R., and Botnick, L. The significance of positive chorionic gonadotropins in apparently pure seminoma of the testis. *Int. J. Radiat. Oncol. Biol. Phys. 5:*887–889, 1979.
62. Goldenberg, D. M., DeLand, F., Kim, E., Bennett, S., Primus, F. J., and Van Nagell, J. R., Jr. Use of radiolabeled antibodies to carcinoembryonic antigen for the detection and localization of diverse cancers by external photoscanning. *N. Engl. J. Med. 298:*1384–1388, 1978.
63. Goldenberg, D. M., Kim, E. E., DeLand, F. H., vanNagell, J. R., Jr., and Javadpour, N. Clinical radioimmunodetection of cancer with radioactive antibodies to human chorionic gonadotropin. *Science 207:*1284–1286, 1980.
64. Goldenberg, D. M., Kim, E. E., DeLand, F., Spremulli, E., Nelson, M. O., Gockerman, J. P., Primus, F. J., Corgan, R. L., and Alpert, E. Clinical studies on the radioimmunodetection of tumors containing alpha-fetoprotein. *Cancer 45:*2500–2505, 1980.
65. Javadpour, N., Kim, E. E., DeLand, F. H., Salyer, J. R., Shah, U., and Goldenberg, D. M. The role radioimmunodetection in the management of testicular cancer. *JAMA 246:*45–49, 1981.
66. Begent, R. H. J., Searle, F., Stanway, G., *et al.* Radioimmunolocalization of tumours by external scintigraphy after administration of 131-iodine antibody to human chorionic gonadotropin. *J. Roy. Soc. Med.* (In press).
67. Mach, J. -P., Forni, M., Ritschard, J., *et al.* Use and limitations of radio-labeled anti-CEA antibodies and their fragments for photo-scanning detection of human colorectal carcinomas. *Oncodev. Biol. Med. 1:*37–48, 1980.
68. Heyderman, E. Multiple tissue markers in human malignant testicular tumours. *Scand. J. Immunol. (Suppl) 8:*119–126, 1978.
69. Talerman, A., van der Pompe, W. R., Haije, W. B., and Boekestein-Tjahjadi, H. M. Alpha-fetoprotein and carcinoembryonic antigen in germ cell neoplasms. *Br. J. Cancer 35:*288–291, 1977.
70. Lange, P. H. Cancer markers in germ-cell testicular tumors. *In Cancer Markers: Developmental and Diagnostic Significance*, Vol. 2, pp. 259–273, edited by S. Sell and B. Wahren. Humana Press, Clifton, N.J., 1982.
71. Wahren, B., Alpert, E., and Esposti, P. Multiple antigens as marker substances in germinal tumors of the testis. *J. Natl. Cancer Inst. 58:*489–498, 1977.
72. Boyle, L. E., and Samuels, M. L. Serum LDH activity and isoenzyme patterns in nonseminomatous germinal (NSG) testis tumors. *Proc. Am. Soc. Clin. Oncol. 18:*278, 1977.
73. Bosl, G. J., Lange, P. H., Nochomovitz, L. E., Goldman, A., Fraley, E. E., Rosai, J.,

Johnson, K., and Kennedy, B. J. Tumor markers in advanced nonseminomatous testicular cancer. *Cancer 47:*572–576, 1981.

74. Edler von Eyben, F. Biochemical markers in advanced testicular tumors: serum lactate dehydrogenase, urinary chorionic gonadotropin, and total urinary estrogen. *Cancer 41:*648–652, 1978.
75. Lange, P. H., Bremner, R. D., Horne, C. H. W., Vessella, R. L., and Fraley, E. E. Is SP-1 a marker for testicular cancer? *Urology 15:*251–255, 1980.
76. Rosen, S. W., Javadpour, N., Calvert, I., and Kaminska, J. Increased "pregnancy-specific" beta-glycoprotein in certain nonseminomatous germ cell tumors. *J. Natl. Cancer. Inst. 62:*1439–1441, 1979.
77. Fishman, W. H., Krishnaswamy, P. R., Fishman, L., Millan, J. L., and McIntire, K. R. Gamma-glutamyl transferase in seminoma patients sera. In Carcino-Embryonic Proteins, Vol. 1, pp. 699–708, edited by F-G. Lehmann, Elsevier/North Holland Biomedical Press, Amsterdam, 1979.
78. Wahren, B., Holmgren, P. A., and Stigbrand, T. Placental alkaline phosphatase, alphafetoprotein and carcinoembryonic antigen in testicular tumors: tissue typing by means of cytologic smears. *Int. J. Cancer 24:*749–753, 1979.
79. Lange, P. H., Millan, J. L., Stigbrand, T., Vessella, R. L., Ruoslahti, E., and Fishman, W. H.: Placental alkaline phosphatase as a tumor marker for seminoma. *Cancer Res. 42:*3244–3247, 1982.
80. Zetter, B. R., and Martin, G. R. Expression of a high molecular weight cell surface glycoprotein (LETS protein) by preimplantation mouse embryos and teratocarcinoma stem cells. *Proc. Natl. Acad. Sci. U.S.A. 75:*2324–2328, 1978.
81. Ruoslahti, E., Jalanko, H., Comings, D. E., Neville, A. M., and Raghavan, D. Fibronectin from human germ cell tumors resembles amniotic fluid fibronectin. *Int. J. Cancer 27:*763–768, 1981.
82. Artzt, K., Dubois, P., Bennett, D., Condamine, H., Babinet, C., and Jacob, F. Surface antigens common to mouse cleavage embryos and primitive teratocarcinoma cells in culture. *Proc. Natl. Acad. Sci. U.S.A. 70:*2988–2992, 1973.
83. Hogan, B., Fellous, B., Avner, P., and Jacob, F. Isolation of a human teratoma cell line which expresses F9 antigen. *Nature 270:*515–518, 1977.
84. Holden, S., Bernard, O., Artzt, K., Whitmore, W. F., Jr., and Bennett, D. Human and mouse embryonal carcinoma cells in culture share an embryonic antigen (F9). *Nature 270:*518–520, 1977.
85. Edidin, M., Ostrand-Rosenberg, S., and Bartlett, P. F. Teratocarcinoma cells and cell surface differentiation. In *Cell Differentiation and Neoplasia*, edited by G. F. Saunders. Raven Press, New York, 1978.
86. Solter, D., and Knowles, B. B. Monoclonal antibody defining a stage-specific mouse embryonic antigen (SSEA-1). *Proc. Natl. Acad. Sci. U.S.A. 75:*5565–5569, 1978.
87. Andrews, P. W., Bronson, D. L., Benham, F., Strickland, S., and Knowles, B. B. A comparative study of 8 cell lines derived from human testicular teratocarcinoma. *Int. J. Cancer 26:*269–280, 1980.
88. Edwards, P., Foster, C., and McIlhinney, R. A. J. Monoclonal antibody to teratoma and breast. *Transplant. Proc. 12:*398–402, 1980.
89. McIlhinney, R. A. J. Cell surface molecules of human teratoma cell lines. *Int. J. Androl. Suppl 4*, pp. 93–110.
90. Ballou, B., Levine, G., Hakala, T. R., and Solter, D. Tumor location detected with radioactively labeled monoclonal antibody and external scintigraphy. *Science 206:*844–846, 1979.
91. Moshakis, B., McIlhinney, R. A. J., Raghavan, D., and Neville, A. M. Monoclonal antibodies to detect human tumours: an experimental approach. *J. Clin. Pathol. 34:*314–319, 1981.
92. Heyderman, E. Immunoperoxidase techniques in histopathology: applications, methods, and controls. *J. Clin. Pathol. 32:*971–978, 1979.
93. Nørgaard-Pedersen, B., Toftager-Larsen, K., Nørregaard-Hansen, K., and Albrechtsen, R. Radioimmunoelectrophoretic detection of alpha-fetoprotein in tumour specimens. *Invest. Cell. Pathol. 3:*147–150, 1980.
94. Woltering, E. A., Know, R. D., Javadpour, N., Soares, T., and Chen, H-C. Detection of human chorionic gonadotropin in fresh and formalin-fixed testicular tumor tissue:

comparison of sensitivity of immunoperoxidase to radioimmunoassay. *Urology 16:*215–218, 1980.

95. Javadpour, N., Woltering, E. A., and Soares, T. Simultaneous measurement of peripheral serum and tumor cytosol levels of human chorionic gonadotropin and alpha-fetoprotein in testicular cancer *Invest. Urol. 18:*11–12, 1980.
96. Heyderman, E., Raghavan, D., and Neville, A. M. The functional pathology of testicular tumours. In *The Management of Testicular Tumours*, edited by M. J. Peckham, Edward Arnold, London (In press).

7

Clinical Staging

Douglas E. Johnson, M.D.

Once the diagnosis of a germ cell tumor of the testis has been established histologically, it becomes imperative that the physician make an accurate assessment as to the extent of the disease (staging). The importance of staging cannot be overemphasized, since it is this knowledge that allows for the orderly planning of appropriate treatment and serves as a guide for prognosis. It is obvious that the degree of accuracy in identifying metastases and documenting the frequency of their occurrence is directly related to the thoroughness with which staging procedures are carried out.

SITES OF METASTASES

Familiarity with the routes of spread and knowledge of the usual sites for metastases are essential if staging is to be complete and accurate. Testicular carcinoma usually spreads initially through the lymphatics in an orderly fashion, and later by vascular dissemination. The primary lymphatic drainage from the right testis is to the interaortocaval, precaval, preaortic, paracaval, right common iliac, and right external iliac nodes, in that order; subsequent drainage is to the para-aortic, left common iliac, and left external iliac nodes. The primary lymphatic drainage of the left testis is to the para-aortic, preaortic, left common iliac, and left external iliac nodes, in that order; subsequent drainage is to the interaortocaval, precaval, paracaval, right common iliac, and right external iliac nodes (Fig. 7.1).[1] Solitary contralateral metastases from the right testis to the left para-aortic nodes may occur, but similar cross-metastases have not been reported in patients with tumors of the left side. The iliac lymph nodes may be involved primarily when the tumor has invaded the epididymis or spermatic cord, and secondarily when para-aortic disease is present. Inguinal metastasis may occur if the tunica albuginea has been invaded or when previous surgery (inguinal herniorrhaphy or orchiopexy) has interrupted the normal lymphatic network. Inguinal-iliac extension is usually unilateral unless previous inguinal or scrotal surgery has been performed.

Distant spread of testicular carcinoma occurs most commonly to the lungs, followed by the liver, viscera, brain, and bone.[2] Sites of metastases from both seminomas and nonseminomatous tumors, as determined by necropsy findings, are shown in Table 7.1. A rather high incidence of

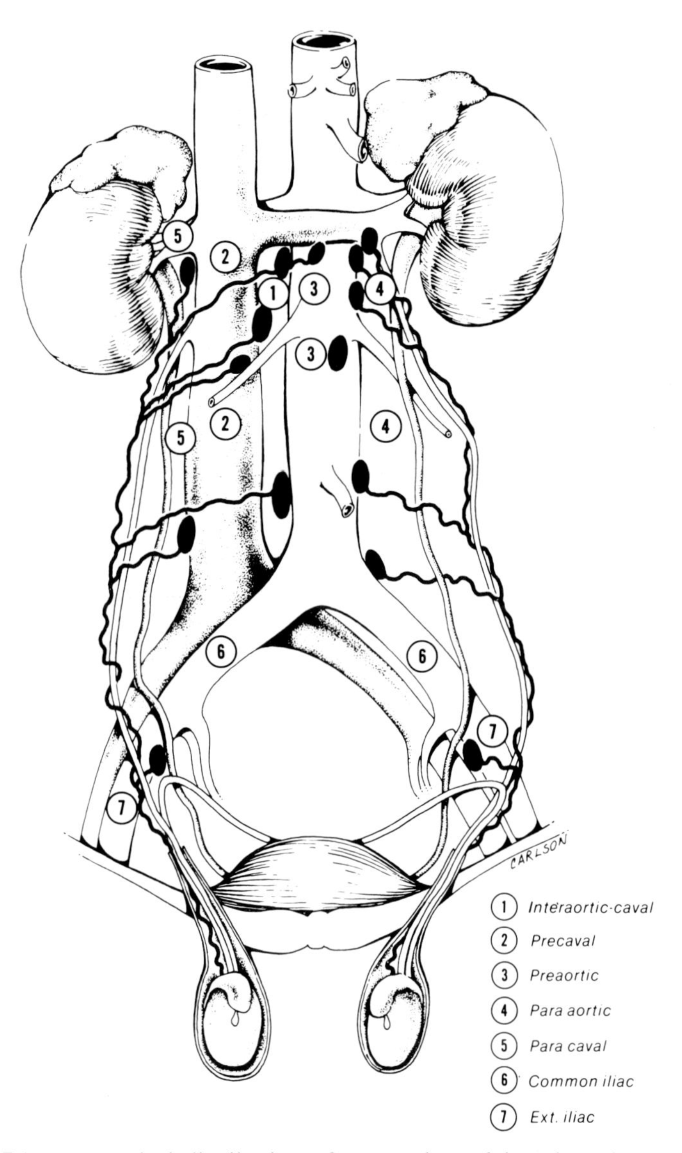

Figure 7.1. Anatomical distribution of retroperitoneal lymph nodes. (Reproduced by permission from R. J. Babaian and D. E. Johnson, *Cancer 45:*1775, 1980.)

osseous metastases (19%) reflects the extensiveness of disease present at necropsy. Osseous lesions are rarely encountered in clinical practice until saturation metastases have occurred late in the disease. Consequently, bone marrow aspiration or biopsy, radioisotope photoscanning, and skeletal surveys are unnecessary as an integral part of the routine staging procedure.

STAGING PROCEDURES

Findings noted at the time of orchiectomy, plus physical examination, radiological procedures (chest x-ray films, excretory urograms, and bipedal lymphangiograms), and laboratory studies (β-chain human chorionic gonadotropin, α-fetoprotein, simultaneous multiple analysis (SMA)) are used initially in assessing clinical stage. Although some investigators have urged that ultrasonography and computed tomography replace lymphangiography because of their lower morbidity, relatively low cost, and ease of performance,[3, 4] comparative studies suggest that these newer procedures are, at best, complementary to, not exclusive of, lymphangiography.[5] In selected instances, inferior venacavography, selective renal venography, and angiography may help in determining the extent of retroperitoneal disease.

Metastases, especially those from nonseminomatous germ cell tumors, may be assessed not only clinically, but also by surgical methods. Various investigators[6-9] have recommended supraclavicular lymph node biopsy as a routine procedure for staging patients with testicular tumors. However, the infrequency with which subclinical metastases have been documented and the potential morbidity of the procedure contraindicate its use in patients without a palpable supraclavicular mass (Table 7.2). Although some investigators are challenging the need for any surgical intervention, retroperitoneal lymphadenectomy remains an important method for determining regional lymph node spread.[10]

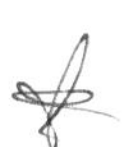

Table 7.1.
Sites of metastases from testicular carcinoma[a]

Site of Metastasis	Seminoma (19 Patients)	Nonseminoma (59 Patients)	Overall (78 Patients)
	%	%	%
Lung	74	93	89
Liver	79	69	72
Brain	32	29	30
Kidney	32	25	27
Gastrointestinal tract	26	27	27
Bone	37	14	19
Adrenal	37	14	19
Peritoneum	32	15	19
Spleen	21	19	19
Pancreas	26	10	14
Pleura	21	8	12

[a] Adapted from Johnson *et al.* Metastases from testicular carcinoma, *Urology* *8*:234, 1976.[2]

Table 7.2.
Incidence of metastases in routine supraclavicular lymph node biopsy

Series	Clinical Extent of Disease	
	Confined to the Testis	Involvement of Regional Nodes
	%	%
Buck *et al.*[6]	0 (15)[a]	16 (25)
Donohue *et al.*[7]	3[b] (39)	8 (12)
Fowler *et al.*[8]	0 (6)	5 (22)
Lynch and Richie[9]	0 (47)	4 (23)
Totals	1 (107)	9 (82)

[a] ( ) Number of patients studied.
[b] One patient had unsatisfactory lymphangiogram and did not undergo lymphadenectomy.

Table 7.3.
TNM (tumor-node-metastasis): American Joint Committee staging definitions[11]

Primary tumor (T)	
TX	Minimum requirements cannot be met (in the absence of orchiectomy, TX must be used)
T0	No evidence of primary tumor
T1	Limited to body of testis
T2	Extends beyond the tunica albuginea
T3	Involvement of the rete testis or epididymis
T4a	Invasion of spermatic cord
T4b	Invasion of scrotal wall
Nodal involvement (N)	
NX	Minimum requirements cannot be met
N0	No evidence of involvement of regional lymph nodes
N1	Involvement of a single homolateral regional lymph node which, if inguinal, is mobile
N2	Involvement of contralateral or bilateral or multiple regional lymph nodes which, if inguinal, are mobile
N3	Palpable abdominal mass present or fixed inguinal lymph nodes
N4	Involvement of juxtaregional nodes
Distant metastasis (M)	
MX	Not assessed
M0	No (known) distant metastasis
M1	Distant metastasis present

Findings at Orchiectomy

Radical (inguinal) orchiectomy is considered to be a biopsy for staging purposes in all cases of testicular carcinoma.[11] Careful processing of the orchiectomy specimen is necessary to assure that all elements within the tumor are recognized and, therefore, the histologic diagnosis is accurate. Equally important in examining the surgical specimen is determining the local extent of the tumor. The pathologists should record whether the tumor is confined within the body of the testis (T1), extends beyond the tunica albuginea (T2), involves the rete testis or epididymis (T3), or invades either the spermatic cord (T4a) or scrotal wall (T4b) (Table 7.3). While lymphatic or vascular invasion within the tumor mass should be noted, evidence is lacking as to whether these findings adversely influence prognosis.[12, 13] Currently, they do not affect staging assignments.

Physical Examination

While it may appear unnecessary to discuss the importance of a thorough physical examination in the careful assessment of a patient's disease status, the fact is that, in the total evaluation of the patient, today's physician often gives only superficial consideration to the physical examination. The patient should be examined only after he has removed all clothing. Examination requires careful inspection and palpation of the patient in both an erect and supine position.

When beginning the examination, the physician should direct careful attention towards detecting the presence or absence of enlarged lymph nodes, especially in the supraclavicular and cervical regions. Although it is more common for the subdiaphragmatic lymph channels to drain into the left supraclavicular lymph nodes, anomalous lymphatic drainage can occur, affecting either the right or both supraclavicular areas.

The breasts should be carefully inspected and palpated for gynecomastia, as its presence usually indicates trophoblastic elements. Auscultation and percussion of the chest may reveal evidence of pulmonary metastases, which can be confirmed by chest roentgenograms. The abdomen should be palpated for abnormal masses as well as for evidence of visceromegaly. Early lymphatic metastases are usually retroperitoneal in position and located on the same side as the affected testis. The inguinal areas should be checked for adenopathy, since these areas may be involved when patients have had prior inguinal or scrotal surgery. (In these latter situations the inguinal lymph nodes are also considered regional rather than juxtaregional or second-station nodes.) Careful attention should also be focused on the contralateral scrotal compartment, as bilateral involvement may occasionally be present. Digital examination of the prostate and a thorough neurological examination conclude the physical examination.

Radiological Procedures

A chest x-ray with supplemental lateral views should be the initial radiographic procedure performed. Full chest tomograms are not obtained routinely at M. D. Anderson Hospital, but are used in selected instances to clarify the nature of suspicious-appearing or indistinct pulmonary lesions. In a study of 76 patients with testicular cancer who were evaluated both by routine posteroanterior and lateral roentgenograms of the chest and by chest tomography, the laminagrams failed to detect a single metastatic lesion not previously found on the routinely performed studies.[14]

Bipedal lymphangiography is the standard procedure for assessing the regional (retroperitoneal) lymph nodes in patients with testicular cancer. Using the rigid criteria of a filling defect within a lymph node and that defect not traversed by lymphatics, false-positive interpretations are rare. Wallace and Jing[15] reported only one instance of a false-positive lymphangiographic interpretation among 81 patients with histologically proven negative lymph nodes. Lymphangiography is currently the only available study that demonstrates internal nodal architecture and, as a result, makes visible small metastatic deposits. On the other hand, false-negative interpretations have been reported in 15–20% of the patients. In these situations the error is usually due to microscopic disease below the 7-mm resolution of the test, but may occasionally result from complete replacement of the lymph node by tumor, which prevents the contrast medium from entering the node for visualization. An excretory urogram performed following lymphangiography may help to confirm metastatic disease and provides a safe and simple method for studying the retroperitoneal areas. Para-aortic and perirenal lymph node involvement may be suspected when displacement or obstruction of the kidney or ureters is present.

Although several physicians have suggested that computed tomography and ultrasonography should replace lymphangiography,[3, 4] Dunrick and

Javadpour,[5] in a prospective study of 63 patients with nonseminomatous testicular cancer examined by computed tomography, bipedal lymphangiography, and inferior venacavography, found that lymphangiography was the most accurate modality for detecting nonbulky tumor. Computed tomography, they determined, was most useful for examining extranodal disease and disease outside the area studied by lymphangiography. They concluded that the combination of lymphangiography followed by computed tomography provided the most accurate assessment of para-aortic metastasis. Inferior venacavography and angiography, while of little help in detecting metastasis, may aid in the precise localization of bulky retroperitoneal disease.[16]

Laboratory Studies

The usual routine laboratory screening procedures (complete blood count, urinalysis, and SMA) should be performed in all patients, but only the SMA helps in staging. Abnormalities of the liver or osseous function demand further investigation, which may require liver or bone scans.

Belville and associates[17] recently reviewed the predictive value of liver scans for detecting hepatic metastases in 104 patients with urologic malignancies who had undergone both liver scans and liver function tests (SMA-12/60 or SMAC-20: Technicon Instruments Corporation, Tarrytown, N.Y.). Positive scans were not reported for any of the 21 patients with testicular cancer. The authors concluded that, on the basis of its low predictive value and high cost/benefit ratio, liver scanning had no routine role in urologic oncology staging and should be discontinued. They found the alkaline phosphatase test to be nearly 10 times as cost-effective in predicting the existence of hepatic metastasis. Combining the alkaline phosphatase determination with the total serum bilirubin and serum glutamic oxaloacetic transaminase determinations available from the SMA provides all the information necessary for screening for hepatic metastases.

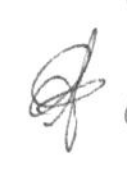

Double-antibody radioimmune assays for both β-human chorionic gonadotropin (β-HCG) and α-fetoprotein (AFP) should be obtained. While most current staging classifications have not made allowances for these biological markers, a persistent elevation of one or both in the serum following the removal of the primary tumor indicates metastatic disease, provided sufficient time has elapsed since surgery to allow levels to return to normal (see Chapter 6). Unfortunately, an elevation of biological marker levels after orchiectomy only indicates the existence of metastasis and does not help to stratify patients according to the location and extent of metastasis. Consequently, biological markers are of limited usefulness in staging.

Investigational Procedures

Using specific antisera AFP and HCG labeled with gamma-emitting ^{131}I, external scintoscans are being developed for the radioimmunodetection and staging of testicular cancer. While these tests are currently investigational, preliminary reports are encouraging.[18–20]

Javadpour[21] has reported using selective venous catheterizations and assaying the α-subunit of HCG to localize metastatic testicular cancer.

The α-subunit of HCG has a half-life of 20 min, which permits localization of a solitary metastasis when the peripheral level of α-HCG is only minimally elevated (less than 4 mg/ml).

As experimental studies continue, additional oncodevelopmental antigens are being discovered. One such new antigen, which appears to have importance in testicular cancer, is pregnancy-specific β-1 glycoprotein (SP-1). SP-1 is the product of the syncytiotrophoblast and its serum concentration tends to parallel HCG levels. However, SP-1 has shown discordance with HCG. In these situations, monitoring SP-1 levels provides information that otherwise would not be obtained. In preliminary studies, Lange *et al.*[22] have shown SP-1 to be a useful additional tumor marker in testicular cancer. Other oncodevelopmental markers that may also prove to help assess metastatic disease include γ-glutamyltransferase (GGT) and the placental-type Regan isoenzyme of alkaline phosphatase.[23]

While current staging procedures are imprecise and classification systems change as our knowledge of testicular cancer is expanded, staging remains the single most important step in the proper treatment of the patient with a testicular neoplasm.

STAGING CLASSIFICATION

Staging classifications for neoplastic diseases have been developed to assist the physician to: (1) prescribe proper therapy, (2) evaluate the results of treatment, and (3) compare the results of therapy from a variety of institutions and locales. Therefore, after all staging procedures have been completed and before beginning definitive therapy, the physician should assign a staging classification. When using a classification or staging system, however, it is important to apply it only to malignant diseases with similar or like biological behaviors and natural histories.

The fundamental basis for most staging systems rests on the belief that survival (cure) is related to the anatomic extent of disease at diagnosis. It is assumed that as the primary tumor increases in size, local invasion occurs, followed by spread to the regional lymph nodes and, later, by distant spread or metastasis[11] (Fig. 7.2). These tenets form the basis for the TNM classification (Table 7.3). While the metastatic process may be an orderly and accumulative sequence of events as suggested by Carter,[12] it involves many complex and, as yet, poorly understood mechanisms.[24]

Types of Staging Classification

Originally, staging classifications were developed solely on the basis of what could be discerned clinically before treatment. Unfortunately, as the years have passed and our diagnostic armamentarium has become more sophisticated, clinicians have become less precise as to what factors constitute the basis for staging classification. The American Joint Committee for Cancer Staging and End-Results Reporting, in developing the current TNM system, has reaffirmed the importance of and necessity for distinguishing between clinical-diagnostic staging (cTNM), surgical-evaluative staging (sTNM), postsurgical treatment-pathologic staging (pTNM), retreatment staging (rTNM), and autopsy staging (aTNM). The

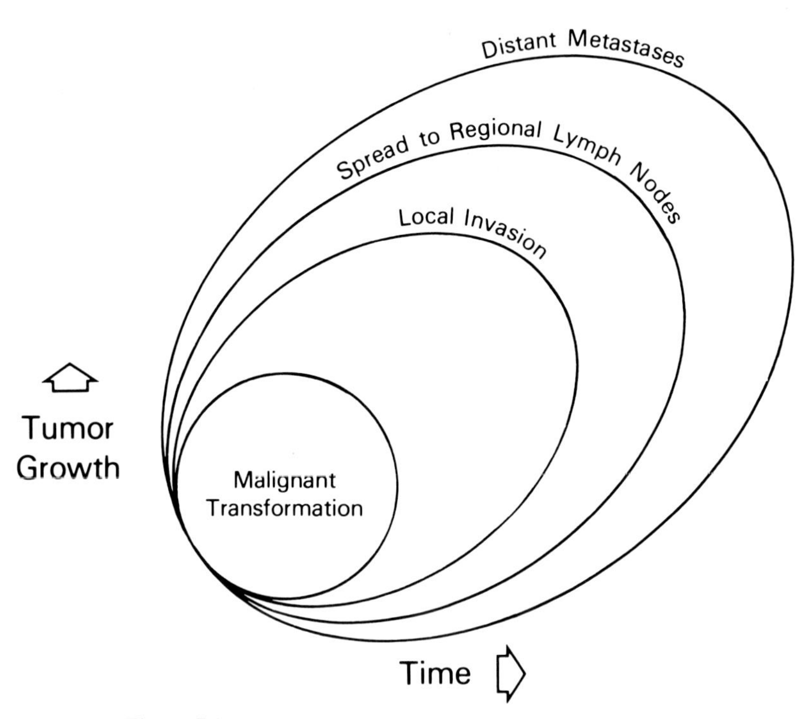

Figure 7.2. Schema for the development of metastases.

clinical-diagnostic stage classification is based on the extent of cancer determined and recorded before definitive treatment is given. The term *surgical-evaluative* is used to identify those instances in which the extent of disease is determined by surgical exploration, biopsy, or both. *Postsurgical treatment-pathologic staging* uses information gathered from the examination of a therapeutically resected specimen. Patients who fail initial treatment, but in whom subsequent therapy is being considered, should be given the additional stage classification of *retreatment staging.* Data from these secondary treatment patients should never be combined with data from a primary treatment series until they have first been separately evaluated and reported. These patients, likewise, should not be deleted or omitted from the original primary treatment series.

Nomenclature

Although numerous staging classifications have been developed and remain in current use (Tables 7.3–7.5), most are a modification and extension of the one proposed by Boden and Gibb[32] in 1951. These investigators separated the extent of the disease into one of three stages: stage I, tumor limited to the testicle with no evidence of spread through the capsule or to the spermatic cord; stage II, clinical or radiographic evidence of tumor extension beyond the testicle but not beyond the regional lymphatic drainage; and stage III, disseminated disease. The ensuing plethora of systems came about due to the interaction of three major factors: (1) differences in treatment among various centers, (2) differences in the methods used by physicians to assess the extent of disease, and (3) differences in the needs among the various specialities (urology, radiotherapy, medical oncology) responsible for the care of these patients.

Since patients with germ cell tumors of the testis can be conveniently divided for treatment planning into those with seminomas and those with nonseminomatous tumors, major differences in staging principles and nomenclature have arisen. Staging of a patient with pure seminoma is usually clinical, whereas staging is usually surgical for patients with nonseminomatous tumors.

Seminoma

Seminomas have an orderly lymphatic spread and, being relatively more radioresponsive than nonseminomatous tumors, are treated primarily with radiotherapy. A clinical-diagnostic staging system is therefore used, determining the extent of disease with the staging procedures previously described.

Since the extent of lymphatic disease influences treatment planning and prognosis, various attempts have been made to subdivide stages II and III (Table 7.4). Stage II has been somewhat arbitrarily subdivided into II-A and II-B according to the size of the retroperitoneal masses, but the definitions of the subgroups differ among institutions. Stage III has likewise been subdivided into various subclassifications that describe the location and extent of metastatic disease. As improved chemotherapeutic programs evolve for this disease, and as combination treatment programs

Table 7.4.
Staging systems for seminoma (clinical)

Stage	Investigator: Blandy *et al.*[25]	Hussey *et al.*[26]	Caldwell *et al.*[27]
I	No clinical or radiological evidence of metastases—assume all cases have "occult" metastases to para-aortic nodes	Cancer confined to testicle	A. Confined to testicle Microscopic evidence of invasion through the capsule or involvement of the epididymis or spermatic cord
II	Demonstrable retroperitoneal lymph node metastases	A. Retroperitoneal nodal metastases <10 cm in diameter B. Retroperitoneal nodal metastases >10 cm in diameter	A. Retroperitoneal nodal metastases <10 cm in diameter B. Retroperitoneal nodal metastases >10 cm in diameter
III	A. Negative para-aortic metastases but metastases in mediastinum or supraclavicular nodes	A. Extension beyond the diaphragm but still confined to the mediastinal or supraclavicular lymphatics	A. Metastases to mediastinal or supraclavicular nodes
	B. Negative para-aortic nodes, but pulmonary metastases C. Positive abdominal nodes, mediastinal or supraclavicular nodes, and lungs	B. Extranodal metastases	B. Metastases more extensive than stage III-A

Table 7.5.
Staging systems for nonseminomatous tumors from different institutions

Stage	Royal Marsden Hospital[28a] Clinical Stage	Mass. General Hospital[3a] Clinical Stage	UCLA Med. Ctr.[29a] Clinical or Surgical Stage	M. D. Anderson Hospital Clinical and Surgical Stage	Univ. So. Calif.[30] Surgical Stage	Memorial Sloan-Kettering[31] Surgical Stage
I (A) Tumor confined within the testis						And adnexa
II (B) Spread to regional lymph nodes	Maximum diameter of metastases:	Maximum diameter of metastases:				
A (1)	<2 cm	<2 cm	Microscopic	Negative lymphangiogram/positive nodes	Minimal disease (<6 nodes)	Microscopically positive
B (2)	2–5 cm	>2 cm	<3 cm	Positive lymphangiogram	Moderate disease (>6 nodes)	Macroscopically positive, completely resected
C (3)	>5 cm	NA[b]	Bulky retroperitoneal	NA	Massive disease	Macroscopically positive, incompletely resected
III (C) Beyond retroperitoneal lymph nodes	Supraclavicular and mediastinal nodes	Supraclavicular and mediastinal nodes		(See Table 7.6)		
A			NA	Supraclavicular nodes	NA	Lymph nodes outside primary area
B			NA	Other sites	NA	Lung metastases
C			NA	NA[b]	NA	Multiple organ metastases
	(IV-extralymphatic metastasis)	(IV-disseminated disease)				

[a] System also used for staging seminoma.
[b] NA, not applicable.

are used earlier in its course, these staging subclassifications may be expected to change.

Nonseminomatous Tumors

The wide differences of opinion regarding the initial or primary therapy to follow inguinal orchiectomy for nonseminomatous tumors (radiotherapy, retroperitoneal lymphadenectomy, chemotherapy, or various combinations thereof)[33] have contributed to the confusion surrounding the evaluative methods used in staging these tumors.

Generally, in the United States, a surgical-evaluative staging system based on the operative and pathologic findings of retroperitoneal lymphadenectomy has been employed. Once disseminated disease has been excluded, and in the absence of massive retroperitoneal disease that can be readily diagnosed by physical examination, excretory urography, and/or computed tomography and ultrasonography, surgical staging is performed. Using the information obtained by retroperitoneal lymphadenectomy, subcategorization for patients with stage II disease is carried out, providing a sound basis for selecting adjuvant chemotherapy.[34]

Clinical staging, relying on lymphangiograpy to assess the retroperitoneal area, has not been widely used in the United States for nonseminomatous tumors due to (1) the lack of available trained personnel to perform and interpret the procedure, (2) an insufficient number of cases at most institutions, which prevents the personnel from becoming proficient at interpretation, (3) disagreement among clinicians as to whether the procedure visualizes the primary sites of lymphatic spread from testicular tumors, and (4) reluctance to use preoperative therapy (radiotherapy or chemotherapy) for patients with either minimal or moderate retroperitoneal lymph node metastases. The literature is voluminous, with reports proving both the proponents and antagonists of the procedure correct! Suffice it here to say that only a few centers in this country, one of which is M. D. Anderson Hospital, rely heavily on the procedure for detecting minimal retroperitoneal metastasis in patients with nonseminomatous germ cell tumors of the testis.

In England, where radiotherapy plays a more dominant role in the treatment of patients with nonseminomatous disease, clinical findings alone, including lymphangiograms, are used for staging.[28] Stage II, metastasis confined to retroperitoneal lymph nodes, has been subdivided into A, B, or C on the basis of metastasis size: metastases with a maximum diameter of <2 cm are categorized II-A; between 2 and 5 cm, II-B; and >5 cm, II-C. The value of this subcategorization in helping to prognosticate and to plan therapy is emphasized by Peckham's[35] report. He demonstrated a cure rate of 80% for patients with II-A disease as opposed to only 35% for patients with stage II-B or greater. Consequently, chemotherapy is recommended as initial therapy for patients with stage II-B, II-C, III, or IV disease.

Shipley,[3] at Massachusetts General Hospital in Boston, has recommended a similar classification but only divides stage II into A and B, using a 2-cm diameter of metastasis as the dividing point. He has suggested that patients with clinical stage I disease be treated primarily with radiotherapy, patients with clinical stage II-A disease be treated with

Table 7.6.
Staging system for stage III disease[a]

III-A	Disease confined to supraclavicular nodes
III-B-1	Gynecomastia, either unilateral or bilateral, with or without elevation of biomarkers. Estrogen levels may be elevated. No gross tumor detectable
III-B-2	Minimal pulmonary disease. Up to five metastatic masses in each lung, with the largest diameter of any single lesion no larger than 2 cm
III-B-3	Advanced pulmonary disease. Any mediastinal or hilar mass, neoplastic pleural effusion, or intrapulmonary mass greater than 2 cm in diameter
III-B-4	Advanced abdominal disease. Any palpable abdominal mass, ureteral displacement, or obstructive uropathy
III-B-5	Visceral disease (excluding lung). The liver is the most common organ involved. Also included are the gastrointestinal tract and brain. Inferior vena cava invasion is considered in this category

[a] Samuels *et al.*[36]

preoperative radiation therapy followed by lymphadenectomy, and patients with more extensive disease be treated initially with multidrug chemotherapy, reserving surgery and/or radiation therapy for control of possible residual disease.

Until recently, little attention was focused on subcategorizing patients with metastatic tumor above the diaphragm. However, as multidrug chemotherapy programs have evolved, it has become very apparent that the extent of metastatic disease is a primary determinant for achieving a complete remission.[36–38] Consequently, it is essential to break down the disease status of patients in any study population in order to compare the merits of one chemotherapy program with another. Samuels *et al.*[36] were the first to propose a staging subclassification based on the extent of metastatic disease (Table 7.6), and it remains the most complete breakdown for patients with stage III disease.

While medical oncologists see patients who present initially with metastasis as well as those who develop metastasis after primary surgical or radiation therapy, usually no attempt is made to separate the primary cases from the secondary cases. Physicians' failure to use a retreatment staging classification when appropriate has contributed to the continued impreciseness of the staging nomenclature and further subverts the general staging principles.

CONCLUSIONS

The minimum assessment of patients with testicular cancer requires a carefully performed physical examination, chest x-ray, excretory urogram, measure of serum markers, and liver function tests as well as a careful review of the findings recorded at the time of orchiectomy. In addition, lymphangiography, computed tomography, and/or ultrasonography should be performed to document the status of the retroperitoneal lymph nodes. Patients with pure seminoma are assigned a *clinical* stage based on these findings, but most patients with nonseminomatous tumors are additionally subjected to a retroperitoneal lymphadenectomy before the assignment of a *surgical stage.*

Staging nomenclature differs widely among institutions, reflecting both strong local prejudices regarding the reliability of the various staging procedures and differing philosophies regarding treatment capabilities. Generally, patients are stratified according to the following guidelines: stage I, disease confined within the testis; stage II, spread beyond the testicle but not beyond the regional lymphatic drainage; and stage III, disseminated disease. Finding that the extent of metastatic disease is the primary determinant for achieving a complete response with multidrug chemotherapy programs has required that multiple subcategories be developed in stage III for comparative and prognostic purposes. Failure, however, to separate primary from secondary cases in reporting results of therapy in these patients has additionally confused the fundamental principles of staging.

While the primary goals of staging (aid in planning treatment, prognosticating, and comparing results of therapy) are currently being satisfied at the local level, failure to achieve a universally acceptable system has severely restricted communications at regional, national, and international levels. The greatest need today is for standardizing: (1) the basic or minimum requirements for staging, (2) staging nomenclature, and (3) methods of reporting results.

REFERENCES

1. Ray, B., Hajdu, S. I., and Whitmore, W. F., Jr. Proceedings: distribution of retroperitoneal lymph node metastases in testicular tumors. *Cancer 33:*340–348, 1974.
2. Johnson, D. E., Appelt, G., Samuels, M. L., and Luna, M. Metastases from testicular carcinoma: study of 78 autopsied cases. *Urology 8:*234–239, 1976.
3. Shipley, W. U. The role of radiation therapy in the management of adult germinal testis tumors. In *Testicular Tumors*, p. 48, edited by L. H. Einhorn. Masson Publishing U.S.A., New York, 1980.
4. Williams, R. D., Feinberg, S. B., Knight, L. C., and Fraley, E. E. Abdominal staging of testicular tumors using ultrasonography and computed tomography. *J. Urol. 123:*872, 1980.
5. Dunrick, N. R., and Javadpour, N. Value of CT and lymphography: distinguishing retroperitoneal metastases from nonseminomatous testicular tumors. *AJR 136:*1093–1099, 1981
6. Buck, A. S., Schamber, D. T., Maier, J. G., and Lewis, E. L. Supraclavicular node biopsy and malignant testicular tumors. *J. Urol. 107:*619, 1972.
7. Donohue, R. E., Pfeister, R. R., Weigel, J. W., and Stonington, O. G. Supraclavicular node biopsy in testicular tumors. *Urology 9:*546–548, 1977.
8. Fowler, J. E., Jr., McLeod, D. G., and Stutzman, R. E. Critical appraisal of routine supraclavicular lymph node biopsy in staging of testicular tumors. *Urology 14:*230–232, 1979.
9. Lynch, D. F., and Richie, J. P. Supraclavicular node biopsy in staging testis tumors. *J. Urol. 123:*39, 1980.
10. Babaian, R. J., Bracken, R. B., and Johnson, D. E. Complications of transabdominal retroperitoneal lymphadenectomy. *Urology 17:*126–128, 1981.
11. American Joint Committee for Cancer Staging and End-Results Reporting of the American College of Surgeons. *Manual for Staging of Cancer 1978.* American Joint Committee, Chicago, 1980.
12. Carter, R. L. Metastasis. In *Biology of Cancer,* p. 74, edited by E. J. Ambrose and F. J. C. Roe. John Wiley, New York, 1975.
13. Johnson, D. E., Gomez, M. D., and Ayala, A. G. Histologic factors affecting prognosis of pure seminoma of the testis. *South. Med. J. 69:*1173–1174, 1976.
14. Woodhead, D. M., Johnson, D. E., Pohl, D. R., and Robison, J. R. Aggressive management of advanced testicular malignancy: experience with 147 patients. *Milit. Med. 136:*634–638, 1971.
15. Wallace, S., and Jing, B. S. Testicular malignancies and the lymphatic system. In *Testicular Tumors,* p. 71, edited by D. E. Johnson. Medical Examination, New York, 1976.

16. Smith, R. B. Diagnosis and staging of testicular tumors. In *Genitourinary Cancer*, p. 448, edited by D. E. Skinner and J. B. deKernion. W. B. Saunders, Philadelphia, 1978.
17. Belville, W. D., McLeod, D. G., Prall, R. H., Mood, M. S., Corcoran, R. J., and Stutzman, R. E. The liver scan in urologic oncology. *J. Urol. 123:*901, 1980.
18. Goldenberg, D. M., Kim, E. E., DeLand, F. H., Spremulli, E., Nelson, M. O., Cockerman, J. P., Primus, F. J., Corgan, R. L., and Alpert, E. Clinical studies of radioimmunodetection of tumors containing alpha-fetoprotein. *Cancer 45:*2500–2505, 1980.
19. Goldenberg, D. M., Kim, E. E., DeLand, F. H., van Nagell, J. R., Jr., and Javadpour, N. Clinical radioimmunodetection of cancer using radioactive antibodies to human chorionic gonadotropin. *Science 208:*1284–1286, 1980.
20. Kim, E. E., DeLand, F. H., Nelson, M. O., Bennett, S., Simmons, G., Alpert, E., and Goldenberg, D. M. Radioimmunodetection of cancer with radiolabeled antibodies to alpha-fetoprotein. *Cancer Res. 40:*3008, 1980.
21. Javadpour, N. Testicular germ cell tumors. In *Principles and Management of Urologic Cancer*, p. 419, edited by N. Javadpour. Williams & Wilkins, Baltimore, 1979.
22. Lange, P. H., Bremner, R. D., Horne, C. H. W., Vessella, R. L., and Fraley, E. E. Is SP1 a marker for testicular cancer? *Urology 15:*251, 1980.
23. Fishman, W. H., Krishnaswamy, P. R., Fishman, L., Millan, J. L., and McIntire, R. K. Gamma-glutamyltransferase in seminoma patients sera. In *Carcino-Embryonic Proteins: Chemistry, Biology, Clinical Applications*, Vol. 2, edited by F. G. Lehmann. Elsevier/North Holland Biomedical Press, New York, 1979.
24. Wood, S., Jr., and Strauli, P. Tumor invasion and metastasis. In *Cancer Medicine,* p. 140, edited by J. F. Holland and E. Frei. Lea & Febiger, Philadelphia, 1973.
25. Blandy, J. P., Hope-Stone, H. F., and Dayan, A. D. *Tumors of the Testicle,* p. 95. Grune & Stratton, New York, 1970.
26. Johnson, D. E., Bracken, R. B., Wallace, S., Samuels, M. L., Hussey, D. H., Miller, L. S., and Ayala, A. G. Urologic cancer. In *Cancer Patient Care at M. D. Anderson Hospital and Tumor Institute,* p. 361, edited by R. L. Clark and C. D. Howe. Year Book Medical Publishers, Chicago, 1976.
27. Caldwell, W. L., Kademian, M. T., Frias, Z., and Davis, T. E. The management of testicular seminomas, 1979. *Cancer 45:*1768, 1980.
28. Hendry, W. F., Barrett, A., McElwain, T. J., Wallace, D. M., and Peckham, M. J. The role of surgery in the combined management of metastases from malignant teratomas of testis. *Br. J. Urol. 52:*38, 1980.
29. deKernion, J. B. (Personal communication, 1980).
30. Skinner, D. G. Management of nonseminomatous tumors of the testis. In *Genitourinary Cancer,* p. 470, edited by D. E. Skinner and J. B. deKernion. W. B. Saunders, Philadelphia, 1978.
31. Barzell, W. E. I., and Whitmore, W. F. Neoplasms of the testis. In *Campbell's Urology,* Vol. 2, p. 1143, edited by J. H. Harrison, R. F. Gittes, A. D. Perlmutter, T. A. Stamey, and P. C. Walsh. W. B. Saunders, Philadelphia, 1979.
32. Boden, G., and Gibb, R. Radiotherapy and testicular neoplasms. *Lancet 2:*1195, 1951.
33. Babaian, R. J., and Johnson, D. E. Management of stages I and II nonseminomatous germ cell tumors of the testis. *Cancer 45:*1775–1781, 1980.
34. DeWys, W. D. Basis for adjuvant chemotherapy for stage II testicular cancer. *Cancer Treat. Rep. 63:*1693, 1979.
35. Peckham, M. J. An appraisal of the role of radiation therapy in the management of nonseminomatous germ-cell tumors of the testis in the era of effective chemotherapy. *Cancer Treat. Rep. 63:*1653, 1979.
36. Samuels, M. L., Lanzotti, V. J., Holoye, P. Y., Boyle, L. E., Smith, T. E., and Johnson, D. E. Combination chemotherapy in germinal tumors. *Cancer Treat. Rev. 3:*185–204, 1976.
37. Samuels, M. L., Johnson, D. E., Brown, B., Bracken, R. B., Moran, M. E., and von Eschenbach, A. Velban plus continuous infusion bleomycin (VB-3) in stage III advanced testicular cancer. In *Cancer of the Genitourinary Tract*, p. 159, edited by D. E. Johnson and M. L. Samuels. Raven Press, New York, 1979.
38. Einhorn, L. H., and Williams, S. D. The management of disseminated testicular cancer. In *Testicular Tumors*, p. 117, edited by L. H. Einhorn. Masson Publishing U.S.A., New York, 1980.

8

Surgical Staging of Testicular Tumors

Donald G. Skinner, M.D.

Testis tumors predictably metastasize through lymphatics to regional lymph nodes located in the retroperitoneum at the periaortic and perivena caval regions just caudal to the renal hilum. Approximately 25% of patients with pure seminoma will have metastasized when first seen for therapy, compared to more than 66% of patients with nonseminomatous tumors who have metastasized at the time of initial presentation. Once the diagnosis of a germinal tumor of the testis has been established by radical orchiectomy, diagnostic evaluation should include a chest x-ray with full lung tomograms to rule out pulmonary metastatic disease and an intravenous pyelogram (IVP) to detect bulk retroperitoneal disease. The hallmark of extensive retroperitoneal nodal disease is lateral deviation of the proximal third of the ureter. Utilization of full lung tomograms allows an approximate 6% increase in detection of early pulmonary metastatic disease and provides a baseline study for future reference should any questions arise concerning the possible presence of metastatic disease. The 6% increased yield may not be cost effective or significantly alter therapeutic plans and, thus, some investigators do not routinely obtain this study. Bilateral pedal lymphangiography is usually obtained in patients with pure seminoma, but has not proven useful in patients with nonseminomatous tumors for four reasons. First, there is a high incidence of false-negatives in patients with minimal disease; second, there is the discomfort morbidity and cost of the procedure; third, surgical staging is performed in each case regardless of the results of the lymphangiogram unless massive abdominal disease is present, thus rendering the test unnecessary, and; fourth, massive disease can be readily detected by careful abdominal palpation together with an IVP or CT scan of the abdomen. The purpose of clinical staging in patients with nonseminomatous germinal tumors of the testis is to distinguish those with advanced disease who require initial chemotherapy from those with early disease who will be treated initially by surgery. If advanced disease is determined on the basis of full lung tomograms, IVP, or physical exam, initial therapy, regardless of cell type, should be chemotherapy. If there is no evidence of advanced disease, patients with pure seminoma are managed by radiotherapy utilizing portals according to the results of the lymphangiogram.

Patients with nonseminoma are then surgically staged by means of a retroperitoneal lymph node dissection. The staging scheme used in the United States is noted in Table 8.1.

Historically retroperitoneal lymphadenectomy was the primary therapeutic option and early operations performed either through flank approaches or transabdominally were limited and fairly ineffective in removing either the entire extent of tumor or in removal of all primary nodes draining the testis. In 1963, Tavel and associates[11] following an autopsy study, reported that even under ideal circumstances, more than 25% of the retroperitoneal nodes were left behind following dissection. This report, together with a significant failure rate of patients with metastatic nonseminomatous germ cell tumors of the testis, treated by surgery only, led most centers treating patients to use postoperative radiation therapy in hopes of better control of retroperitoneal disease. During the 1970s, however, development of truly effective chemotherapy drugs[5, 6] and improved surgical approaches to the retroperitoneal area led to a reappraisal of the use of surgical staging. Careful scrutiny of the work of Tavel and associates led to the realization that mobilization of the great vessels with ligation of the lumbar arteries and veins could allow removal of all retroperitoneal nodes. Clinical reports from several centers during the 1970s indicated that a properly performed node dissection could effectively control retoperitoneal disease obviating the need for postoperative radiation therapy.[4, 7, 9] In fact, a collation of data reported from three centers utilizing surgery and chemotherapy without radiation therapy indicated that only 1/227 consecutive patients with pathologic stage A or B nonseminomatous germ cell tumors of the testis treated between 1974 and 1978 developed retroperitoneal recurrence.[9] Furthermore, a recent review of our experience has led to the conclusion that a properly

Table 8.1.
Pathologic staging scheme for testicular cancer according to the ABC designation, modified Walter Reed scheme utilizing I, II, and III, or the TNM designation

Stage			Definition
A	I	N–0	Tumor confined to testis; no evidence of spread beyond the confines of the testis
B_1	IA	N–1, N2A	Evidence of minimal retroperitoneal lymph node metastases, detected by retroperitoneal lymph node dissection (fewer than six positive nodes); no node greater than 2 cm in diameter
B_2	IIB	N2B	Evidence of moderate retroperitoneal lymph node spread (more than six positive nodes) or any node larger than 2 cm in diameter
B_3	IIC	N3	Massive retroperitoneal lymph node involvement, but without evidence of spread above the diaphragm or to solid visceral organs. This diagnosis is made clinically on the basis of a palpable abdominal mass. If extensive retroperitoneal lymph node involvement is encountered surgically, but was not detected prior to surgery, the pathhologic stage designation remains B_2, IIB or N2B
C	III	M+	Metastatic tumor noted above the diaphragm or involvement of solid visceral organs, brain, or bone

performed retroperitoneal node dissection not only controls retroperitoneal disease but, on the basis of pathologic staging, allows selection of the least toxic chemotherapeutic agent or combination, tailored to the specific needs of an individual patient to allow maximum survival.[7, 9] Since 1974, 96% of all patients with stage A and B disease remain alive and tumor free.[9]

We prefer the thoracoabdominal approach for nearly all retroperitoneal tumors and utilize it in the management of renal cell carcinoma and renal pelvic tumors, in addition to node dissection for testis tumors. We have found it particularly useful in the management of massive retroperitoneal disease including primary tumors as well as extensive metastatic disease from testicular primaries. The thoracoabdominal approach was originally reported and utilized by Sweet[10] in 1947 for the resection of a large carcinoma originating in the fundus of the stomach. Subsequently Chute and associates[1] adopted its use for resecting large renal cell carcinomas and Cooper and associates[2] first described the transthoracic approach for retroperitoneal node dissection in the management of testicular tumors. Since 1970, we have modified the technical aspects of the operation to facilitate a completely retroperitoneal method for standard procedures, or combined it with an intraperitoneal approach for massive disease or complicated situations.[8] Figure 8.1 illustrates the anatomic boundaries to be dissected.

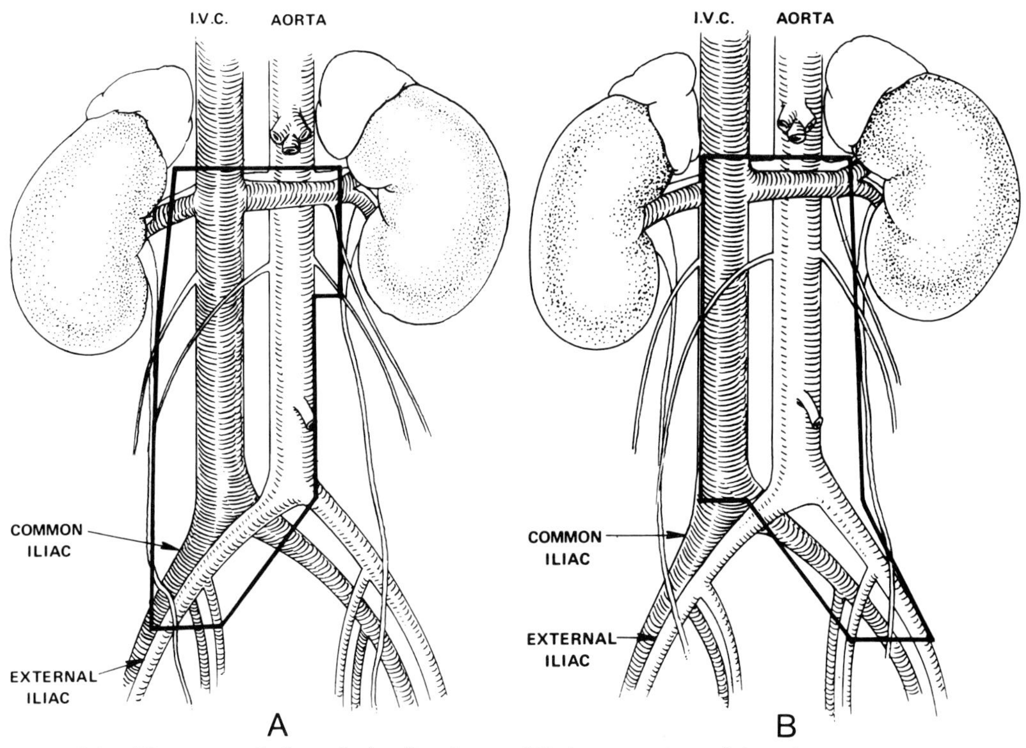

Figure 8.1. The anatomic boundaries for the modified retroperitoneal lymph node dissection. *A*, the limits of dissection for right-sided tumors. *B*, the limits of dissection for left-sided tumors. (Adapted from B. Ray *et al.* Distribution of retroperitoneal lymph node metastases in testicular germinal tumors. *Cancer*, *33:*340, 1974.)

PREOPERATIVE PREPARATION

Preoperative preparation is fairly routine. In patients over 50 years of age, prophylactic digitalization is usual unless there is a specific contraindication. Our practice is to give 0.5 mg of digoxin early the day before surgery followed by 0.25 mg that afternoon and 0.125 mg the evening before surgery. Overnight hydration utilizing Ringer's lactate is routine.

ANESTHESIA

For the past several years we have studied the use of controlled sodium nitroprusside-induced hypotensive anesthesia in the group of young patients undergoing node dissections for testicular tumors. A recent review of the group of patients in whom this technique was utilized compared to a similar group operated by the same surgeon in whom standard normotensive general anesthesia was used, revealed a significant advantage to the hypotensive group in terms of blood loss and the need for blood replacement. The average blood loss in 25 patients with pathologic stage B disease undergoing the thoracoabdominal retroperitoneal node dissection utilizing controlled hypotensive anesthesia was 920 ml compared to an average blood loss of 1341 ml in 32 stage B patients undergoing the same operation by the same surgeon under normotensive conditions ($P < 0.001$). Blood replacement, intraoperative plus postoperative requirements, also differs markedly and significantly favors the hypotensive group. Patients were matched stage-for-stage to eliminate bias due to extent of disease.

PATIENT POSITION

Patient position is extremely important and attention to details facilitates all phases of the operation. Patients should be positioned on the ipsilateral side of the operating table with the brake of the table located immediately above the superior iliac crest. The down leg is flexed 90° and the hip approximately 30°. The ipsilateral shoulder is then torqued approximately 20° off the horizontal and the ipsilateral arm brought across the chest to be placed in an adjustable arm rest. The pelvis remains nearly supine, perhaps rotated approximately 10° off the horizontal. A sheet roll is then placed longitudinally under the ipsilateral back and a similar roll is placed under the contralateral abdomen. The table is then fully hyperextended and the patient secured with wide adhesive tape applied to the shoulders, hips and leg. The ipsilateral leg remains extended along the ipsilateral side of the table supported by a pillow (Fig. 8.2).

SURGICAL PROCEDURE

A 9th rib-excising incision is generally utilized beginning at the midaxillary line, extending across the costochondral junction to the epigastrium and is then directed inferiorly as a paramedian incision. For a routine radical nephrectomy, the incision extends across the epigastrium to the

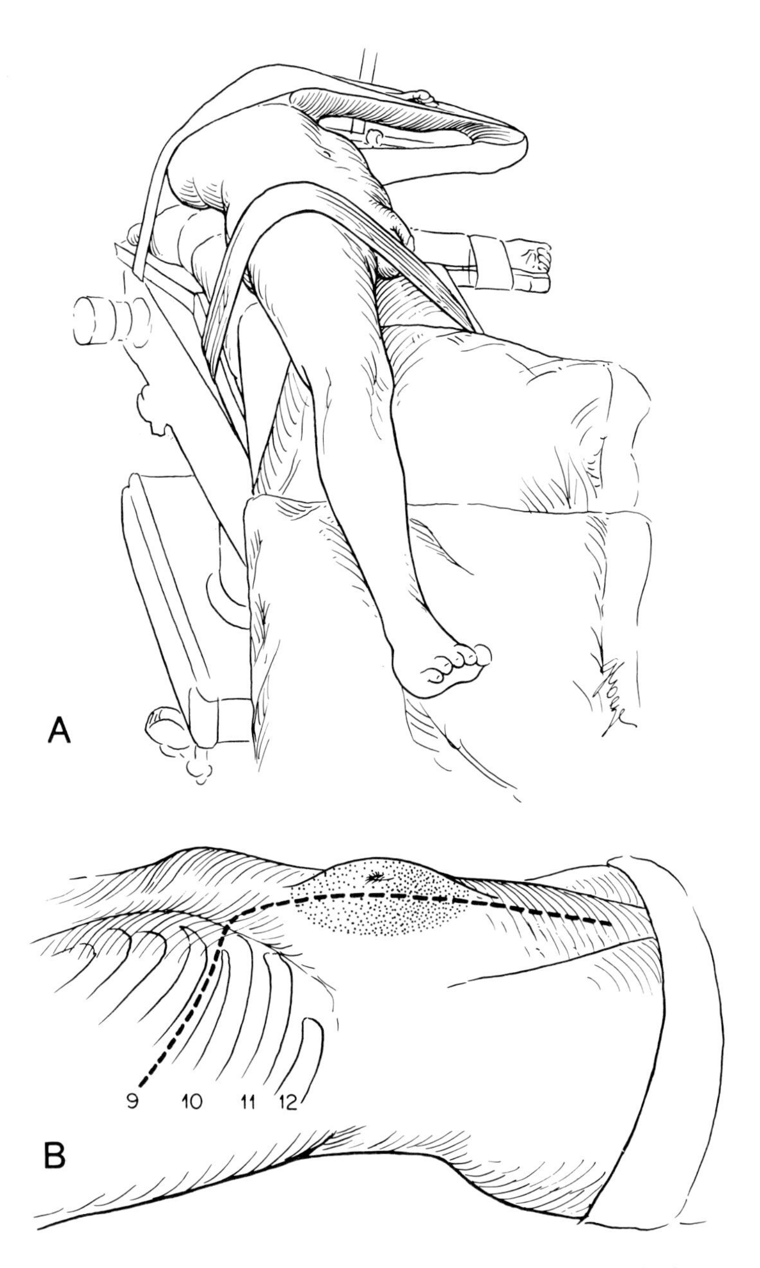

Figure 8.2. Proper positioning of the patient for the modified thoracoabdominal approach. *A*, note that the pelvis is nearly supine and that the shoulders are angled approximately 30°, with the patient placed as close to the ipsilateral side of the table as possible. *B*, note that the abdominal portion of the incision extends high into the epigastrium and then is directed inferiorly as a paramedian incision. (Adapted from D. G. Skinner. Considerations for management of large retroperitoneal tumors: use of the modified thoracoabdominal approach. *Journal of Urology*, *117*:605, 1977.)

contralateral costachondral junction and the paramedial extension is not necessary. For large tumors a T-shaped incision is utilized by dropping a paramedian incision or midline extension inferiorly off the horizontal epigastrium incision. For very large tumors, or tumors associated with a vena caval tumor thrombus, when control of the vena cava above the diaphragm or at the level of the right atrium is desired, a higher incision is used resecting the 8th or 7th rib.

I prefer a rib resection to an intercostal incision as a careful comparison reveals no difference in pain or the postoperative requirement for analgesics; it is rapid, easy to close, and allows wider exposure without fracturing adjacent ribs.

The muscles overlying the rib and the periosteum are incised using the cautery and a subperiosteal resection is performed.

The anterior rectus fascia is incised, the rectus muscle retracted laterally, and the rectus muscle transected in the epigastrium. This prevents denervation of the rectus with resultant diastasis and weakness of the abdominal wall.

The costochondral junction is then divided after bluntly passing a Mayo scissors under the cartilage into the abdominal cavity. This is an important step as it identifies the plane between the muscle and fascia of the abdominal wall and the peritoneum. Since all abdominal muscles and the diaphragm insert into the ribs and/or costochondral junction, this maneuver is the key to developing a retroperitoneal plane. At this point, the peritoneum can be dissected off the abdominal muscles and fascia by a combination of blunt and sharp dissection. Medially, at the region where the lateral abdominal muscles fuse to form the aponeuroses of the anterior and posterior rectus sheath, the peritoneum is quite adherent, and sharp dissection may be necessary to dissect it off the posterior rectus fascia. In mesomorphic or endomorphic individuals, dissection is facilitated because of the thin fatty areolar layer between the peritoneum and posterior rectus fascia. A small peritoneotomy is not uncommon medially but usually the peritoneum can be dissected completely off the remaining posterior rectus fascia medially, the transverse abdominal muscle laterally, the diaphragm superiorly, and the quadratus lumborum posteriorly. The posterior rectus fascia is then divided longitudinally and any peritoneotomies closed. The pleura is then incised through the posterior periosteum and the diaphragm split posterior and parallel to the direction of its fibers. A self-retaining Finochietto retractor is then placed utilizing the holes in the retractor blades to secure each protruding costal cartilage. A careful palpation of the ipsilateral lung should be performed in search of unsuspected pulmonary metastases together with a close inspection of the mediastinum and supraclavicular regions.

The next step is the development of the plane between the anterior surface of Gerota's fascia and the posterior parietal peritoneum. This is best initiated superiorly where one can usually readily identify the plane between the cephalad extension of Gerota's fascia and the peritoneum as it attaches to the diaphragm. It should be remembered that posteriorly the peritoneum passes over the apical portion of the kidney and adrenal to attach to the diaphragmatic muscles. The key to developing the plane between the anterior surface of Gerota's fascia and the posterior parietal peritoneum is identification of the thin, completely avascular, fibroareolar tissue which separates the two. There are only three major vessels that penetrate through Gerota's fascia into the peritoneum below the insertion of the hepatic veins into the vena cava: the celiac artery, the superior mesenteric artery, and the inferior mesenteric artery. Therefore, this plane can be followed across the midline to the contralateral side. The most important landmark to be identified during this dissection is the origin of the superior mesenteric artery—easily identified by following the inferior mesenteric vein to its junction with the splenic vein to form the portal vein. Medial to this junction is the origin of the superior mesenteric artery passing anteriorly directly over the left renal vein. This anatomic relationship is extremely important to the understanding of retroperitoneal anatomy and is essential to the safety of the superior mesenteric artery (Fig. 8.3).

Once the retroperitoneum has been elevated off the anterior surface of Gerota's fascia across the midline, the inferior mesenteric artery is ligated and divided except in elderly individuals when a more limited approach is usually warranted with preservation of the inferior mesenteric artery. Ligation of the inferior mesenteric artery allows elevation of the colonic mesentery which then provides a complete bilateral access to the retroperitoneum below the origin of the superior mesenteric artery.

The next step depends upon the pathology and the desired operation. The following description of a left thoracoabdominal radical retroperitoneal lymph node dissection for testicular tumors will be presented in detail followed by modifications for right-sided lesions. Once the inferior mesenteric artery has been divided and the mesentery of the descending colon elevated off the anterior surface of Gerota's fascia, one traces the inferior mesenteric vein to its junction with the splenic vein. Immediately medial to this will be the origin of the superior mesenteric artery. One will also note that as one palpates the aorta in a cephalad direction, the superior mesenteric artery will come off anterior and hinder further cephalad palpation. Immediately below this, or inferior to this, is the left renal vein crossing over the aorta.

At this point the origin of the superior mesenteric artery is skeletonized. Several large lateral arteries or lymphatics coming from the mesentery run parallel with the superior mesentery artery and should be secured with hemoclips to prevent significant loss of lymphatic fluid. Dissecting out the origin of the superior mesenteric artery allows identification of the left crus of the diaphragm which surrounds the aorta at this location. Located on this crus is the celiac ganglion which is usually clipped and divided.

Gerota's fascia is then dissected from its cephalic attachments to the diaphragm, dividing between hemoclips several arterial and venous communications between the adrenal and phrenic vessels. This completely frees Gerota's fascia and the adrenal from the crus of the diaphragm and the diaphragm itself.

Gerota's fascia is incised immediately over the left renal vein which is widely mobilized. This necessitates ligation of the spermatic vein, ligation of the adrenal vein, and ligation of the posterior ascending lumbar vein. Once the renal vein has been dissected and retracted caudally with a vein retractor, the lymphatic and fibroareolar tissue overlying the aorta is divided and dissected laterally allowing identification of the renal artery or arteries. These vessels should then be dissected out as far as feasible into the renal hilum. At this point it is usually best to incise Gerota's fascia lateral to the kidney and dissect it off the renal capsule. Gerota's fascia should be divided directly over the renal vein in such a way that

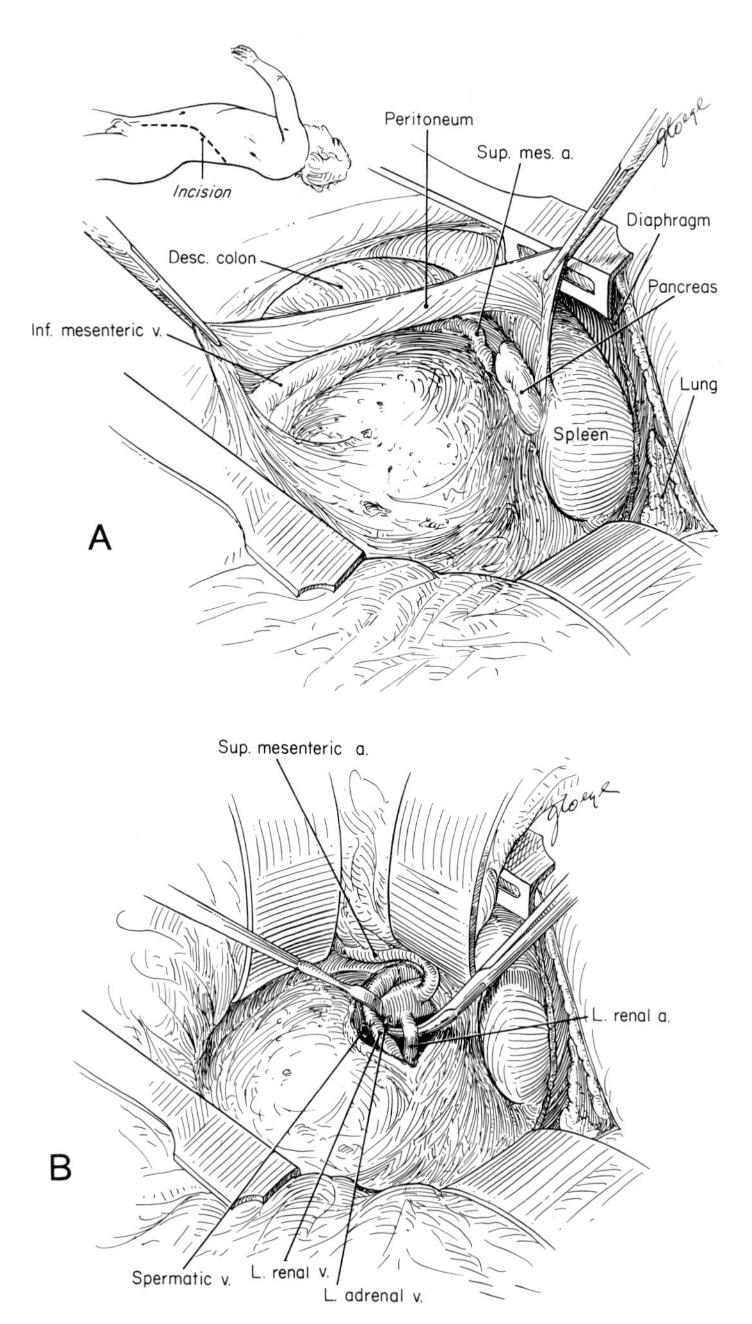

Figure 8.3. Diagram illustrating the development of the plane between the anterior surface of Gerota's fascia and the posterior parietal peritoneum. *A*, peritoneum may or may not be entered depending on the surgeon's preference and the degree of tumor burden. In learning the technique of this operation, initially it may be useful to open the peritoneum inasmuch as this allows the surgeon accurately to determine the plane between the lateral peritoneal reflection and the anterior surface of Gerota's fascia. Definition of this plane is one of the important aspects of this operation, its proper identification is heralded by the findings of avascular fibroareolar tissue separating the two surfaces. Once this plane is identified it is further developed medially beyond the great vessels by both sharp and blunt dissection. The inferior mesenteric vein can be traced to its junction with the splenic vein immediately identifying the origin of the superior

half of Gerota's fascia will pass anterior to the renal pedicle and the other half posterior. This allows further safe dissection of the renal hilum. The ureter needs to be carefully protected and should now be dissected out.

Once the kidney has been completely dissected, the fibroareolar tissue directly overlying the aorta is further incised all the way distally to the aortic bifurcation. The inferior mesenteric artery is relegated at its origin from the aorta. The aorta is then further skeletonized and all lumbar arteries ligated and divided, completely mobilizing the aorta. There are usually three pairs of lumbar arteries distal to the renal pedicle. These are best secured with silk ligatures rather than hemoclips since the hemoclips may catch on gauze sponges and be dislodged.

Dissection continues over the top of the left renal vein to the vena cava and then down the contralateral side of the vena cava. It is usually possible to sweep all fibroareolar tissue over the top of the vena cava to the ipsilateral side necessitating ligation of only the ipsilateral lumbar veins. The dissection continues down the vena cava to the insertion of the right spermatic vein where the dissection proceeds more medially down to the point where the right common iliac artery crosses over the vena cava.

At this point the origin of the right renal artery is further dissected from the aorta and this represents the upper limits of dissection on the contralateral side. The right renal artery is dissected out to the point where it crosses the crus of the diaphragm and all fibroareolar and lymphatic tissue is swept medially and inferiorly. This is the location of the contralateral sympathetic chain and if there is no gross evidence of extensive disease one tries to preserve these ganglia. The aorta can then be elevated by means of a vein retractor and all fibroareolar tissue is swept medial over the intervertebral ligaments to the ipsilateral side.

The spermatic cord is then dissected out of the internal ring. For germinal testicular tumors it is generally not necessary to dissect the external iliac artery beyond the point of its origin, as the bifurcation of the common iliac usually represents the distal limits of dissection. All fibroareolar tissue is then swept from the hypogastric and common iliac vessels toward the residual specimen. Great care must be taken not to injure the ureter in this process, and it should be retracted laterally. Once the distal limits of the dissection have been further defined, all fibroareolar tissue is then swept off the aortic bifurcation and the sacral promentory and the entire specimen is then removed.

Careful inspection should then be made to make sure that all bleeding is well controlled.

I routinely inspect the origins of all lumbar arteries and further secure them with medium hemoclips. I also secure the inferior mesenteric artery with a hemoclip.

---

mesenteric artery, the most important landmark for both right- and left-sided tumors. *B*, immediately below (caudal and posterior) the origin of the superior mesenteric artery is the left renal vein. Gerota's fascia should be opened over the renal vein with ligation of the gonadal vein, the adrenal vein, and the normally present lumbar vein that enters posteriorly, which facilitates retraction of the renal vein to expose the left renal artery at its origin from the aorta. (Adapted from D. G. Skinner. *Urologic Clinics of North America*, 5:253, 1978.)

It is not necessary to fix the kidney, as it adheres quite rapidly to the bare muscular surface. A No. 32 chest tube is routinely inserted. Five milileters of an 0.75% solution of bupivacaine hydrochloride is injected into the intercostal neurovascular bundles of the 7th, 8th, 9th, 10th, and 11th ribs. This can be easily done by percutaneous injection with a finger placed within the thorax to make sure the needle is properly placed. Care must be taken not to inject the solution intravascularly. The diaphragm is closed with a running 0 Dexon suture in two layers. Closure of the thoracic part of the incision can be facilitated by a figure 8 suture through and though No. 1 Dexon sutures securing all of the muscular layers of the chest in one layer. Medially, the diaphragm should be incorporated in several of these sutures. The posterior fascia is closed with a running 0 Dexon suture and the anterior fascia with an interrupted figure 8 0 Dexon sutures.

We routinely give mannitol at the time of dissection around the renal pedicle or before initiation of hypotensive anesthesia, as this seems to prove beneficial in maintaining an excellent urine output throughout the procedure and in reducing the amount of arterial spasm due to dissection of the pedicle.

For right-sided tumors the dissection starts along the vena cava at the insertion of the lowest hepatic vein. The vena cava is circumferencially dissected free and the adrenal vein ligated. I routinely remove the ipsilateral adrenal. The vena cava can then be widely mobilized to allow sweeping of all fibroareolar tissue as well as the celiac ganglion off the right crus of the diaphragm behind the vena cava toward the ipsilateral kidney.

For massive retroperitoneal disease it is best to initiate the procedure as an intraperitoneal operation. One then frees the ascending colon and the mesenteric attachments to the small bowel from the retroperitoneum. This This allows the entire colon as well as small bowel to be elevated on the superior mesenteric artery pedicle and placed in a bowel bag on the chest. This provides wide exposure to the most massive retroperitoneal disease. Again, the landmarks are the same and the safety of the superior mesenteric artery must be maintained. For extensive tumors involving the vena cava it is usually best to plan to resect the vena cava distal to the insertion of the renal veins and, in some cases, it is necessary to remove the ipsilateral kidney. Details of this approach have been described in detail.

COMPLICATIONS AND COMMENTS

Since the operation is performed retroperitoneally, postoperative ileus is minimal, and most patients are discharged from the hospital by the 7th to 9th postoperative day. Several comments seem appropriate, however, in helping reduce possible complications and facilitating the procedure and convalescence.

The cisterna chyli commonly originates between the aorta and vena cava just caudal and posterior to the origin of the right renal artery. Failure to ligate the cisterna may result in a chyle fistula, with considerable loss of lymph and protein during the postoperative period. This usually resolves spontaneously during the postoperative period and does not result in chylous ascites unless proximal lymphatic obstruction due to tumor is present.

Bleeding from an avulsed lumbar vessel may occur, but can usually be avoided by individual ligation and division of each pair distal to the renal pedicle. Placement of hemoclips on the distal portion of the vessel facilitates this part of the operation, but it is best to ligate the origins of lumbar arteries and veins from the aorta and vena cava, because clips may be dislodged later in the procedure causing troublesome bleeding behind the great vessels. Occasionally, bleeding from a torn lumbar artery or vein will develop despite all precautions, in which case use of an Allis forcep clamp is helpful and 4-0 arterial silk sutures should be available at all times.

Concern over possible devascularization of the spinal cord is not warranted, provided no lumbars are ligated above the renal pedicle. The spinal cord ends at the level of the first lumbar vertebral body. Its nutrient arteries—the longitudinal, anterior, and posterior spinal arteries—arise from the vertebral arteries and receive additional blood from the aortic intercostal and high lumbar arteries through radicular branches. The main lower radicular artery providing collateral blood supply to the anterior spinal artery is called the arteria radicularis magna or artery of Adamkiewicz. This artery originates from the thoracic aorta in 50% of patients and from the lumbar region in the other 50%. However, it has been demonstrated that in those patients in whom the arteria radicularis magna originates in the lumbar region, there is an important radicular artery from the lower thoracic aorta, which is constantly present and provides adequate collateral circulation to the anterior spinal artery. Although paraplegia following aortic replacement procedures for abdominal aortic aneurysms was not reported before 1960, and DeBakey's group has reported no neurologic deficits in 1432 consecutive abdominal aortic aneurysm resections, 28 cases of paraplegia following abdominal aortic surgery have been reported in the world literature through March 1975. A review of these 28 cases reveals, however, that 18 were associated with ruptured aneurysms and prolonged hypotension. Permanent paraplegia occurred in only 1 of the 10 patients undergoing elective abdominal aortic aneurysm resection, the remaining patients recovering function. All 28 patients had evidence of extensive atherosclerosis. We believe that the evidence supports our contention that extensive aortic mobilization and ligation of lumbar arteries or aortic replacement is a safe and necessary part of the surgical resection of large retroperitoneal tumors.[8] In our own personal experience we have seen no neurologic deficits in more than 180 patients.

Metastatic retroperitoneal tumors seldom invade the walls of the vena cava or aorta but they may encase it. Efforts to resect these extensive retroperitoneal tumors are probably warranted, provided extensive metastatic disease is not present above the diaphragm and adjuvant chemotherapeutic agents are available. In these cases the entire vena cava below the insertion of the renal vein can be removed, and when the aorta is involved as well, aortic bypass should be considered to allow an en bloc resection of tumor. Bypass may be preferable to sharp dissection to avoid the possibility of tumor spill and hemorrhage from the injured aortic wall.

Ureteral injuries may occur when least expected, usually just before removal of the retroperitoneal specimen when the surgeon is dissecting tissue off the ipsilateral iliac region. Because the ureter has been skeletonized during this procedure, it is best to perform a vesicopsoas hitch and to reimplant the ureter above the level of the iliac vessels. Compromised blood supply makes primary ureteroureterostomy dangerous, particularly if the injury has occurred in the middle or upper third of the ureter. Nephrectomy is strongly recommended in this situation, provided the opposite kidney is normal, or a possible autotransplant and ureteral reimplantation can be considered.

Occasionally, a polar vessel to the kidney will be ligated inadvertently during a retroperitoneal lymph node dissection. It is generally best to do nothing about this, since all collateral renal circulation is removed with the dissection, and secondary hypertension is very unusual.

Retroperitoneal drains are not necessary, but chest tubes should be employed routinely to avoid the reported 30–35% incidence of hemopneumothorax with consequent prolonged hospitalization. In general, the tubes are maintained on suction until significant drainage ceases and then are placed on water seal for 24 h before removal. Accumulation of pleural effusion may necessitate thoracentesis or, rarely, the reinsertion of a chest tube. This problem can be avoided, however, by meticulous closure of the diaphragm.

Postoperative pain may be minimized by the administration of bupivacaine as an intercostal block at the time of surgery.[3]

Other postoperative complications from retroperitoneal lymph node dissection are similar to those with any major surgical procedure. Several points, however, should be emphasized. With the modified unilateral or bilateral dissection, the sympathetic ganglia are removed unilaterally. This results in a unilateral sympathectomy with a warm ipsilateral leg due to peripheral vasodilatation as compared with the normal but relatively cool contralateral extremity. An occasional frantic call from the Intensive Care Unit can be resolved if the contralateral distal pulses are predictably intact.

Occasionally diarrhea may result from ischemia to the large bowel after ligation of the inferior mesenteric artery, but this is rare in young patients and usually successfully managed conservatively without long-term sequelae.

Ejaculatory impotency or retrograde ejaculation commonly results from bilateral retroperitoneal lymph node dissection and is seen in approximately 65–70% of patients undergoing that dissection. This results from resection of the lumbar sympathetic ganglia or division of the sympathetic nerves where they cross over the sacral promentory at the level of the aortic bifurcation. The possibility of this late sequelae must be discussed with the patient preoperatively, but it should also be placed in proper perspective relative to the overall merits of the node dissection. Furthermore, there is evidence that many patients with testicular tumors may be infertile before any therapy is initiated. Many of these patients have atrophic contralateral testis with semen analysis revealing severe oligospermia with poor morphology and motility. Semen analysis prior to therapy may eliminate this long-term complication as being meaningful to the overall management plan. In those patients who have good quality as well as quantity of semen prior to therapy, semen cryopreservation may allow successful subsequent artificial insemination.

In summary, retroperitoneal lymph node dissection is a well established urologic procedure. The thoracoabdominal approach is ideally suited for maximum exposure to the retroperitoneal area. Complications from this procedure can be minimized by careful surgical technique and a thorough knowledge of the anatomy of the retroperitoneum. It is, nonetheless, a major operative procedure and should be undertaken only by those thoroughly trained in major surgical technique and totally familiar with retroperitoneal anatomy.

Other approaches to the retroperitoneum, described elsewhere in this book, have proven equally effective in pathologic staging and control of retroperitoneal disease. Pathologic staging (placing patients in groups A, B_1, B_2, B_3, and C) allows selection of a specific chemotherapeutic approach that has achieved a high cure rate associated with minimal morbidity in terms of hospitalization or lost time from work. While the future may offer a more limited node sampling procedure in an effort to preserve fertility, current evidence suggests that it is the patients with the most limited microscopic disease that benefits most from meticulous surgical staging and may, thereby, avoid recurrence and the need for intensive platinum, vinblastine sulfate and bleomycin combination chemotherapy. This point should be emphasized in lieu of the lack of sensitivity of biochemical tumor markers for minimal disease and our inability to carefully assess and monitor the retroperitoneal nodes. A meticulous surgical staging procedure currently allows selection of the least toxic chemotherapeutic agent or combination tailored to maximum survival of the individual patient, eliminates retroperitoneal recurrence and remains a most important factor for dictating therapeutic plans.

CONCLUSION

The 1970s saw dramatic changes in the management of nonseminomatous germ cell tumors of the testis which resulted in a tumor-free survival of 96% for all patients with stage A and B disease and a tumor-free survival in excess of 70% for patients with advanced disseminated disease. Biochemical tumor markers are helpful in the management of advanced disease and in evaluating clinical suspicion of tumor recurrence, but they have a more limited value in patients who initially present with early stages (A and B) of nonseminomatous germ cell tumors of the testis, since their influence on the therapeutic regimen is minimal and the treatment failure rate in optimally managed patients is so low.

Improved chemotherapy utilizing platinum, vinblastine sulfate and bleomycin is largely responsible for the remarkable improvement in survival, but a meticulous lymphadenectomy remains the most important determinant in selecting the least toxic chemotherapeutic adjuvant, eliminating local retroperitoneal recurrence and obviating the need for radiation therapy.

REFERENCES

1. Chute, R., Soutter, L., and Kerr, W. S., Jr. Value of theracoabdominal incision in removal of kidney tumors. *N. Engl. J. Med. 241:*951, 1949.
2. Cooper, J. F., Leadbetter, W. F., and Chute, R. The thoracoabdominal approach for retroperitoneal gland dissection: its application of testis tumors. *Surg. Gynecol. Obstet. 90:*486, 1950.
3. Crawford, E. D., Capparell, D. B., and Skinner, D. G. Intercostal nerve block with thoracoabdominal incisions. *J. Urol. 121:*290, 1978.
4. Donohue, J. P., Einhorn, L. H., and Perez, J. M. Improved management of nonseminomatous testis tumors. *Cancer 42:*2903, 1978.
5. Einhorn, L. H., and Donohue, J. P. Improved chemotherapy in disseminated testicular cancer. *J. Urol. 117:*65, 1977.
6. Samuel, M. L., Holoye, P. Y., and Johnson, D. E. Bleomycin combination chemotherapy in the management of testicular neoplasia. *Cancer 36:*318, 1975.
7. Scardino, P. T., and Skinner, D. G. Germ cell tumors of the testis: improved results in a prospective study using combined modality therapy and biochemical tumor markers. *Surgery 86:*86, 1979.
8. Skinner, D. G. Considerations for management of large retroperitoneal tumors: use of the modified thoracoabdominal approach. *J. Urol. 117:*605, 1977.
9. Skinner, D. G., and Scardino, P. T. Relevance of biochemical tumor markers and lymphadenectomy in management of nonseminomatous testis tumors: current perspective. *J. Urol. 123:*378, 1980.
10. Sweet, R. H. Carcinoma of the esophagus and the cardiac end of the stomach. *JAMA 135:*485, 1947.
11. Tavel, F. R., Osius, T. G., Parker, J. W., Goodfriend, R. B., McGonigle, D. J., Jassie, M. P., Simmons, E. L., Tobenkin, M. I., and Schulte, J. W. Retroperitoneal lymph node dissection. *J. Urol. 89:*241, 1963.

9

Historical Perspectives on Node Dissection

William J. Staubitz, M.D., F.A.C.S.

Retroperitoneal lymphadenectomy is recognized and accepted today as an effective treatment for testis tumor. The first radical operation for malignant teratomas was credited to Kocher[17] in 1882. This was not a retroperitoneal lymphadenectomy as we practice today, but an attempt to remove large metastatic masses from the retroperitoneal space. It was recognized even then that malignant tumors of the testicle treated by simple castration alone is a highly fatal disease. Kober[16] in 1899 reported a mortality of 85% in 113 cases treated by orchiectomy only. From 1882 to the present, or 100 years, the operation has been modified, abandoned, revived on several occasions and ultimately perfected. It is the purpose of this chapter to review and trace the highlights of the development of radical retroperitoneal lymphadenectomy over this past century.

Most[23] in 1899 described the normal lymphatic drainage of the testis which is regarded as a major contribution to the understanding of the natural history of testicular cancer. He showed that cancer of the testicle metastasizes first and primarily to a limited zone of the lumbar lymph nodes which lie on the aorta for the left testicle and on the vena cava for the right. Communication between these two groups does occur but only secondarily. Cuneo[7] in 1901 reported his findings concerning the primary lymphatic drainage of the testes and traced their path on the right side from the renal pedicle to the iliac bifurcation adjacent to the vena cava and on the left to the nodes adjacent to the aorta from the renal pedicle to the iliac bifurcation.

This discovery by both Most[23] and Cuneo[7] changed the surgical approach to therapy of testis tumors. Prior to their reports, surgeons such as Kocher[17] in 1885 and later Bland-Sutton[2, 2a] were removing large retroperitoneal masses of metastatic testis cancer with little attention to the testis lymphatic drainage. After the publication by both of these anatomists, surgeons redirected their efforts to the lumbar lymphatic chain.

Hinman[13] in 1923 reporting on his own experience with retroperitoneal lymphadenectomy for malignant teratoma of the testis indicated that the evolution of the radical operation could be divided into three periods:

"1. Attempts to remove clinically appreciable abdominal metastases.
2. Realization of the gravity of such procedure, its futility and attempts to perfect the method.

3. Development of the present retroperitoneal lymphadenectomy made possible by exact knowledge of the lymphatic drainage of the testicle."

In the first period, beginning in 1882, the first surgeon was Kocher[17] followed by Bland-Sutton,[2] and several others.

In the second period Stimson[30] (1897) proposed a high excision of the cord and inguinal glands.

In the third period, Roberts[24] in 1901 is credited with the first retroperitoneal lymphadenectomy for malignant testis tumor in this country. He presented his paper before the American Surgical Association on June 3, 1902. The patient on which this first operation was performed was 68 years old who had developed a mass in the left testicle in May, 1901. A left orchiectomy was performed in July 1901, and a pathological diagnosis of squamous cell carcinoma was made. In September 1901 a small nodule was noted in the inguinal incision. On October 16, 1901, Dr. Roberts made a median incision from the umbilicus to the pubis, and later extended the incision to the anterior superior spine of the left ilium. Upon entering the abdominal cavity, he divided the peritoneum over the aorta and dissected the fatty tissue over the aorta at its bifurcation and carried the dissection to a point approximately 2 inches above the aortic bifurcation. He described this dissection as time consuming and difficult due to the large frame and fat of the patient. A postoperative fecal fistula developed 2 weeks later and several attempts to close this failed. The patient died on December 8, 1901 from sepsis and peritonitis. The pathological findings in the four excised lumbar lymph nodes showed metastatic disease in two of the four nodes removed.

The American literature contained no substantial series of cases until 1919 when Hinman[14] reported on six cases and reviewed the literature. Forty-six cases had been reported and most of these originated in Europe. Cuneo[8] of France is credited with performing the first successful resection of the lumbar gland-bearing area on August 26, 1906. The resection included four enlarged lymph nodes, one of which contained metastatic disease. The patient was followed for 3 years and remained free of disease. He then was lost to follow-up. Other surgeons reporting their results during this early period were Raymond Gregiore[12] and Maurice Chevassu.[4–4b]

The beginning of radiation therapy as an effective treatment modality began early in the 1920s. Remarkable cures were reported following the use of radium packs for large abdominal masses. Barringer and Dean[1] reported their experience with 36 cases of teratoma of the testes. A radium pack was used with a dose factor of 12,000 mCi hours at 6 cm distant. Of the 36 cases, 3 were listed as operable, without evidence of local or metastatic disease, 8 were inoperable with metastatic involvement, 19 patients had postoperative recurrence of disease, and 6 were classified as prophylactic irradiation. These six patients were referred after operation before metastasis had been noted. The overall results of radiation therapy in these 36 cases were: 11 alive and well, 14 died of disease, and 11 were lost to follow-up.

With the success of radiation therapy, the radical surgical approach was practically abandoned in the 1920s and 1930s. A few papers appeared in the American literature concerning radical surgery for testis tumors.

Hinman[13] in 1923 and 1933[15] updated his original paper of 1919,[14] adding several more cases of his own and reviewed the literature. Cahill[3] in 1941 reported his experience with the radical operation. Of the 18 patients having this operation 15, or 83%, were alive for more than 1 year, 3 for as much as 10 years.

It was not until 1948 when Lewis[19, 20] reported on his experience at the Walter Reed Army Hospital during World War II that radical surgery for testis tumor had its renaissance. Lewis was in a very fortunate position at Walter Reed Army Hospital. The induction of millions of young men into the Armed Service, and the concentration of treatment of testis tumors to this hospital, provided Lewis with an extremely large number of patients with testis tumors, a malignancy that most urologists would normally see only a few times a year. In addition, the hospital had on its staff Dr. Nathan B. Friedman, a radiologist, and Dr. Robert A. Moore, a pathologist, both of whom provided expertise in this area of oncology. This team of three highly qualified individuals, with over 900 cases of testis tumors to work with, were able to develop the first logical classification of testis tumors; they randomized various forms of treatment, one of which was a radical retroperitoneal lymphadenectomy for nonseminomatous testis tumors.

Lewis[19, 20] fashioned his unilateral retroperitoneal lymphadenectomy after that used by Hinman.[13-15] Several incisions were described by Hinman but he preferred that which paralleled the lower border of the 12th rib coursing anteriorly and inferiorly to the region of the internal inguinal ring (Fig. 9.1). This approach provided exposure of the major portion of the aorta and inferior vena cava, as well as the vessels within the pelvis (Fig. 9.2). Lewis modified this unilateral lymphadenectomy by extending the incision to the tip of the 11th rib, affording greater exposure in the region of the renal pedicle. Lewis stated that ". . . crossed metastases below the renal pedicle have not been observed by us except when there is tremendous involvement of the precaval nodes from right testis tumor."[19, 20] He therefore felt a unilateral dissection was adequate. Of the 169 radical retroperitoneal resections performed in the series of 250 patients reported in 1948, there was no mortality, four had complications, and 58 (34%) had metastatic lymph nodes removed.

The radical operation utilized during the early period, and even to the time of Lewis, was used on all testis tumors regardless of histological type. As more experience was gained with the use of the radium pack, it was soon discovered that seminoma responded extremely well to this form of treatment and most of the x-ray successes were with this type of tumor. Hinman[15] in his publication of 1933 states that "It seems fairly well established that seminoma is radiosensitive, but that the teratoma is radioresistant." Furthermore he states "It is still an open question whether in a case of pure seminoma, with or without clinical evidence of metastases, radical resection should be attempted or entire trust put in deep x-ray therapy."[15] Lewis[19] in his report of 1948 made the following statement "Personally, I would like to have a radical orchiectomy for any type of testis tumor. It may not be indicated for seminoma because of the radiosensitivity of that tumor, but I have in mind the possibility of inclusion of some more malignant elements unrecognized in the routine

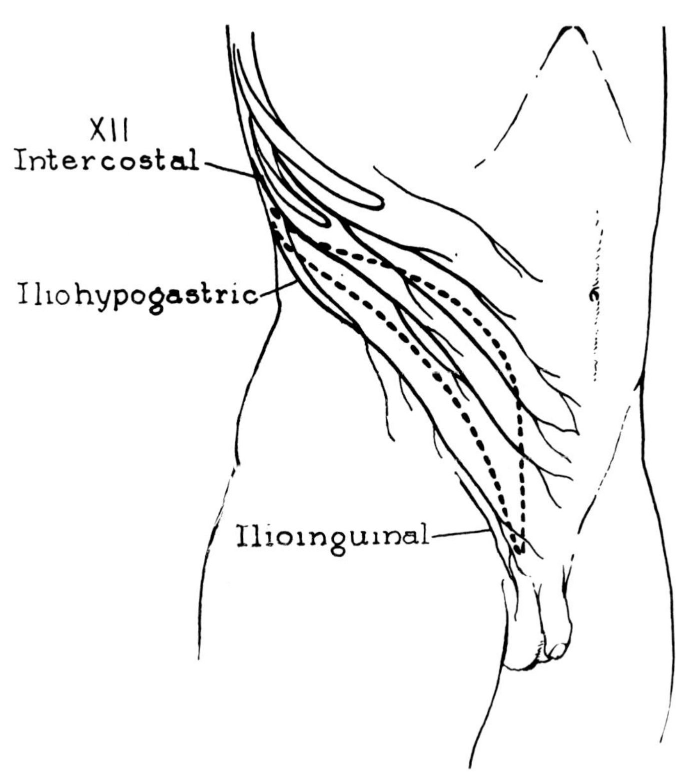

Figure 9.1. Line of incision from Frank Hinman's article February, 1933.[15] (Reproduced by permission from F. Hinman. Tumors of the testis. *Surgery, Gynecology, and Obstetrics*, 56:451, 1933.)

section." Lewis[19] described a radical orchiectomy consisting of removal of the testis with its tunics, the epididymis, vas, entire spermatic cord, and the retroperitoneal lymph chain from the inguinal ring to the renal pedicle. In his conclusions Lewis[19] states that "For seminoma, simple orchiectomy plus radiation therapy is probably sufficient." The experience at Walter Reed Army Hospital more or less established the future therapy of seminoma as simple orchiectomy with external irradiation to the lymph-bearing areas. Few if any retroperitoneal lymphadenectomy were used subsequently in the therapy of seminoma.

Many who adopted the Lewis operation for retroperitoneal lymphadenectomy experienced difficulty in dissecting lymphatic tissue in relation to the renal pedicle, particularly if there was metastatic disease in this area. Chute *et al.*[5] encountered this difficulty and used the thoracoabdominal route to perform a radical retroperitoneal lymphadenectomy on five patients with testis tumor. He originally used this surgical approach for large renal tumors and found it gave excellent exposure of the renal pedicle and areas well above the renal vessels.

Cooper *et al.*[6] in 1950 reported their experience with four patients using the thoracoabdominal approach. They concluded that ". . . the adaption of the thoracoabdominal approach for retroperitoneal gland dissection in carcinoma of the testis has provided excellent exposure of the renal pedicle and infradiaphragmatic area in comparison to previous conven-

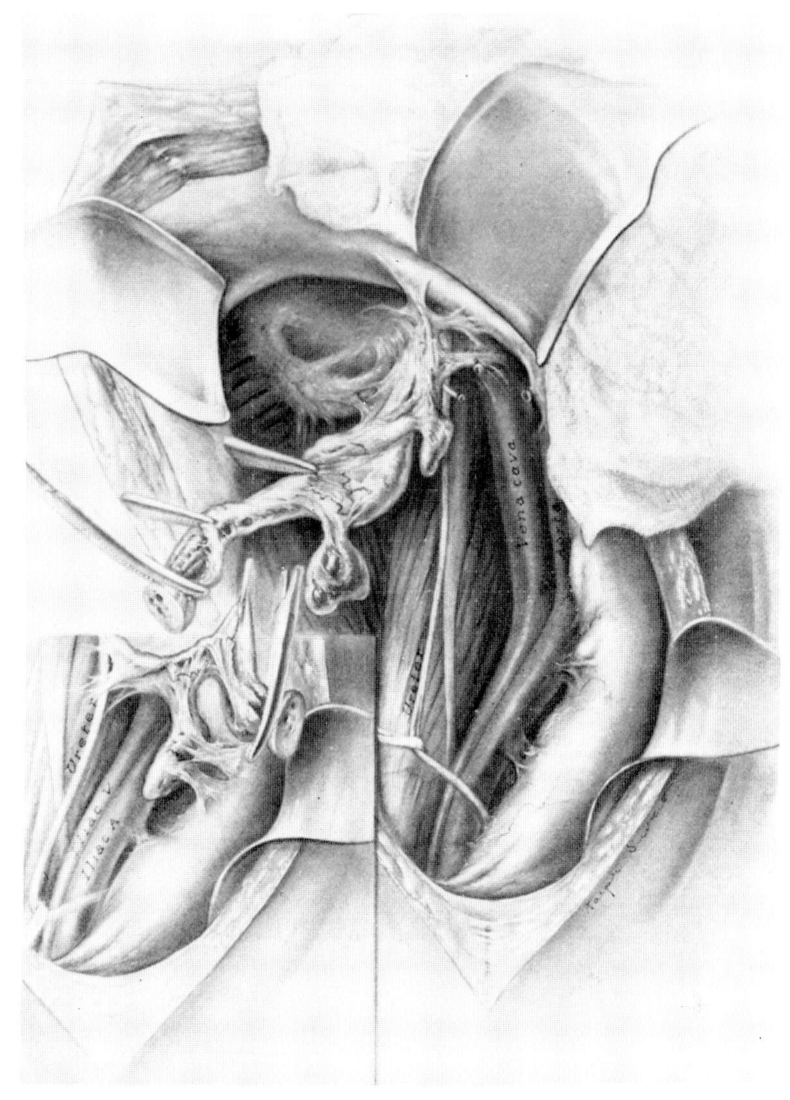

Figure 9.2. Completion of operation from Frank Hinman's article February, 1933.[15] (Reproduced by permission from F. Hinman. Tumors of the testis. *Surgery, Gynecology, and Obstetrics, 56:*452, 1933.)

tional incisions of the type originally described by Hinman and Chevassu."

Others who adopted this combined chest and abdominal route were Staubitz *et al.*[26] and Dowd.[10] With increased interest in the use of the radical retroperitoneal lymphadenectomy for nonseminomatous testis tumor, important clinical observations were made indicating that there is in fact contralateral metastatic node involvement. Lowry *et al.*[21] found in autopsy studies of 34 patients dying with testis tumors that bilateral retroperitoneal node involvement with metastatic disease occurred in patients. Leadbetter[18] reported that 5 of 19 patients in his series had evidence of contralateral node involvement.

Citing these reported experiences of bilateral retroperitoneal lymph node involvement with metastatic disease and supported with their own experience of three cases of bilateral involvement in a total of 19 cases, Mallis and Patton[22] adopted a bilateral retroperitoneal lymphadenectomy employing the transperitoneal approach. Using a midline incision extending from the xyphoid to the symphysis pubis, these authors described their technique as follows: "The transverse colon is brought out of the abdominal cavity and placed on the chest. The small bowel is completely exteriorized to the right. The posterior peritoneum is opened between the aorta and vena cava. This exposes the retroperitoneal area. Dissection is then begun above the left renal vessels and, using both blunt and sharp dissection, the nodes and surrounding tissue are removed *en bloc* from around both renal pedicles, the vena cava and the aorta. The dissection is carried down to and including the bifurcation of the iliac vessels." Others reporting their experience with bilateral retroperitoneal lymphadenectomy for testis tumors using the transperitoneal route were Stehlin *et al.*[29] and Staubitz.[27]

At this point in time, 1958, the majority of radical retroperitoneal sites of nonseminomatous testis tumor removal were given postoperative irradiation. There was some question, especially among radiologists as to whether or not the radical operation was really necessary. The radiotherapists emphasized that with the improved equipment now available a more effective dose of radiation could be delivered to the retroperitoneal area. In addition they claimed that it was now possible to control the scattered irradiation and hence cut down the involvement of adjacent bowel and kidneys.

In an effort to truly evaluate the therapeutic value of a retroperitoneal lymphadenectomy for nonseminomatous testis tumors, Staubitz and associates[28] in 1958 embarked on a prospective study at the Roswell Park Memorial Institute in Buffalo, N.Y. A transperitoneal approach was used to perform a bilateral retroperitoneal lymphadenectomy. No adjuvant therapy was used either pre- or postoperatively. In 1970 this study was completed. It showed that with a transperitoneal bilateral retroperitoneal lymphadenectomy only, the 5-year survival of 65 patients was 86% for stage I and 70% for stage II.

This prospective study clearly and undisputedly established the clinical value of a retroperitoneal lymphadenectomy for testis tumor. This study, in addition, shows that with retroperitoneal lymphadenectomy alone, 70% of the patients with metastatic lymph node disease can be cured.

With the establishment of radical lymphadenectomy as a useful operation for the treatment of nonseminomatous testis tumor, several surgeons endeavored to improve the operation. Two types of surgical approaches were ultimately accepted as superior to the several types proposed by a number of groups. The two being the transabdominal route and the classic thoracoabdominal approach whose proponents claimed an adequate bilateral dissection was possible with this transthoracic technique.

Donahue[9] in 1977 described his modification of the transperitoneal approach in which he extended the retroperitoneal dissection above the renal pedicle to the base of the diaphragm. He names this a bilateral suprarenal-hilar dissection. By dividing the inferior mesentery vein, the pancreas can be mobilized and retracted off the anterior surface of

Gerota's fascia. This exposes the area of the superior mesenteric artery, and dissection is started in this area, carried down around the aorta and cephalad between the aorta and either crus of the diaphram. The tissue is divided as high as possible at the base of the diaphram. The dissection is then carried down to the renal vessels. Donahue[9] states that "in our series, one of every four patients with tumor-containing infrahilar nodes also had tumor in the suprahilar nodes."

Modifications were also made in the thoracoabdominal operation in an effort to perform a more thorough bilateral lymphadenectomy, as well as to facilitate the removal of large retroperitoneal metastases.

Skinner[25] in 1977, described his modification of the original thoracoabdominal procedure. He made the incision in the midaxillary line as high as the 8th rib and divided the costochondral junction. Fraley[11] also utilized the bed of the 8th or 9th rib and carried the incision medially across the ipsilateral rectus muscle. The incision is extended across the contralateral rectus as necessary.

SUMMARY

It became well established as far back as 1899 that treatment of testis tumors by simple orchiectomy alone was inadequate and carried a mortality of 85%. In addition, this disease occurred most frequently in young males whose loss to society at an early age was profound. As a result of these two sinister facts, a concerted effort over a period of 100 years has been carried out by dedicated and concerned physicians and surgeons to improve the survival of patients suffering from this disease.

The following individuals or groups whose contribution have led to phenomenal achievements of survival success can be listed in reference to the time of their accomplishment.

1. Kocher in 1882 first removed large retroperitoneal metastatic masses in an effort to prolong life of the patient.
2. Most in 1899 and Cuneo in 1901 described the lymphatic drainage of the testis and thereby laid the foundation for an effective retroperitoneal lymphadenectomy.
3. Roberts in 1901 performed the first radical operation for testis tumor in this country.
4. Cuneo in 1906 is credited with performing the first successful resection of the lumbar lymph glands.
5. Hinman in 1919 published his experience with 6 cases and established the need and effectiveness of the radical operation.
6. Lewis in 1948 brought about a renaissance of radical retroperitoneal lymphadenectomy after it had been abandoned because of high operative mortality. He accomplished this by taking advantage of a very large number of patients at his disposal with testis tumors, and proved that the radical operation could be performed without mortality and with few postoperative complications.
7. Chute and associates in 1949 introduced the thoracoabdominal surgical approach which facilitated a more thorough dissection.
8. Mallis and Patton in 1958 introduced the concept of a transabdominal bilateral lymphadenectomy. This technique made it possible to remove the retroperitoneal lymph nodes on both the ipsilateral as well as the contralateral sides with one operation.

9. Staubitz and associates[26] in 1958 established the therapeutic value of a bilateral retroperitoneal lymphadenectomy as a necessary and effective modality. This surgical technique used alone without the assistance or addition of either pre- or postoperative adjuvant treatment. They[28] proved that a bilateral retroperitoneal lymphadenectomy alone can cure 70% of patients with retroperitoneal metastatic disease.
10. Donahue in 1977 added a suprahilar dissection to the transabdominal route. This enabled him to dissect as high as the base of the diaphram.

The efforts and contributions of the above, as well as of many others, have improved the quality of life and the survival of patients with testis tumors. The survival rate has been raised from 15% a century ago to over 90% in 1980. Today with the successful application of effective chemotherapy to supplement the retroperitoneal lymphadenectomy, there is strong evidence that survival of nonseminomatous testis tumor may approach 100%.

REFERENCES

1. Barringer, B. S., and Dean, A. L. Radium therapy of teratoid tumors. *JAMA 77:*1237–1240, 1921.
2. Bland-Sutton. An improved method of removing the testicle, and spermatic cord for malignant disease. *Lancet 2:*1906, 1909.
2a. Bland-Sutton. The "radical" operation of the testicle. *Lancet 1:*606, 1912.
3. Cahill, G. G. Testicular tumors. *Trans. Am. GU Surg. 33:*301–309, 1941.
4. Chevassu, M. Tumeurs de testicule. Thesis of Paris, 1906. Les diagnostic clinique des cancer du testicule. *Presse Med. 17:*363, 1910.
4a. Chevassu, M. Le traitement chirurgical des cancer du testicule. *Rev. Chir. 41:*628–886, 1910.
4b. Chevassu, M. Deux Cas d'epitheliome du testicule traites par la castration et l'ablation des ganglion lombo-aortiques. *Bull. Soc. Chir. Lief. 50B:*414–532, 1887.
5. Chute, R., *et al.* The value of the thoracoabdominal incision in the removal of kidney tumors. *N. Engl. J. Med. 241:*951–960, 1949.
6. Cooper, J. F., Leadbetter, W. F., and Chute, R. The thoracoabdominal approach for retroperitoneal gland dissection: its application to testes tumors. *Surg. Gynecol. Obstet. 90:*486, 1950.
7. Cuneo, B. Note sur les lymphatiques du testicule. *Bull. Soc. Anat. (Paris) 71:*105, 1901.
8. Cuneo, B. Quoted by Hinman, F. The radical operation for teratoma testis. *Surg. Gynecol. Obstet. 28:*495–508, 1919.
9. Donahue, J. P. Retroperitoneal lymphadenectomy: the anterior approach including bilateral suprahilar dissection. *Urol. Clin. North Am. 4:*509–521, 1977.
10. Dowd, J. B. Surgery of testicular tumors. *Surg. Clin. North Am. 42:*779, 1962.
11. Fraley, E. E. Surgical treatment of stage 1 and state 2 nonseminomatous testicular cancer in adults. *Urol. Clin. North Am. 4:*453–463, 1977.
12. Gregoire R. Considerations sur l'etat des ganglions dans le cancer du testicule. *Arch. Gen. Chir 2:*1, 1908.
13. Hinman, F., *et al.* The radical operation for teratoma testis. *Surg. Gynecol. Obstet. 37:*429–451, 1923.
14. Hinman, F. The radical operation for teratoma testis. *Surg. Gynecol. Obstet. 28:*495–508, 1919.
15. Hinman, F. Tumors of the testis. *Surg. Gynecol. Obstet. 56:*450–461, 1933.
16. Kober, G. M. Sarcoma of the testicle. *Am. J. Med. Sci. 117:*535, 1899.
17. Kocher. Frankheiter de maennl geschlechlsongane. *Deutsche Chir. Lief, 50B:* 414–532, 1882.
18. Leadbetter, W. F. Treatment of testis tumors based on their pathological behavior. *JAMA 151:*275–280, 1953.
19. Lewis, L. G. Testis tumors: report of 250 cases. *J. Urol. 59:*763–772, 1948.
20. Lewis, L. G. Radical operation for tumors of the testis. *JAMA 137:*828–832, 1948.

21. Lowry, E. C., *et al.* Tumors of the testicle analysis of 100 cases: preliminary report. *J. Urol. 55:*373–384, 1946.
22. Mallis, N., and Patton, J. F. Transperitoneal bilateral lymphadenectomy in testes tumors. *J. Urol. 80:*501–503, 1958.
23. Most. Ueber die lymphagefaesse des hoden. *Arch. F. Anat. u. Enlwicklungsgesch.* p. 113, 1899.
24. Roberts, J. B. Excision of the lumbar lymphatic nodes and spermatic vein in malignant disease of the testicle. *Ann. Surg. 36:*539–549, 1902.
25. Skinner, D. G. Considerations for management of large retroperitoneal tumors: use of the modified thoracoabdominal approach. *J. Urol. 117:*605, 1977.
26. Staubitz, W. J., *et al.* Management of testicular tumors. *JAMA 166:*751, 1958.
27. Staubitz, W. J., *et al.* Surgical management of testicular tumors. *NY State J. Med. 59:*3959–3963, 1959.
28. Staubitz, W. J., *et al.* Surgical treatment of nonseminomatous testes tumors. *Cancer 32:*1206–1211, 1973.
29. Stehlin, J. S., Jr., *et al.* Lymphadenectomy *via* the transperitoneal (anterior abdominal) approach for cancer of the testis. *Am. J. Surg. 97:*756–765, 1959.
30. Stimson, J. C. A new approach for malignant disease of the testicle. *Med. Rec. NY, 52:*623, 1897.

10

Transthoracic Retroperitoneal Lymphadenectomy for Testicular Cancer

Elwin E. Fraley, M.D.

There is no one best way to do an extended retroperitoneal dissection for nonseminomatous germ cell-derived testicular cancer, and any surgeon of consequence knows the importance of this axiom. The correct surgical approach must be determined in the light of the patient's body build; previous treaments, including operations; the experience and beliefs of the surgeon; and the precise nature of the retroperitoneal disease. Thus, anyone contemplating operating on the retroperitoneum for testicular cancer should know the technical variations of both the transabdominal (Chapter 11) and the transthoracic approaches.

This chapter will describe only the transthoracic approach and the variations that we have found essential in the management of patients with these neoplasms. The operation we use is designed to remove the tissues from the posterior mediastinum, the suprahilar regions, and both sides of the great vessels down to the level of the inferior mesenteric artery. Usually the dissection then becomes unilateral and is extended to the level of the bifurcation of the common iliac vessels. All connective, lymphatic, and autonomic tissue in this region is removed, as is the ipsilateral adrenal gland. It is especially important to dissect the renal hilum free of all lymphatics, because this is one of the primary landing areas for metastases from testicular tumors.

INDICATIONS

There is little doubt that the transthoracic approach is used less widely now than is the transabdominal approach, probably for the following reasons. First, it is widely thought that it matters little whether one does a suprahilar or infrahilar dissection, especially for low stage disease; and therefore many surgeons do not emphasize the type of dissection described herein, whatever the approach. In addition, many who believe that a thoroughgoing dissection proximal to the renal vessels is important also believe that this can be done transabdominally. Second, it is the opinion of many that a retroperitoneal dissection can be done more quickly transabdominally. Third, it is the impression of many surgeons that there is less postoperative morbidity with the transabdominal technique. Finally, many urological surgeons have no training in chest surgery and consequently avoid it.

What, then, are the major advantages of the transthoracic approach? First, if one accepts the need for suprahilar dissection, I believe that the operation is facilitated, especially in extremely robust patients, by the transthoracic approach. In fact, I find the dissection above the right adrenal gland and dorsal to the vena cava, proximal to the short hepatic veins, to be very difficult with the transabdominal approach, even in a thin patient. Therefore, I favor the transthoracic approach or some modification thereof in the large, barrel-chested patient and the obese patient, especially for right-sided tumors. Second, I have found no important difference in the amount of time required to do this operation by the transthoracic as compared with the transabdominal route, because the exposure of the posterior mediastinum and suprahilar regions is more complete with the transthoracic route, for reasons illustrated herein. Furthermore, time usually is not the most important consideration in these patients, most of whom are young and otherwise healthy. However, from a practical standpoint most surgeons will choose the operation that they do most efficaciously unless there is a compelling reason to use an alternative, more time-consuming technique. Third, the transthoracic approach makes it possible to inspect the ipsilateral lung and to palpate the mediastinum, which, at least theoretically, improves the accuracy of staging by operation. Also, not infrequently, in patients being operated on for more advanced disease, resections of pulmonary metastases can be carried out at the same time as the retroperitoneal dissection.

There is one contraindication to the transthoracic operation: previous radiation therapy. It is my impression that these patients too often have prolonged drainage from the chest postoperatively. The same caveat may apply to patients who have had prolonged chemotherapy, but this is less certain.

PREOPERATIVE PREPARATION

Because this is primarily a chapter on surgical technique, the problems of preoperative staging and indications will not be discussed. Reviews of these subjects and discussions of our philosophy regarding them have been published recently.[1, 2]

Little needs to be said about most aspects of the preoperative preparation. There are, however, three points worth mentioning. First, we advocate the use of preoperative and intraoperative intravenous infusion of Lasix and mannitol to induce a sustained diuresis. The type of meticulous dissection done in the renal hilum often causes severe renal artery spasm and renal ischemia, which often is alleviated by the combined use of sustained diuresis and intraoperative vasodilators applied directly to the renal arteries. A second important part of preoperative preparation is explaining to the patient that he probably will be sterile postoperatively, at least for a few years, because of aspermia (dry ejaculation). Many patients find this difficult to accept, but it can be pointed out that perhaps as many as half of them will recover fertility spontaneously and that progress is being made in drug treatment to restore ejaculation.[3] Also, it is only fair to point out that alternative treatments (chemotherapy and radiation) also may cause sterility. Unfortunately, there are few data on the incidence, but our experience with Velban, bleomycin, and cisplatin suggests that at the very least this treatment causes oligospermia in most patients and that at worst it causes azoospermia in most. Further, it is not known whether destruction of germ cells by chemotherapy is reversible, and this will not be known for some time. Perhaps it also is worth noting that testicular cancer frequently is associated with atrophy of the germ cells remaining outside the tumor, and many patients are severely oligospermic before any treatment is given.[4]

Another fact worth emphasizing is that these patients should have their bowels prepared by mechanical cleansing for at least 2 days before surgery. Enemas should be avoided, especially the night before surgery, because the large bowel can be overdistended with air and fluid, making the operation difficult.

OPERATIVE TECHNIQUE

The position of the patient that is most suitable for the transthoracic operation and the site of the incision are both shown in Figure 10.1. We use a T-type incision, the vertical component of which usually is made in the midline. We divide the ipsilateral rectus muscle and a portion of the contralateral rectus muscle, the extent being determined by the amount of exposure needed. In some cases, particularly in slender patients with left-sided cancers, we extend the transverse component to the costochondral junction and do not open the chest. This modification gives much the same exposure as does the transthoracic approach.

The peritoneum is identified, and the space between the dorsal peritoneum and Gerota's fascia is developed (Fig. 10.1). On the right side, this is continued until the duodenum and head of the pancreas are seen. They are dissected free and retracted medially with a Kocher maneuver. On the left side, the small bowel and the tail of the pancreas are dissected free and retracted medially in the same manner. The ipsilateral adrenal gland and suprarenal tissues will then be visible. During the dissection, all lymphatic tissue must be removed from the peritoneum, especially in the region where it is in close contact with the spermatic vessels.

Posterior Mediastinal and Suprahilar Dissection

The adrenal gland and perirenal tissues are dissected free from the diaphragm, and the chest is opened. Usually, only a small distal segment of rib needs to be removed. The diaphragm is then opened with a curvilinear incision that stops opposite the 12th thoracic and 1st lumbar vertebrae. (A common mistake is to divide the diaphragm in a straight

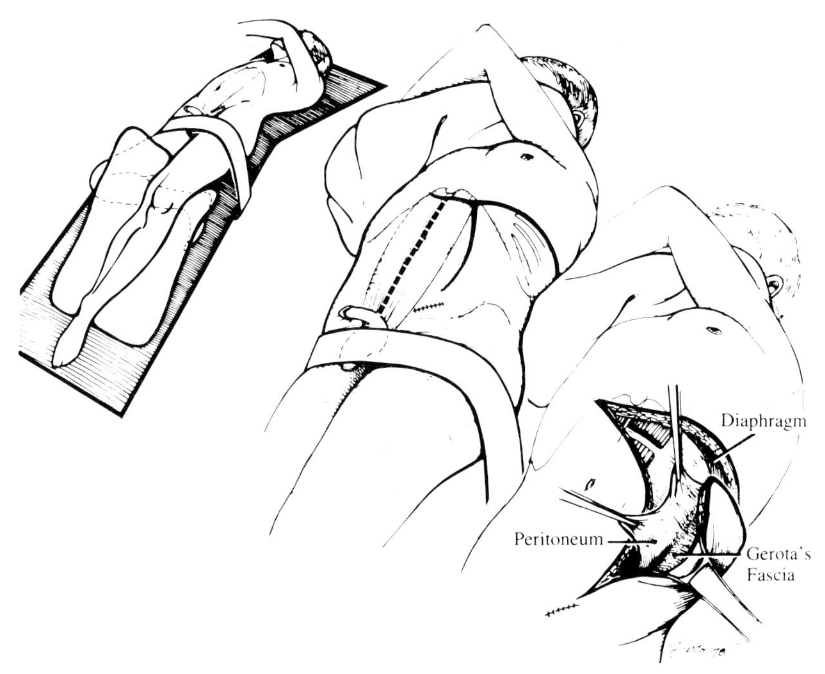

Figure 10.1. (Figs 10.1–10.7 are each reproduced by permission from E. E. Fraley, C. Markland, and P. H. Lange. Surgical treatment of Stage I and Stage II nonseminomatous testicular cancer. *Urol. Clin. North Am. 4*:453–463, 1977. ©W. B. Saunders Co. Used with permission of the copyright holder.)

line perpendicular to the psoas muscle so that the incision ends midway in the 11th or 12th rib. This restricts the exposure, because the chest cannot be spread adequately.) At this time (but not before) a standard chest retractor or ring retractor can be inserted to enhance the exposure of the suprarenal area.

When the dissection is being done on the left side, the next step is to identify the left crus of the diaphragm and pass the index finger underneath it parallel to the vertebral bodies, pushing the aorta away so that the crus can be opened for 3–5 cm. The aorta is then lifted to exposure the lymphatic and connective tissues of the posterior mediastinum.

The dissection of posterior mediastinum should include the tissue from around the pair of lumbar arteries proximal to the celiac axis; the arteries themselves are not divided. A right-angle clamp is used to pull the tissues toward the operator. They should be clipped before they are transected to help prevent postoperative lymphatic fistulas. When the posterior mediastinum has been cleared of all connective and lymphatic tissue, the contralateral fibrous diaphragmatic crus will be visible (Fig. 10.2).

The aorta and the origins of the celiac and superior mesenteric arteries are dissected free, with the lymphatic and connective tissue being removed down to the level of the renal arteries (Fig. 10.3). The tissues proximal to the contralateral renal vessels can be reached by elevating the aorta and inferior vena cava, usually using rubber drains as retractors.

For right-sided tumors, the same type of dissection is performed. However, the diaphragmatic crus cannot be opened until all tissues have been removed from around the inferior vena cava proximal to the right

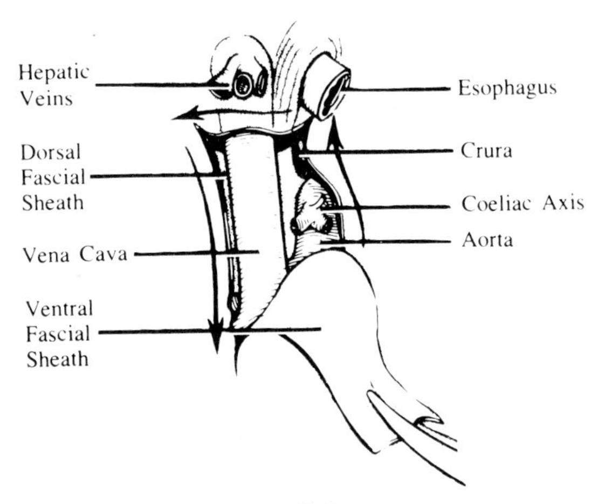

Figure 10.2.

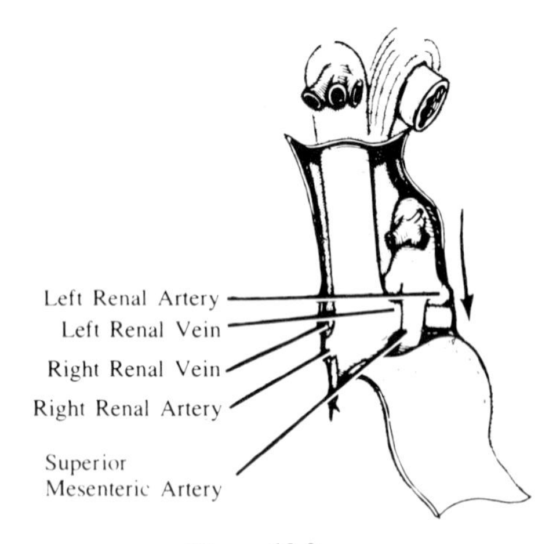

Figure 10.3.

renal vein. This usually involves removal of the main adrenal vein and the periadrenal tissues, after which the vena cava can be retracted medially to expose the right diaphragmatic crus. Sometimes the short hepatic veins must be ligated to gain additional exposure.

Renal Hilar and Infrahilar Dissection

The next step after the suprahilar dissection is completed is the removal of a bloc of tissues extending from just proximal to the renal vessels down along both sides of the great vessels to the inferior mesenteric artery. Initially, we make vertical incisions over the ipsilateral great vessel (aorta or vena cava). Another incision is made at a right angle along the ipsilateral renal vessels and over the kidney so that all of Georta's fascia can be removed from around the kidney and all tissues can be dissected from around the renal artery and vein (Fig. 10.4). We also remove the ipsilateral adrenal gland, because it and the periadrenal tissues may house metastases and because this makes the dissection easier (Fig. 10.5). However, some surgeons leave the adrenal gland; this point of technique is one of personal preference.

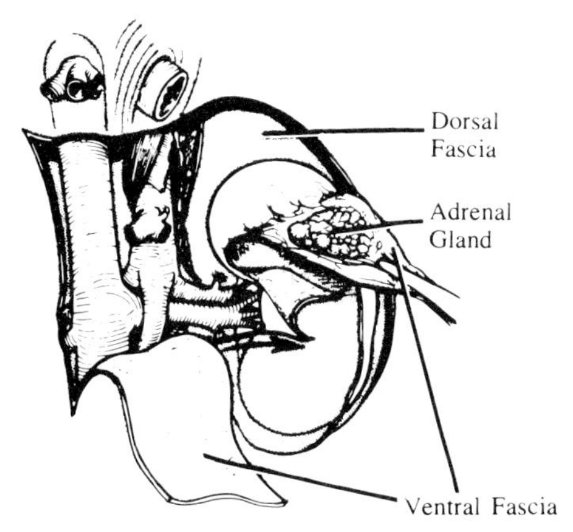

Figure 10.4.

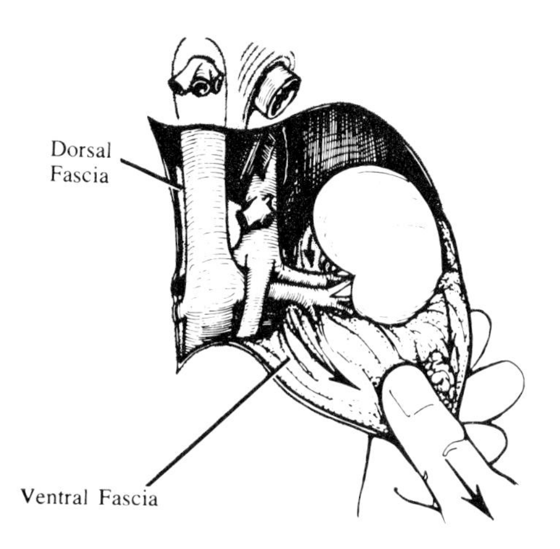

Figure 10.5.

In dissecting the renal hilum, special care must be taken to identify the adrenal blood supply originating from the main renal artery and to ligate the adrenal vessel as far from the renal vessels as possible. Otherwise, bleeding from the adrenal vessel may be difficult to control without damaging the renal artery, especially if it occurs on the left. Throughout the dissection of the renal hilum, we apply vasodilators (2% Xylocaine and 1% papaverine) liberally to the renal vessels to help prevent spasm and renal ischemia.

All lymphatic and connective tissues are excised from around the great vessels from the posterior mediastinum to the inferior mesenteric artery (Fig. 10.6). Dissection underneath these vessels is facilitated by retracting them with rubber drains. The lumbar veins can be divided, but we usually preserve most of the lumbar arteries. The tissues can be removed easily *en bloc* without sacrificing these vessels.

Lymphatic and connective tissue is removed on the ipsilateral side from the inferior mesenteric artery to the bifurcation of the common iliac vessels. Care is taken to preserve the sympathetic and autonomic tissue at the bifurcation of the great vessels in the presacral area. We have postulated that it is because we usually do not extend the bilateral

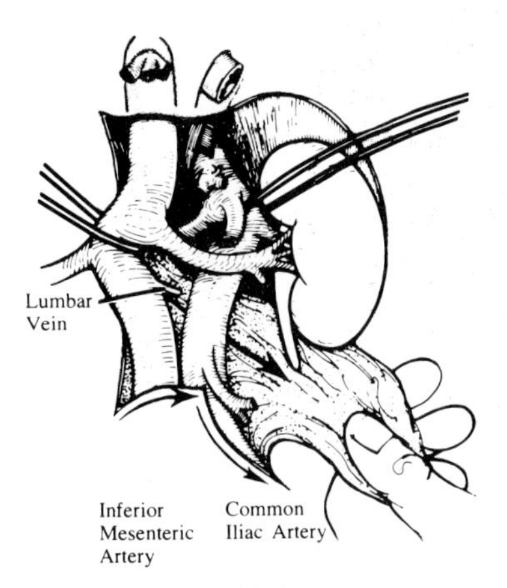

Figure 10.6.

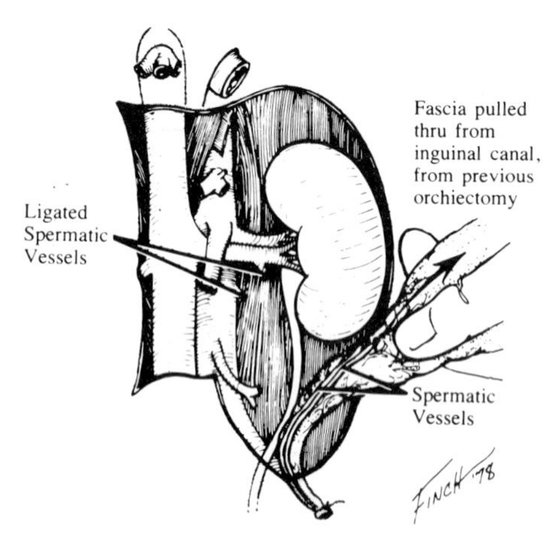

Figure 10.7.

dissection distal to the inferior mesenteric artery that many of our patients eventually regain antegrade ejaculation.[3] However, if many tumorous lymph nodes are seen, we do a more extensive dissection in this region, because the chances that there has been retrograde tumor spread are high.

Care is taken to remove the ipsilateral spermatic vessels and lymphatic tissues, which should have been ligated during orchiectomy with an easily identifiable suture (Fig. 10.7). If there is any question about whether the spermatic cord has been removed completely, the orchiectomy incision should be reopened to make certain.

Modifications

The procedure just described will have to be modified if there is extensive tumor in the retroperitoneum. In patients who have already had retroperitoneal operations or chemotherapy, the ipsilateral kidney and ureter may have to be removed in operations for residual disease. It is far better in most cases to sacrifice the kidney than to compromise the cancer operation.

Another modification is useful in obese patients. In some of these men, it is necessary to open the peritoneum to exteriorize the bowels to get adequate exposure. Such an operation combines features of the transthoracic and transabdominal approaches.

COMPLICATIONS

Although extended retroperitoneal surgery is safe, as evidenced by the fact that we have had no deaths in well over 150 cases, the procedure is not without complications.

The two most frequently encountered major complications in our series are pancreatitis and injury to the renal pedicle resulting in immediate or delayed nephrectomy. Pancreatitis is thought to be caused by the intraoperative traction on the pancreas and appears to us to be more of a problem with the transabdominal approach and in patients who have had chemotherapy. In most cases, it is manifested only by elevations in the serum or urinary amylase or both, although, in a few cases, the patient has symptomatic pancreatitis that prolongs hospitalization. To avoid injury to the renal arteries, I believe that the dissection should be started on the aorta proximal to the arteries and that the renal hilar dissection should be carried out with the aid of both a headlight and operating loops (2× magnification).

Other complications that occur with this operation are, for the most part, common to all surgical operations, with the possible exception of a persistent lymphatic fistula that may occur if the suprahilar and mesenteric lymphatics are not ligated. These fistulas can lead to either chylothorax or a chylous ascites.

DISCUSSION

One of the technical points that warrant discussion is the extent of retroperitoneal dissection necessary for effective treatment of germ cell-derived testicular cancer by operation. As we have emphasized many times, we believe that it is important to begin the dissection proximal to the renal vessels, because the most common landing area for the metastases is in the lymph nodes in the renal hilum around the great vessels. If one starts the dissection at the renal hilum, the proximal margin around the tissues most likely to contain cancer is very narrow. For the same reason, we advocate bilateral dissection. The call for the bilateral, suprahilar dissection also is supported by clinical experience. For example, those series in which the bilateral, suprahilar dissection has been done have produced the best survival figures, especially for patients with low stage disease. Second, Donohue[5] demonstrated that microscopic metastases may exist in the suprahilar nodes even when the infrahilar nodes are tumor free. Third, we have observed several patients referred for tumor recurrences in the retroperitoneum, and almost all had had infrahilar dissections, some of which also were only ipsilateral. Fourth, the rate of retroperitoneal recurrence after a thoroughgoing bilateral, suprahilar dissection is extremely low. In fact, in our series we have had only one documented retroperitoneal recurrence, and this was in the ipsilateral renal hilum.

Another technical point that deserves emphasis is the opening of the crus of the diaphragm at the outset of the dissection. First, this is very easy to do and, second, it certainly makes the dissection of the aorta and the suprahilar region safer, because it makes the area easier to see. In particular, there is less tissue surrounding the aorta after it passes through the diaphragm. Thus, the surgeon can easily enter the tissue plane on the aorta and dissect distally, identifying in succession the celiac axis, the superior mesenteric artery, and the renal arteries. In addition, once the crus is opened, it is easy to identify the main lymphatic trunks that lie on the anterior spinal ligaments so that they can be clipped or ligated, thus helping to prevent postoperative lymphatic fistulas. This technique also has applications in other urological operations where access to the suprarenal aorta is necessary. For example, this approach facilitates placing a vascular clamp well above the renal arteries, either for certain types of renal vascular operations (*e.g.* transaortic endarterectomy) or to achieve lower-torso avascularity when dealing with large renal tumors.[6]

One of the arguments most often advanced against the use of retroperitoneal dissection in the treatment of testicular cancer is that it causes infertility. Some authors have even introduced the term "ejaculatory impotence" to describe the dysfunction that occurs after retroperitoneal dissection, so it is understandable why the casual reader may think that some of these patients are impotent as well as infertile. However, we know of no patient who has lost the ability to achieve a satisfactory erection and experience orgasm as a result of a retroperitoneal dissection as described herein. In addition, if the operation is done as described and the dissection is not carried down past the inferior mesenteric artery on the contralateral side, thus preserving the autonomic nerves in the presacral area, approximately half of the patients will have spontaneous return of antegrade ejaculation within 3 months to 3 years after the operation. Of those who do not, many can have ejaculation restored with various combinations of drugs. In fact, from all available data on infertility and sexual dysfunction after various treatments for testicular cancer, it appears that patients treated by operation alone have higher fertility rates than do those treated primarily by chemotherapy alone, radiation alone, or some combination thereof; and all operation-only patients can expect to be potent and able to experience orgasm. The anatomic basis of these results was described by us recently.[3]

A paper on technique is not necessarily the appropriate forum for discussing whether retroperitoneal dissection will continue to be the cornerstone of treatment for nonseminomatous germ cell-derived testicular cancer. The reader should know, however, that there are those who advocate abandoning this operation, especially for clinically low stage disease. They argue that modern staging techniques are accurate to the point where patients with clinical stage I disease can be followed expectantly, reserving chemotherapy alone or chemotherapy and operation until the clinical situation dictates. There are a few clinical trials in progress testing this approach. Of course, one significant aspect of this disease is that any form of treatment can generate clinically useful information in a short time, so the value of this or similar protocols should be known within 3–5 years.

In the meantime, the following arguments support the continued use of retroperitoneal dissection. First, those series in which operation has been the principal treatment have produced the best overall survival rates for patients with pathologic stages I and II cancers.[2, 5, 7] Second, operation is the most cost-effective treatment, with the lowest morbidity and mortality, and thus is well tolerated by patients. Third, patients with testicular cancer have severe psychological problems as a consequence of their disease, and noncompliance thus is not uncommon whatever the treatment. It seems likely to us that some patients treated only by orchiectomy and follow-up will have advanced disease, sometimes fatal disease, because they will not have returned regularly for examination. Fourth, operation has the fewest long-term side effects. In this regard, it should be remembered that the long-term effects of the present chemotherapy regimen are entirely unknown. How many patients will have progressive renal failure? How many will have serious vascular complications? Will they have an increased incidence of second cancers? These are all legitimate questions to which no one yet knows the answers. Thus, retroperitoneal dissection should remain a part of the treatment for nonseminomatous testicular cancers unless and until carefully controlled clinical trials prove that the patients can be managed just as effectively and efficiently by other means.

CONCLUSION

Not enough emphasis has been given to the difficulty of retroperitoneal dissection. It is a dangerous operation that can result in the loss of vital organs, other horrifying complications, and even death, especially in the wrong hands. It requires experience and surgical versatility and should be done only in a medical center where it is part of a multidisciplinary approach to the treatment of testicular cancer.

REFERENCES

1. Fraley, E. E., Lange, P. H., Williams, R. D., and Ortlip, S. A. Staging of early nonseminomatous germ-cell testicular cancer. *Cancer 45:*1762–1767, 1980.
2. Fraley, E. E., Lange, P. H., and Kennedy, B. J. Medical progress: germ-cell testicular cancer in adults. *N. Engl. J. Med. 301:*1370–1377; 1420–1426, 1979.
3. Narayan, P., Lange, P. H., and Fraley, E. E. Ejaculation and fertility after extended suprahilar retroperitoneal lymphadenectomy for testicular tumor. *J. Urol.* (Submitted).
4. Skinner, D. G. Management of nonseminomatous tumors of the testis. In *Genitourinary Cancer*, pp. 470–493, edited by D. G. Skinner and J. B. deKernion. W. B. Saunders, Philadelphia, 1978.
5. Donohue, J. P. Retroperitoneal lymphadenectomy: the nterior approach including bilateral suprarenal-hilar dissection. *Urol. Clin. North Am. 4:*509–521, 1977.
6. Cummings, K. B., Li, W-I., Ryan, J. A., Horton, W. G., and Paton, R. R. Intraoperative management of renal cell carcinoma with supradiaphragmatic caval extension. *J. Urol 122:*829–832, 1979.
7. Skinner, D. G. Non-seminomatous testis tumor: a plan of management based on 96 patients to improve survival in all stages by combined therapeutic modalities. *J. Urol. 115:*65–69, 1976.

11

Transabdominal Lymphadenectomy

John P. Donohue, M.D.

INTRODUCTION

The role of retroperitoneal lymphadenectomy (RPLND) in the management of nonseminomatous testicular cancer is changing.

First, the support of RPLND as an accurate staging method becomes progressively weaker if the *sole rationale* for RPLND is staging alone. Improvements in clinical noninvasive staging continue to accumulate at such a rate that the false-negative experience, combining all available modalities including lymphangiography, approaches 10–20%. Furthermore, the availability of highly effective combination chemotherapy in the event of clinical relapse makes careful observation without RPLND in clinical stage I cases a promising alternative. In this text, we shall hear of the early experience in one such program which has proven encouraging.[14] More years of experience will be necessary, however, to assure that survival, particularly in treated relapsers, will be maintained.

Yet, the decade of the 1970s has revealed that "staging RPLNDs" are associated with superb survival figures. Analysis of these figures suggests, however, that a key to these improved survivals is the very same rescue by combination chemotherapy in people who clinically relapse. A current basic question, yet unanswered, is "Can we say that those estimated 10–20% who relapse following clinical (nonoperative) staging alone will all be cured by chemotherapy?" Probably not, given the reported morbidity and mortality of combination chemotherapy (1–2% for PVB (cisplatin, vinblastine, bleomycin)) used for salvage of relapsing patients with early stage disease. Furthermore, human nature being as it is, compliance in follow-up will not be perfect; some relapsers will not report until they have more advanced disease. Cure with drugs and surgery in this group is much less certain (50–80%). Until we can know a cure is assured at relapse, RPLND in clinically negative patients (admittedly a staging and nontherapeutic procedure in the event of negative nodes) and possible adjuvant treatment in the event of positive nodes remains appropriate, given its low morbidity and high survival figures. But, if clinical studies can still increase in specificity and sensitivity to confidence levels approaching 100% and if chemotherapy can reliably rescue virtually all relapsers, "staging RPLND" may indeed pass from the scene.

At the same time, we shall see RPLNDs done more for persistent or questionable masses following combination chemotherapy. Our experience thusfar[7] suggests this "cytoreductive surgery" after chemotherapy for massive of disseminated disease should be a full RPLND and not merely a biopsy.

So, on the one hand, low stage disease (clinical stage I) may be managed without RPLND in the future but, on the other hand, clinically advanced disease (bulky stage II_B plus and stage III) will ultimately become operable thanks to chemical cytoreductive effects of improved chemotherapy. Such partial remissions can be converted to complete remissions (with no measurable disease) by thorough excisional surgery. Should persistent malignant elements be found in the excised tissue, these patients become candidates for salvage chemotherapy. They enjoy good prognosis for survival (80%) if their residual tumor was completely resected with negative margins.[3]

Clearly the role of the surgeon is shifting from staging early disease to operating for persistent tumor postchemotherapy for more advanced disease.

GENERAL COMMENTS

Chapter 10 describes the anterolateral or thoracoabdominal approach to retroperitoneal lymphadenectomy. This chapter shall describe the alternative anterior or transabdominal midline approach. The rationale and technique of the anterior approach for a retroperitoneal lymphadenectomy has been well described by Patton and Mallis,[13] Van Buskirk and Young[21] and more recently by Staubitz et al.,[20] Whitmore,[23] and Young.[25] The thoracoabdominal approach to the retroperitoneum for staging testis tumors was championed by Leadbetter.[1, 19] He preferred the thoracoabdominal approach which affords good exposure at and above the ipsilateral renal hilum. This approach has been followed with some modifications by Skinner[18] and by Fraley et al.[11]

Some years ago we wished to learn if the midline approach could be developed to allow the same excellent exposure of the suprarenal hilar zones on both sides. Postmortem dissections of the retroperitoneum were done through a midline incision from xiphoid to pubis. Using specialized techniques to mobilize and elevate the pancreas, we were able to assure ourselves that excellent bilateral dissections could be done with high exposure at and above each renal hilum.

PRIMARY DIAGNOSIS

Before discussing the technique for retroperitoneal lymphadenectomy, one comment on primary diagnosis is in order. A prevailing theme in reviewing all series of testis tumors is the delayed diagnosis. Not only does it at times present in an asymptomatic fashion, but at other times it is delayed when symptoms mimic epididymitis. A helpful way of distinguishing epididymitis from testis tumors is the digital separation of the testis anteriorly from the adnexal delivery structures posteriorly. Please note how the epididymis can and should be separated (Fig. 11.1). Sliding the fingers back over the gonad will assist detection of a firm tumor in the testis tubules which are ensheathed in the tunica albuginea. Studious application of this technique in all patients will standardize gonadal examination and increase appreciation of smaller testicular tumors.

Teaching techniques employing this principle above (i.e. digital separation) are being promulgated in many areas with promising results on early diagnosis. We have found this quite effective in the midwest regional program.

SPECIAL PREOPERATIVE PREPARATION AND MEDICAL NOTES

These patients are prepared, as a donor for renal transplantation would be, with overnight intravenous hydration. We use no antibiotics preoperatively or postoperatively.

The bladder is catheterized at the time of draping in surgery. The catheter is usually removed on the second postoperative day. The patient is in the supine position with the right arm suspended from an ether screen or with both arms extended. Topical 1% Xylocaine is used on the renal vessels during the dissection. Emphasis is placed on the intraoperative administration of colloid to replace large third-space losses of lymph

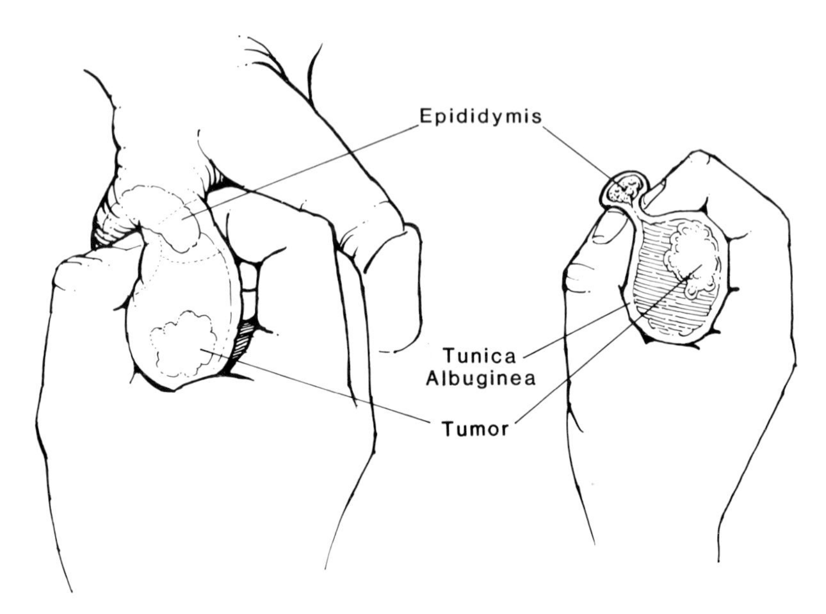

Figure 11.1. Technique of scrotal exam. The preferred technique is the digital separation of the testis anteriorly from the adnexal delivery structures posteriorly. Please note how the epididymis can and should be separated. Sliding the fingers back over the gonad will assist detection of a firm tumor in the testis tubules which are ensheathed in the tunica albuginea. Studious application of this technique in all patients will standardize gonadal examination and increase appreciation of smaller testicular tumors.

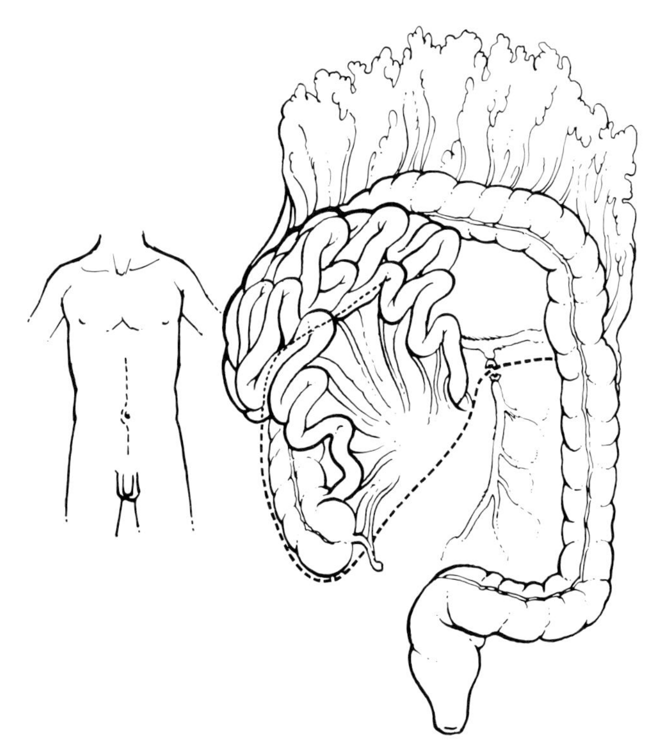

Figure 11.2. Basic mesenteric divisions: right mescolon into the foramen of Winslow, root of small bowel to ligament of Treitz; division of the inferior mesenteric vein and right colic mesentery to renal upper pole. The bowel is then separated from Gerota's fascia below it and placed in a plastic bowel bag on the patient's chest.

during the dissection. Otherwise, falsely high, misleading hematocrit values may follow. An increased need for crystalloid also is apparent, as the losses from the intravascular space into the large, raw third space created in the retroperitoneum can produce significant contraction of effective blood volume. Often, transfusions of whole blood are unnecessary in uncomplicated cases if enough colloid replacement is given.

Preoperative emphasis on pulmonary physiotherapy is given in order to assist the patient postoperatively in this regard. Again, no prophylactic antibiotics are used. If fever develops, appropriate cultures and investigations are made and then the drug is selected, but this is rarely necessary.

TECHNIQUE

Exposure

The incision is midline, xiphoid to pubis. Drapes are sewn in place and an 11-inch circular plastic wound protector is used; then two Balfour abdominal retractors are placed. The abdomen is explored carefully by palpation. Then the basic mesenteric divisions are made in order to mobilize the entire small bowel and right colon (Fig. 11.2) so that they can be placed on the patient's chest in a plastic bowel bag. First, the hepatic flexure is taken down and then the mesocolon is incised from the foramen of Winslow to the cecum. It is important to extend this posterior peritoneal incision through the base of the foramen of Winslow, which covers the anterior surface of the vena cava, because later dissection must extend above this area.

After the right mesocolon is divided, the incision is turned around and the root of the small bowel is incised cephalad to the ligament of Treitz. This incision is carried along the root of the bowel until the inferior mesenteric vein is encountered. This vein must be divided in order to carry the incision in an oblique manner further cephalad, still further into the left upper quadrant, paralleling the inferior border of the pancreas. If the inferior mesenteric vein is not divided, it will restrict the exposure in this area. When the inferior mesenteric vein is divided, the pancreas can be mobilized fully and retracted off the anterior surface of Gerota's fascia. Then the anterior surface of Gerota's fascia is separated bluntly and sharply from the undersurface of the bowel and the pancreatic head and body, as well as the duodenum and cecum. All of this is now completely mobilized and the bowel is placed on the chest in a bowel bag. We no longer recommend a routine appendectomy (the appendiceal stump leaked in one of our cases producing massive peritonitis and abscess

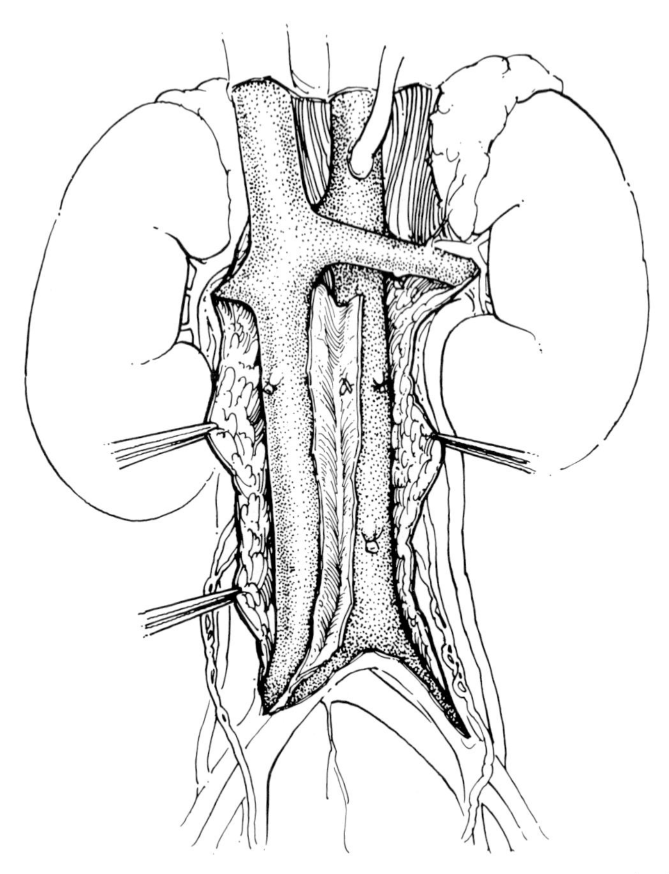

Figure 11.3. The infrahilar aortocaval dissection involves the anterior longitudinal splitting of the nodal and vascular adventitia over the vena cava and aorta, its lateral rotation, and the "squaring out" posterolateral nodal tissue.

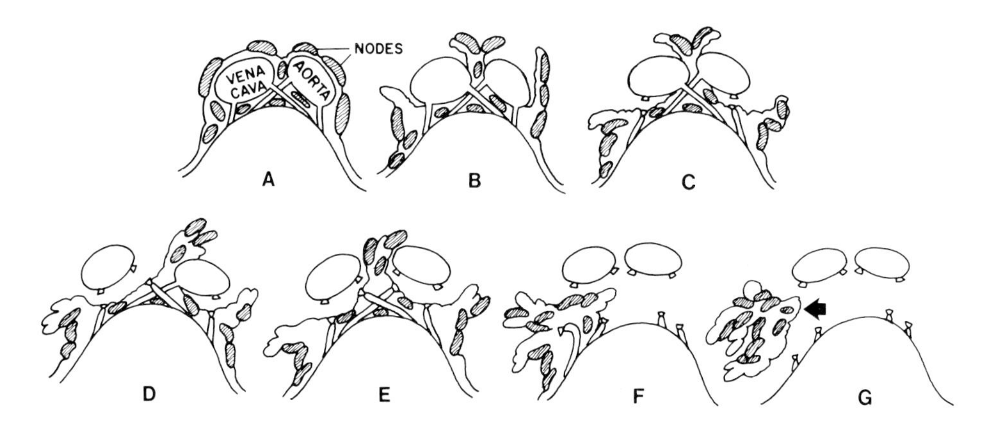

Figure 11.4. An axial view (*A*) showing the anterior split of the nodal package in the subadventitial plane (*B*) and its rotation off the vena cava and aorta after the division of each lumbar vessel (*C–E*). Then the specimen is removed from the posterior body wall by ligating and sharply dividing all the lumbar vessels and ganglia as they emerge from the foramina (*F, G*). The specimen (*arrow*) is easily rotated under the mobilized great vessels after these posterior attachments are divided.

formation.) The retroperitoneum is a rich culture medium postoperatively; all potential sources of contamination should be avoided.

Infrarenal Dissection (Aortocaval Dissection)

This portion of the procedure has been well described in several communications. Basically, the nodal package is split anteriorly down over the inferior vena cava and aorta. The specimen is then rotated off the vessels. This author believes that it is important to divide every lumbar vessel, both aortic and caval, so as to get complete mobilization and central vascular control. Another important maneuver is the squaring out of the upper corners of the nodal package at each renal hilum and taking it down off the posterior body wall at the foramen of L2–L3 (Figs. 11.3 and 11.4). The lateral borders of the dissection are the ureters; the psoas fascia is stripped down parallel to this. The gonadal vein is divided on the left from the renal vein, or on the right from the inferior vena cava. The involved gonadal vein is then followed down to its origin in the groin and dissected out separately and submitted to the pathologist separately.

Care is taken to obtain the divided stump of the spermatic cord with its original ligatures, if at all possible. The vas deferens is clipped and divided so that the distal portion can be submitted with the spermatic vein and cord stump. On the left side, this is then tunneled under the left colic mesenteric artery. The aortic dissection is continued distally by dividing the inferior mesenteric artery. The left colic mesentery is then further mobilized off Gerota's fascia and the splanchnic nervous and venous connections are clipped where necessary to mobilize this thoroughly and, hence, expose the iliac areas from the medial approach without having to divide the left mesocolon. The left ureter is then easily seen over the pelvic brim. As noted earlier, the nodal packages are rotated off the anterior surfaces of both vessels, the dissection being advanced in the subadventitial planes. This allows easy exposure of each lumbar artery and vein and their division between 2-0 silk ligatures. Now the great vessels are completely mobilized (Figs. 11.5 and 11.6). The only thing holding the unfurled nodal package is its posterior and lateral attachments.

Each lumbar artery and venous penetration into the posterior body wall is divided between clips or ligatures. Bleeding venous tributaries are often controlled by Bovie coagulation or additional suture ligature (Fig. 11.5). Once the posterior attachments are divided at the foramina, the nodal package can be wiped off the anterior spinous ligaments with a gauze sponge and drawn under the vessels either medially or laterally. Again, it is convenient for our nodal analysis to submit the aortocaval package of nodes separately and then, later, to submit the two iliac dissections separately. (Formerly, the entire specimen was obtained *en bloc* and laid out on a predrawn template for the pathologist. There were some errors in nodal location once the tissue was placed in formalin, because occasionally the tissue would float off the paper template.)

The iliac dissections extend several centimeters beyond the bifurcation of the hypogastric artery on either side. The same principle of nodal rotation beneath the vessels is employed. The anterior division of the

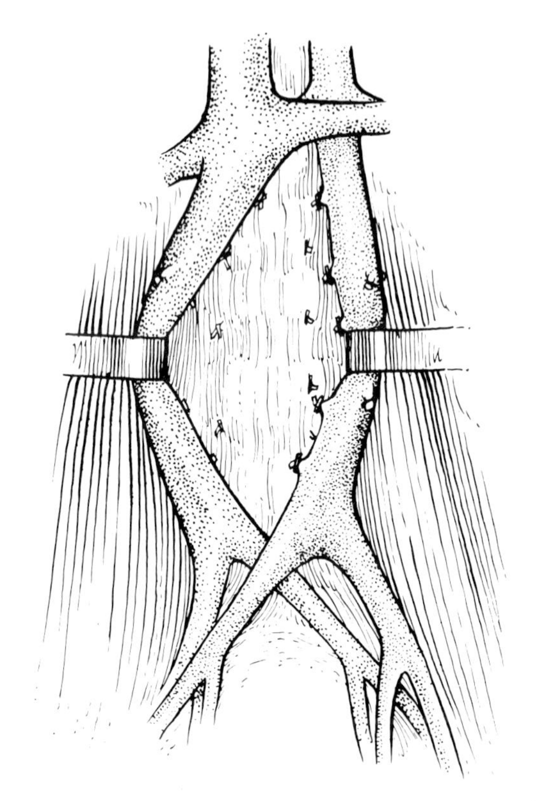

Figure 11.5. At the conclusion of the dissection, the anterior spinous ligaments and medial psoas muscle are seen stripped bare. The lumbar vessels are tied off on the body wall as well as on the great vessels. Each foramen is clear of nodal tissue. Fully mobilized great vessels allow thorough inspection.

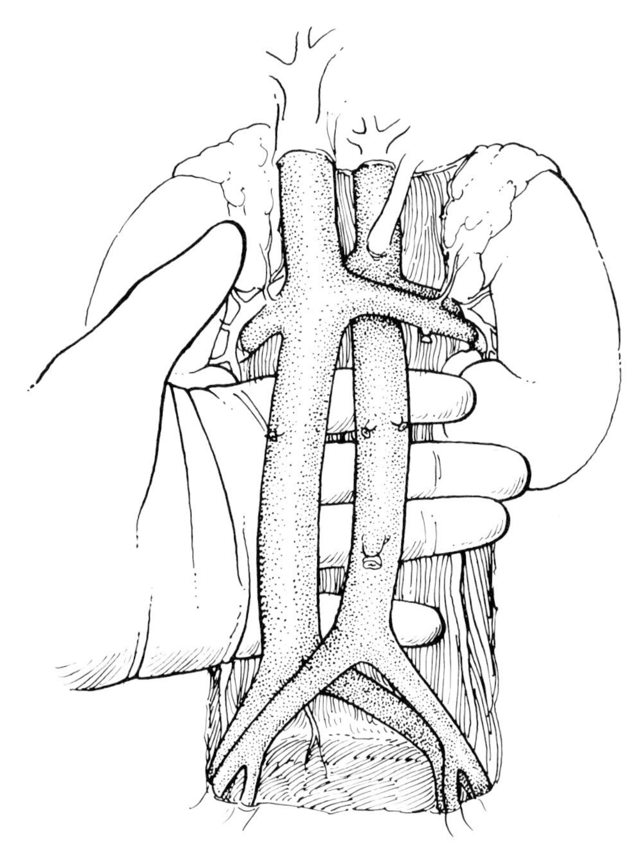

Figure 11.6. The aorta and the inferior vena cava can be manipulated easily during and after the dissection when all the lumbar vessels and the inferior mesenteric artery have been divided. Hemostasis is easily secured with this exposure and vascular mobility. Complete clearance of nodes and removal of bulky tumor deposits are achieved better with this central vascular control.

arteries and veins is carried out and the tissue is rotated below these after the division of any lumbar attachments. It is helpful to depress the psoas muscle in retractors because the nodal chain in the paravertebral area here is often large but not clearly visible without retraction of the psoas. Again, the right iliac and left iliac nodal packages are submitted separately.

The wound is then thoroughly inspected and irrigated. When tumor invasion of the nodes is grossly evident, we irrigate with distilled water, which might lyse any tumor cells that might have been spilled in the wound during dissection. Then we close the mesenteric attachment with running 0 chromic catgut beginning at the left posterior colonic mesentery in the left upper quadrant and proceeding below the pancreas to the ligament of Treitz. Closure is then carried down, closing the root of the small bowel to the cecum up to the foramen of Winslow. We believe that this helps to prevent postoperative bowel complications and that it limits the escape of bloody lymphatic fluid into the peritoneal cavity. The omentum is drawn down over the bowel. The position of the Levin tube is checked. The midline incision is closed with interrupted No. 1 Ethibond sutures placed in the manner of Tom Jones. Buried knots are tied below the fascia to avoid uncomfortable nodules in the subcutaneous tissue in thin patients.

Suprarenal Hilar Dissection

This portion of the dissection refers to nodes above the level of the renal artery extending for several centimeters both above and below the crura of the diaphragm. The lymphatic drainage of the retroperitoneum above the renal vessels is largely retrocrural as it moves into the cisterna chyli just above this level. The cisterna is between the aorta and cava on the anterior spinous ligaments at the L1, to T11 levels. Most of the major lymphatic drainage from the retroperitoneum moves cephalad through this posterior route. There are also smaller nodes and lymphatics on the surface of the crura and medial to each adrenal gland, intermingled with nerves and ganglia. While the major nodes below the level of the renal veins lie mostly anterior and lateral to the great vessels, these assume a posterior lateral relationship to the aorta above the renal vessels. CT scans confirm this as the locus of most bulky suprahilar metastases; they can be seen lying below the crura of the diaphragm on axial views extending to the posterior mediastinum in the chest.

Earlier communications[4] have demonstrated the impracticality of dissecting the suprarenal hilar zones in patients with no gross disease. Our experience has been largely negative in analysis of nodal tissue taken from this zone in patients with stage II_A disease. No patient with right-sided primary tumor and a grossly unimpressive retroperitoneum had positive suprahilar nodes. In like manner, only three patients with left-sided primaries and stage II_A disease had suprahilar nodes; two of these three had their nodes lying just above the renal artery in what could be called the renal hilum. There was only one patient with all negative infrahilar nodes who had a discrete node well above the renal artery medial to the left adrenal. Therefore, on a "net yield" basis, such an extended dissection in patients without gross disease is unnecessary and unwarranted.

Table 11.1.
SECAG:[a] randomized trial, stage II NSGCT

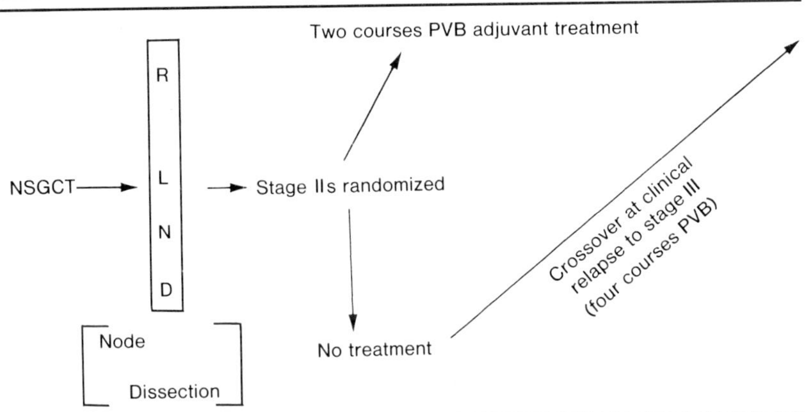

[a] The abbreviations used are: SECAG, Southeastern Cancer Study Group; NSGCT, nonseminomatous germinal testis tumor; and PVB, cisplatin, vinblastine, bleomycin.

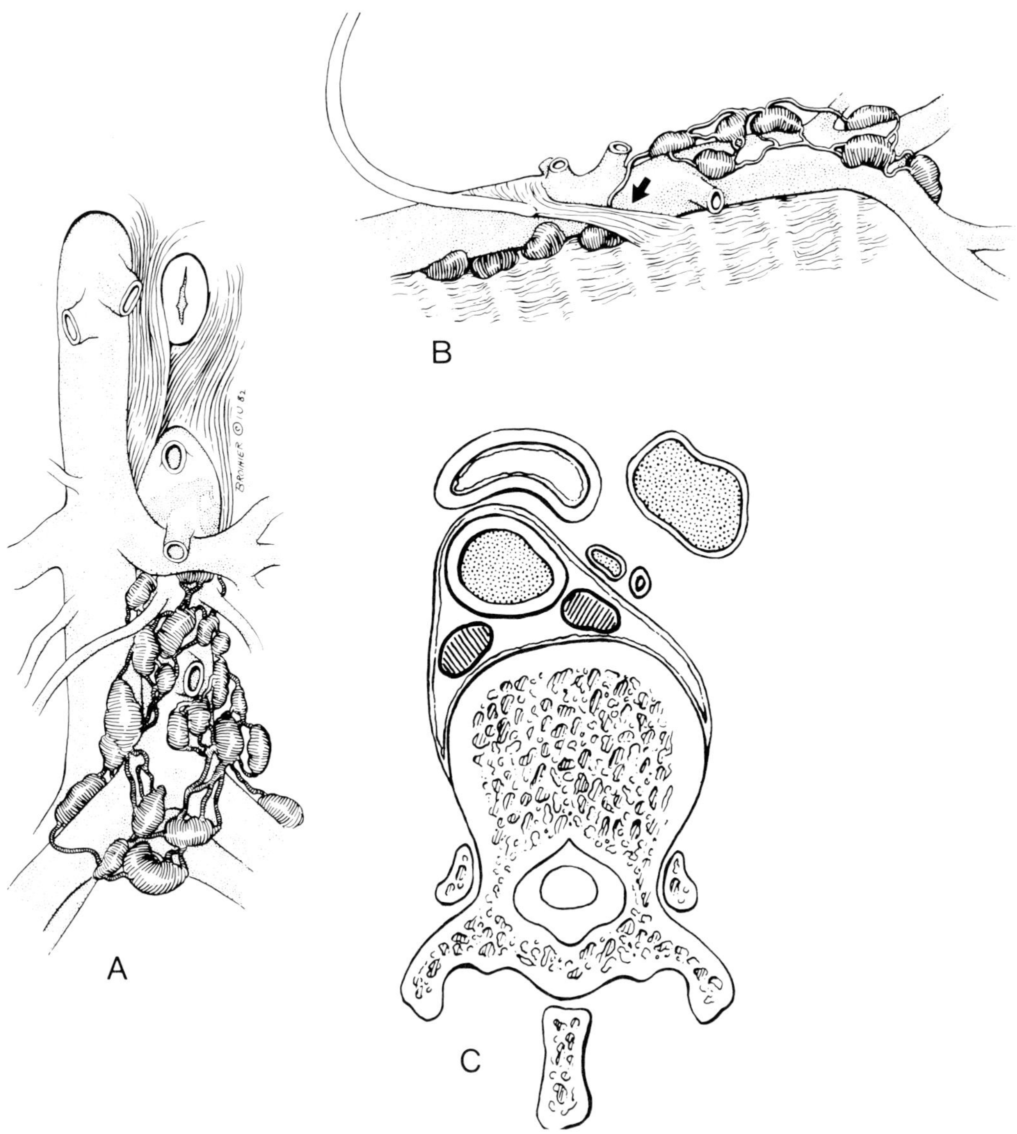

Figure 11.7 A–C. Reveal the anatomy of the most common form of suprahilar nodal involvement. Below the renal vein, most of the nodes are pre- and para-aortic as pictured and readily seen from anterior exposure. However, above the hilum of the kidney, the nodes are retrocrural and para-aortic. *A*, an anterior view with the shaded nodes indicating retroaortic involvement. *B*, a lateral view with the posterior and cephalad flow of lymph shown passing retrocrural and retro- and para-aortic. *C*, an axial view of the relationships of the crura above the aorta with the nodes in the posterolateral relationship to the aorta and below the crura.

On the other hand, patients with gross disease in the retroperitoneum, particularly those with multiple grossly enlarged nodes (larger than 3 cm in diameter) had positive suprahilar nodes (either gross or microscopic) in about one out of four cases. Of course, those patients with massive disease had positive involvement in this area by direct extension of their nodal tumor which was centralized below the hilum, but extended above it. Table 11.1 lists the distribution of positive nodes in the retroperitoneum as correlated with side of the primary lesion and extent of disease (II_A, II_B, II_C). It can be seen that in early stage disease (II_A) suprahilar involvement is a rarity and contralateral involvement is also rare. Therefore, in grossly negative retroperitoneal dissections, the modified bilateral dissection as proposed by Ray *et al.*[15] should suffice.

In cases where there is *gross* disease, a suprahilar dissection can be developed as described below.

In recent times we have found it convenient to save the suprahilar dissection until the infrahilar (main aortocaval) dissection is done. The major suprahilar nodes are posterior at the foramina and medial to the crura of the diaphragm (Fig. 11.7). Their exposure and removal is facilitated by prior complete aortic and caval mobilization, renal vascular dissection, and removal of infrahilar nodal tissue from the posterior body wall. The extension of nodal tissue from infrahilar to suprahilar zones is

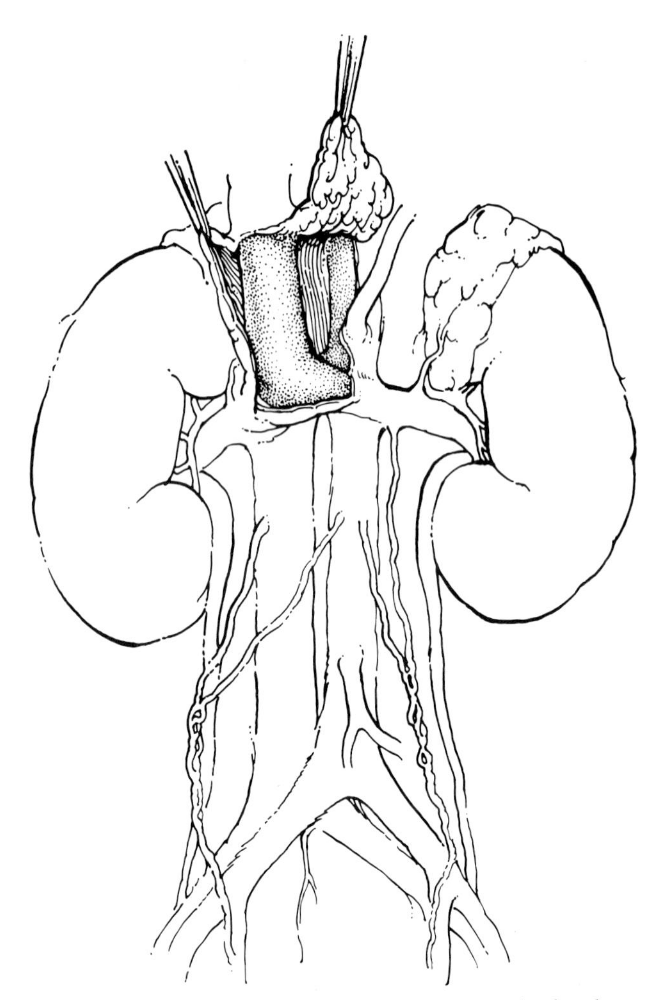

Figure 11.8. The right suprahilar dissection (unnecessary in the absence of gross disease) extends up the aorta from the superior mesenteric artery, onto the crus of the diaphragm, over to the medial aspect of the right adrenal gland about 4–6 cm above the right renal artery, then down the medial border of the right adrenal gland to the right renal artery and along the renal artery back to the aorta. The major nodes are retrocrural.

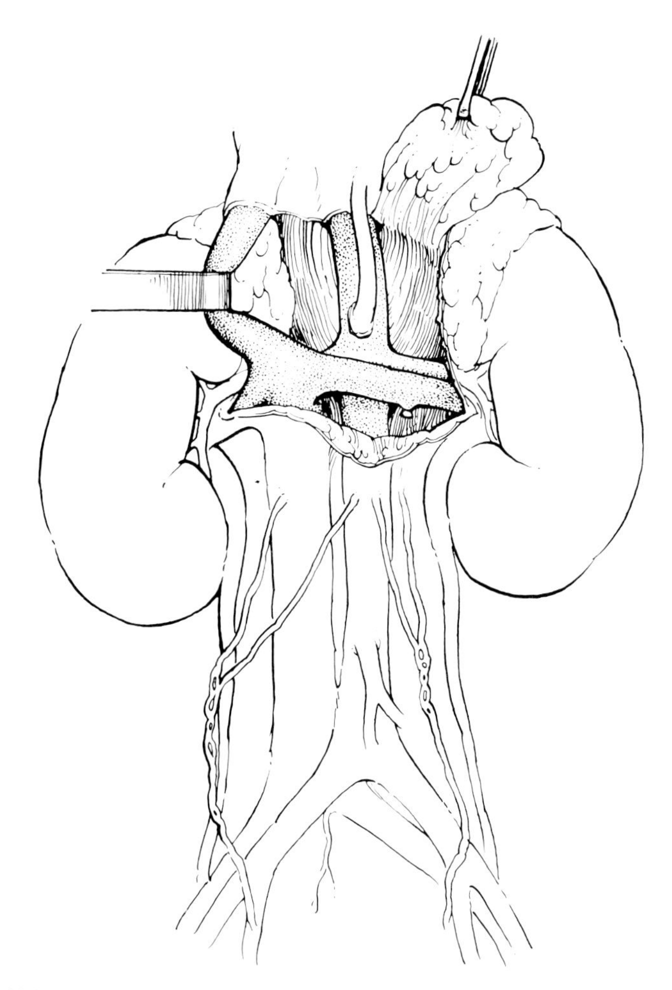

Figure 11.9. The left suprahilar dissection (unnecessary in the absence of gross disease) extends from the superior mesenteric artery up the left side of the aorta, onto the crus and up 4–6 cm above the left renal artery. The left renal vein and artery are mobilized caudad, the adrenal vein is divided, and the adrenal gland is rotated cephalad after all its medial attachments are divided between clips. The tissue is taken off the crus and foramina by sharp dissection between clips. The crus is elevated and nodes below removed. Large nodes may require crural splitting for removal.

then readily appreciated by elevating the aorta and renal vessels in vein retractors (Fig. 11.5). Also the crural muscle fibers can be seen to cover these nodes. The crural muscle can be retracted or split to gain access to the occasional large node here. Usually they can be grasped in broad Russian or Shingley forceps and extracted from this space with care taken to secure approximate lymphatic channels in vascular clips. The dissection on the surface of the crura begins at the base of the superior mesenteric artery. With the head and body of the pancreas padded and elevated by two deep Harrington retractors, both the right and left crus can be dissected clean. The basic technique relates to clipping along the base of the superior mesenteric artery and celiac artery, then across and along the dorsum of each respective renal artery and then laterally along the border of the adrenal (Figs. 11.8 and 11.9). This small wedge of tissue contains fat lymphatics, ganglia, and lymph nodal tissue. But, these are not the major nodes draining the testis. As noted earlier, the major nodal tissue is below the surface of the crus and posterolateral to the aorta (Fig. 11.7).

CYTOREDUCTIVE SURGERY FOLLOWING CHEMOTHERAPY

There are several special considerations of a technical nature when approaching the patient pretreated with combination chemotherapy for cytoreduction of masses and/or disseminated disease. Preoperative considerations are assessment of the bulk and location of the tumor by CT scan. This will direct the choice of incision. The very large persistent lesion in the hilar or suprahilar region is best approached by thoracoabdominal incision on the ipsilateral and involved side. If the disease is very extensive and equally bulky across the midline, the incision can be carried transabdominally as well. Also, preoperative pulmonary function studies and pO_2 values on room air are very useful in assessing the patient's postoperative blood gases. Many patients tolerate relatively low pO_2s postoperatively because it represents their preoperative status quo. It is important to get them off the ventilator as soon as possible and to avoid excessive hydration with crystalloid[6, 12] and excessive oxygenation (fraction of inspired oxygen (fiO_2)) which is damaging to pneumocytes. If not managed properly, these patients become wed to the ventilator and can die of a pulmonary death.

At surgery, the bowel is reflected in the usual manner and set aside in

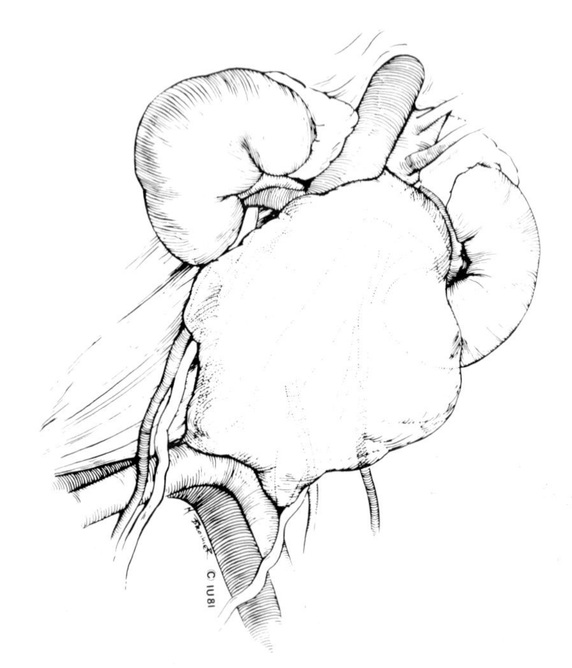

Figure 11.10. Schematic representation of tumor in retroperitoneum following PVB chemotherapy. There still may be extensive tumor disease involving the great vessels, ureters, etc. The bowel and mesenteric divisions are made as usual so as to expose the tumor in its entirety.

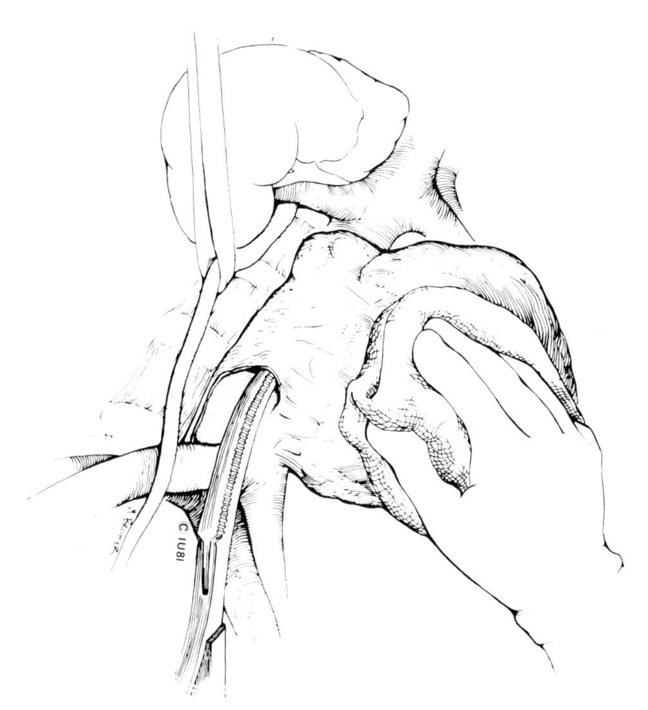

Figure 11.11. The tumor can be dissected off of the vena cava usually in the subadventitial plane below the fibrous capsule of the tumor. When it is extremely dense, subadventitial dissection can assist caval extraction from the tumor. If tumor grows through the wall of the cava, the cava itself can be resected provided it is below the level of the renal veins.

a bowel bag for optimal exposure of the retroperitoneal mass lesion. We have demonstrated in an earlier report, the immense variety of histologic subtypes in these tumor masses.[7] A mere biopsy will be insufficient in providing accurate tissue diagnosis. Therefore, a full RPLND should be done for ideal clearance of potential tumor and complete histopathology sampling.

In order to do a complete RPLND in a retroperitoneum occupied by bulky disease, it is often necessary to dissect either below or on the adventitia of the great vessels and reflect the tumor off in this manner. Usually sharp dissection with scissors or scalpel blade will effectively roll off a tumor, provided it is gently retracted with right-angle clamps, or such, attached to the adventitia and tumor capsule (Figs. 11.10–11.13). Again, the inferior mesenteric artery and the lumbar arteries are best divided prospectively after ligature and clipping. This gives the vessels mobility and allows resection from the posterior body wall more safely. The tumor mass can usually be separated from the ureter and the kidney (Fig. 11.13). At times however, these structures are inseparably bound within the tumor mass and are best removed *en bloc* with the tumor, provided the contralateral renal unit is established as functional and is not also involved with tumor. Our experience suggests that a plane of cleavage can often be established in the subadventitial plane, especially when dealing with the vena cava (Fig. 11.11). However, the aorta in certain cases is so diseased by virtue of tumor involvement of the wall

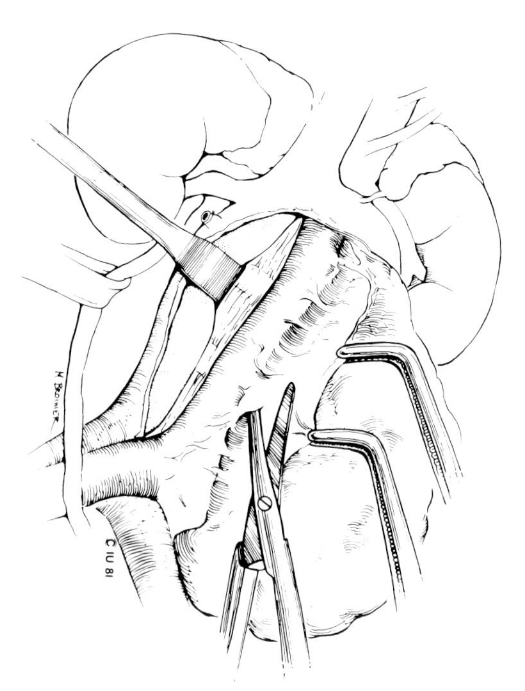

Figure 11.12. The tumor is now dissected free of the cava and the aorta is being dissected free of tumor. Here it is important to preserve the adventitia of the aorta if possible. Subadventitial dissection may leave a very weakened wall which can rupture spontaneously and also which is difficult to repair. An effort to leave adventitia on the aorta is shown in this diagram.

and by postchemotherapy changes that it is quite "cheesy" and does not suture well. Therefore, it is best to leave an additional layer on the aortic side of the dissection so that fibrous tissue can support sutures placed in the aorta (Fig. 11.12). Hence, pre- and para-aortic dissection should be in the extra-adventitial plane to provide this extra support to hold suture ligatures when needed. Should the situation prove technically impossible, or should the aorta give evidence of weakness or rupture, it should be replaced with Dacron interposition tube graft or branched graft if the iliac vessels are also involved. The author has done this on three occasions in such instances. The venous side, however, is less of a problem. As long as the renal veins can be spared, the cava can be resected with impunity below this level and we often do if it is quite involved with tumor. In such cases, we try to spare iliac lumbar contributions whenever possible.

Results

At the time of this writing, some 300 patients have been staged with retroperitoneal lymphadenectomy as just described. Crude 3-year survival rates are available for 194 patients.[5, 9, 24]

These patients can be roughly divided into two groups. The first group can be assigned to the "pre-PVB" era (before cisplatin, vinblastine, bleomycin). There were 30 patients with stage I disease, 3 of whom subsequently developed stage III disease with pulmonary metastases. All three were salvaged by the use of single agent chemotherapy (actinomycin-

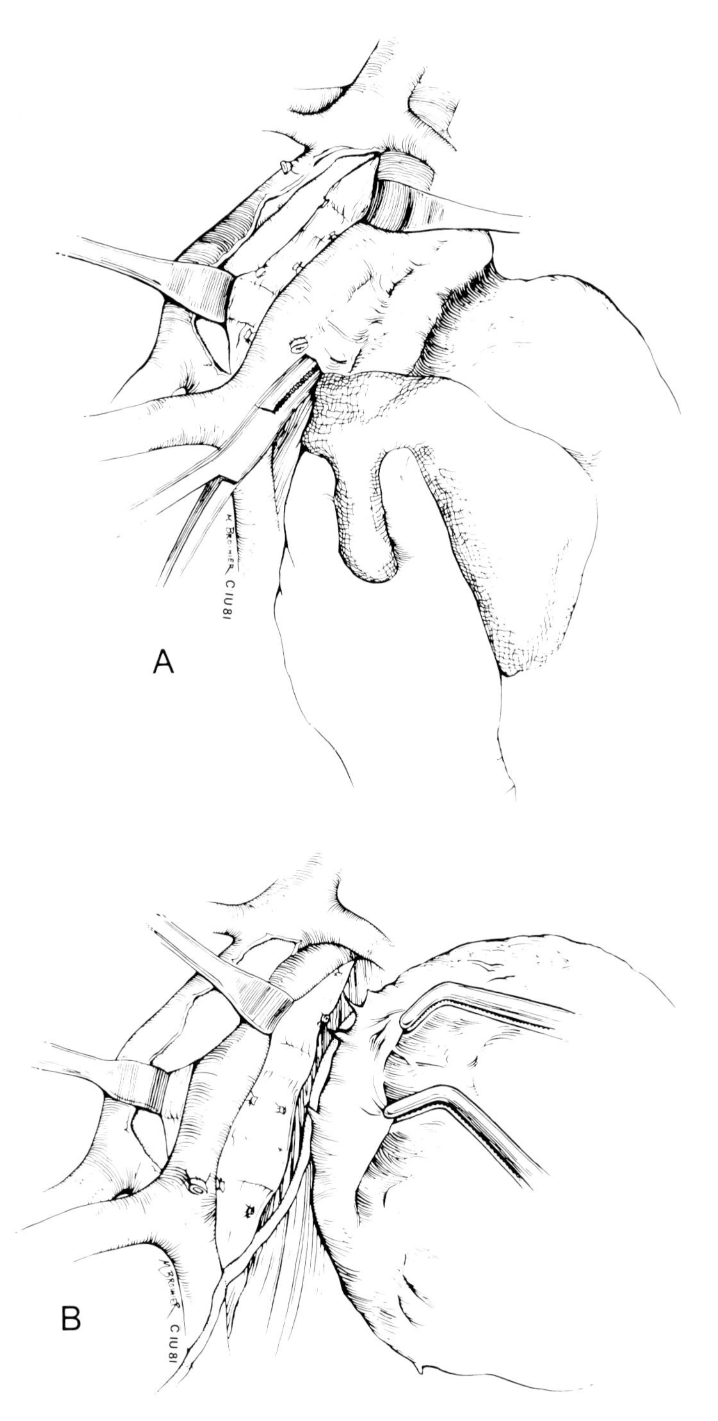

Figure 11.13 A and B. The ureter is dissected out from the tumor after appropriate lumbar arterial divisions. This allows dissection of the tumor off the posterior body wall and the foramina. Please note (*B*) that right angle clamps holding this tumor fibrous capsule or vessel adventitia help in providing traction on the tumor specimen.

D, pulmonary lobectomy and, in one instance, local chest radiotherapy). These 30 patients continue well and disease free. Another 28 patients were proven to be stage II with nodal involvement in the retroperitoneum. Twenty-four of these 28 (86%) survive, all clinically tumor free. Their management in those days consisted of monthly chest radiographs and actinomycin-D, 1 mg intravenously daily for 4 consecutive days at monthly intervals for the first year postoperative. Therefore, 54 of the 58 patients with stage I or II disease still survive all clinically tumor free for a cumulative survival rate of 93% in this early group of patients.[5] (Table 11.2)

The second group represents the "post-PVB" era (after the introduction of cisplatinum, vinblastine, bleomycin for treatment of clinical relapse,[8, 9] *i.e.* stage III disease). This group of 136 patients have also been reported.[24] Again, these patients are divided into two major groups; histologic stage I and histologic stage II. The stage II patients were treated in three different ways. One group was treated with surgery alone and followed expectantly. Another group was treated with single-drug adjuvant actinomycin-D, monthly for 1 year; and the third stage II group was treated with adjuvant PVB as a pilot study. (Table 11.3) The dosages of platinum, vinblastine and bleomycin have been reported elsewhere.[2]

All stage I patients continue alive and well. None received adjuvant chemotherapy after retroperitoneal lymphadenectomy. Of the 57 stage I patients, there were 4 relapses at 3, 4, 10 and 22 months postoperatively. Each was salvaged with PVB chemotherapy at the time pulmonary metastases became evident. Presently, all 57 patients are in complete remission with no evidence of disease. Of the stage II patients, 24 were treated with surgery alone. There were seven relapses (29.1%) all of whom were treated with PVB at time of discovery. Twenty-three enjoy NED (no evidence of disease) status. One died of unrelated causes and at postmortem was tumor free. Another 31 patients were treated with adjuvant actinomycin-D. There were 15 relapses (48.4%) although the incidence of advanced disease seemed no higher in this group than in the surgery alone group. Thirty patients enjoyed NED status (96.8%) and one died of progressive metastatic disease after initial partial remission. The third subset in stage II was a small pilot group given adjuvant PVB. Seven such patients have been followed for a minimum of 24 months and all remain continuously NED. We have reported these in more detail.[2] (Table 11.3) In summary, our "post-PVB" era survival in stage I remains 100%

Table 11.2.
Indiana RPLND[a] results

Era	Survival	
	Stage I	Stage II
Pre-PVB	(%)	(%)
1965–1974	30/30 (100)	24/28 (86)
Post-PVB		
1974–1978	57/57 (100)	60/62 (96.7)

[a] The abbreviations used are: RPLND, retroperitoneal lymphadenectomy; and PVB, cisplatin, vinblastine and bleomycin.

Table 11.3.
1974–1978 Stage I and II NSGTT[a] Indiana

Stage	No. of Patients	Treatment after RPLND	Relapse	Cure with PVB	Survival
Stage I	57	None	4	4	57/57 (100)
Stage II	55	Actinomycin D (31)	15	13	53/55 (96)[b]
Stage II		None (24)	7	7	
Stage II	7	PVB (7)	0		
					60/62 (96.7)

[a] The abbreviations used are: NSGTT, nonseminomatous germinal testis tumor; RPLND, retroperitoneal lymphadenectomy; PVB, cisplatin, vinblastine, bleomycin.
[b] One dead, unrelated cause, mental institution.

and in stage II is 96.7%. (Table 11.2) compares pre- and post-PVB eras.

Therefore, currently we are anticipating in a group study whereby our stage II patients either receive adjuvant chemotherapy (PVB in doses noted above for two courses) as opposed to observation with cross-over to PVB treatment only in the event of clinical relapse (Table 11.1). In such a case, their PVB treatment would be a four-course program.

Thorough retroperitoneal lymphadenectomy provides accurate pathologic staging. Therefore, it offers more true information on the disease status and possibly will assist in optimal assignment of therapy.[17, 24] For example, our current adjuvant study is based on accurate histologic information as opposed to merely clinical noninvasive data which, in our experience, is significantly falsely negative.[16] Although the future of retroperitoneal lymphadenectomy is still unclear and improvements in noninvasive staging will doubtless continue, it would seem unlikely that completely accurate staging can be obtained without surgical dissection and histologic nodal examination.

Commentary

From 1965–1980, our position had been to do thorough bilateral RPLND including bilateral suprahilar dissection. After analysis of our own data, this position has been modified.[4] For example, the merits of a bilateral dissection *versus* a unilateral dissection were debatable. The report by Ray *et al.*[15] of their standard infrahilar dissections indicates that contralateral spread is rare in the face of tumor-free ipsilateral nodes. Our own experience confirms this.[4] Perhaps one purpose of the unilateral dissection was to preserve ejaculation. It appears that the majority of patients are still unable to ejaculate even after this form of dissection. Also, the fact that contralateral spread sometimes occurs, particularly in the face of multiple ipsilateral nodal involvement with tumor, suggests the possible merit of a thorough bilateral dissection in such cases.

The merits of a suprahilar dissection in combination with the standard hilar and infrahilar approach were still less well known. Admittedly, it is rare that a patient would have disease in the suprahilar nodes in the face of tumor-free infrahilar nodes (it happened in only 1 of our 100 stage II patients). But, it is not rare to have the suprahilar nodes involved when the infrahilar nodes contain gross tumor; in our series, one of every four patients with gross tumor in infrahilar nodes also had tumor in the suprahilar nodes. This involvement took several forms, *i.e.* direct extension of bulk disease, microscopic involvement, or occasional discrete nodal enlargements (Figs. 11.14–11.20). It seems reasonable then, in such cases, to clear out the nodal drainage pathways of the testis completely if we are to stage and treate with surgery as thoroughly as possible. The frequency of suprahilar nodal involvement is directly proportional to the number of nodes involved below the hilum. While stage II_A disease has from 0% (right side) (Table 11.4) to 7–14% (left side) (Table 11.5) positive suprahilar nodes, stage II_B has from 13–33% (right) and 16–42% (left) positive suprahilar nodes. Hence, the value of routine bilateral suprahilar dissection in a grossly normal retroperitoneum is doubtful. On the other hand, it seems useful in stage II_B and II_C disease (*i.e.* "B-3" bulky disease).

Questions are often asked about the value of total vascular mobilization by dividing all the lumbar vessels. In our series, there have been no spinal cord complications from this procedure. Ferguson *et al.*,[10] in a literature review, reported 28 cases of paraparesis following total infrarenal aortic replacement for aneurysm in older males. But this study relates to an older group of patients who had lost their primary anterior descending spinal blood supply because of atherosclerotic cardiovascular disease in the thoracic aorta and its branches and which had been depending on their lumbar arteries for collateral circulation. In our younger patients this is not a problem. We believe that vascular mobilization is necessary

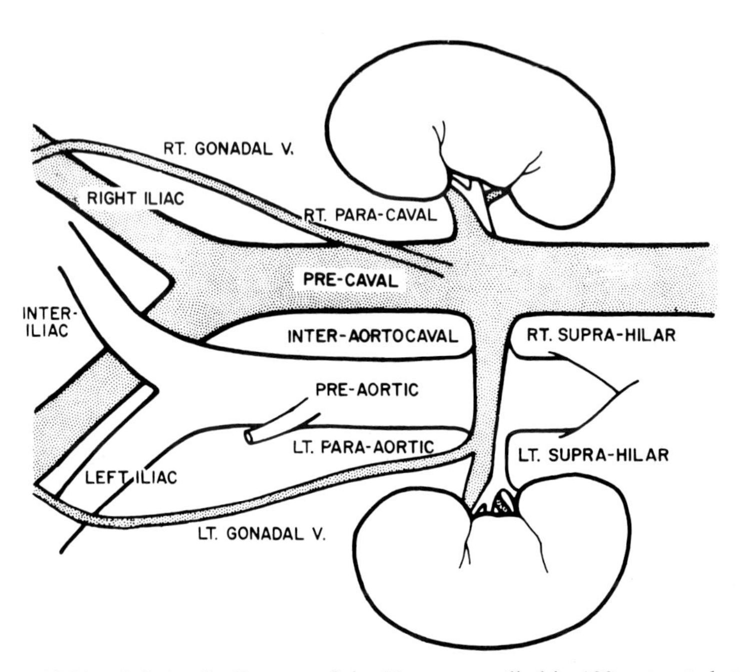

Figure 11.14. Schematic diagram of the 11 zones studied in 100 untreated stage II cases. The specimen was separated into these components and submitted as 11 parts to a single whole. This assisted our analysis of the distribution of positive nodes in testis cancer.

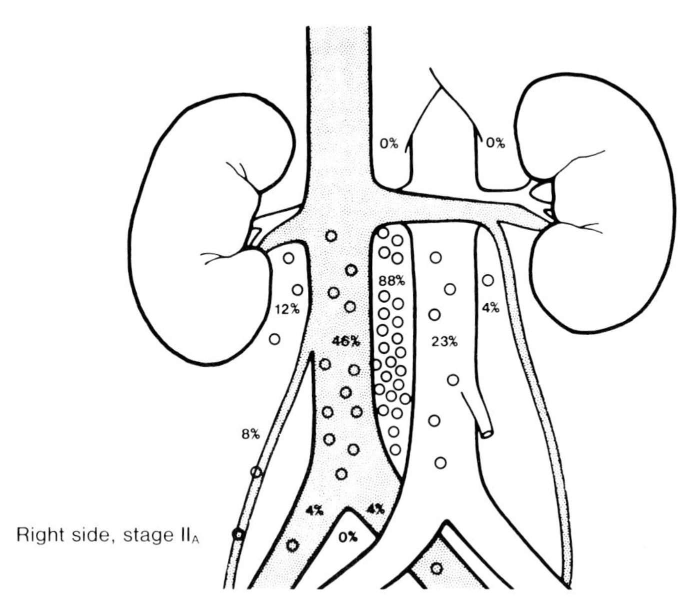

Figure 11.15. (*Circles* represent locations of positive nodes) Right-sided stage II_A patients had an overwhelming preponderance of interaortocaval nodes as positive. Also, precaval nodes were frequently involved. Please note the absence of suprahilar nodal involvement by tumor in right-sided stage II_A cases. Also, note the rarity of contralateral and iliac involvement.

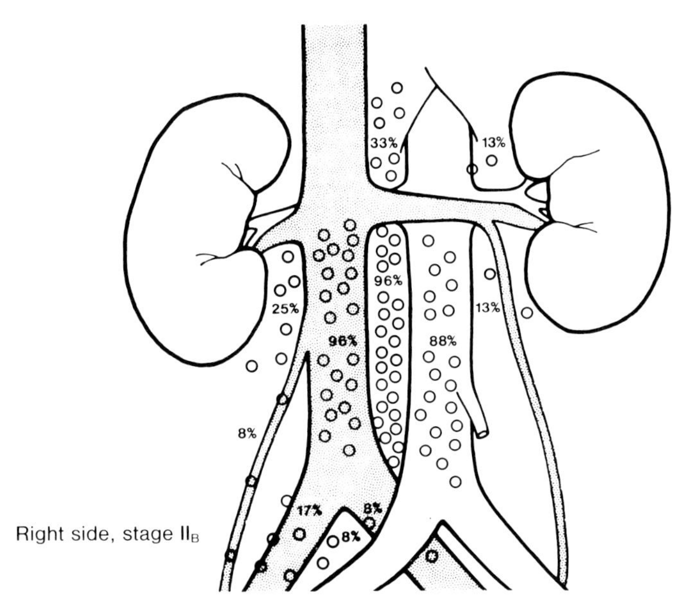

Figure 11.16. Right-sided stage II_B nodal distribution was considerably more widespread. The suprahilar zones were more often involved as preaortic right paracaval and iliac zones.

because lateral views and dissection studies have shown that there are as many nodes and lymphatics behind the great vessels and posterolateral to them as there are above them, particularly high in the retroperitoneum. Also, the lymphatics occupy each lumbar foramen and there are many

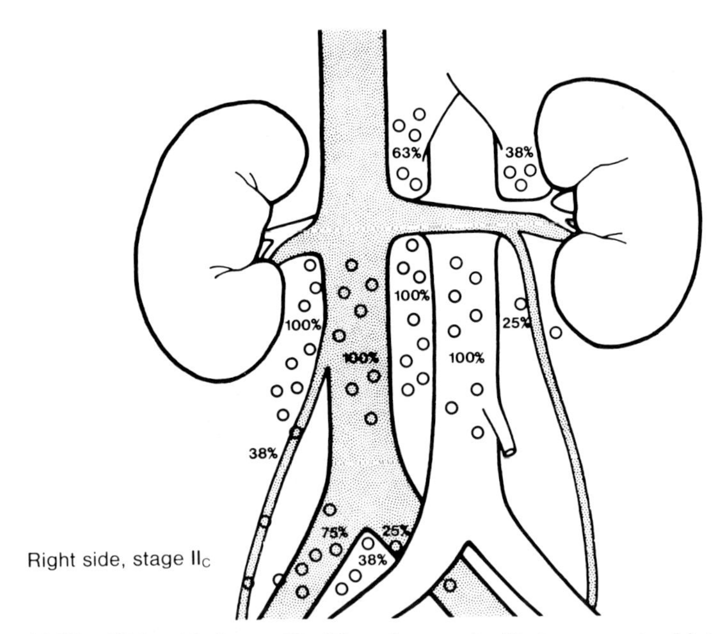

Figure 11.17. Right-sided stage II_C. These large palpable tumors extend into the suprahilar zone by virtue of their size and direct extension. Also, there is retrograde flow of lymph in these large obstructed systems creating many more positive iliac nodes.

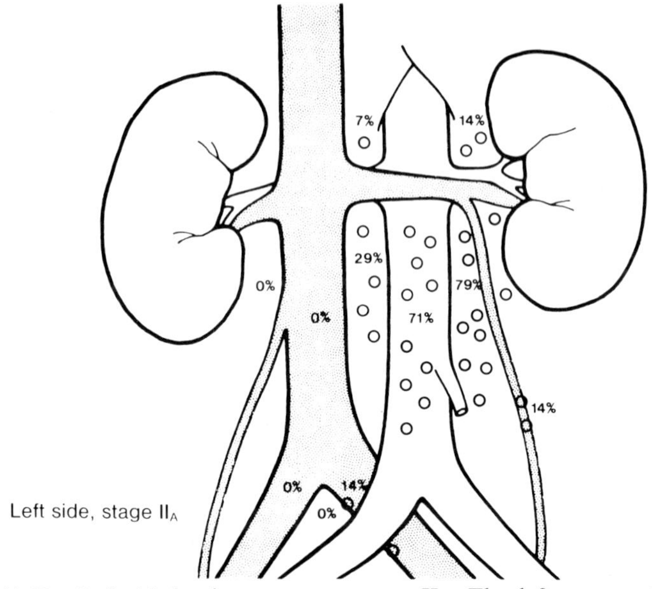

Figure 11.18. Left-sided primary tumor, stage II_A. The left para-aortic zone below the renal vein and the preaortic zone are most commonly involved. Please note the absence of contralateral caval, paracaval and iliac involvement. A few cases have suprahilar nodes involved, but these were para-aortic and just above the level of the renal arteries.

tumor-containing nodes found in these foramina in patients with stage II disease.

Still another area of controversy that should be mentioned concerns the role of radiotherapy in the management of these patients. In brief, it can be said that the need for radiotherapy as treatment for nonseminomatous testis cancer is contracting sharply in the face of great advances in chemotherapy. In our earlier experience, radiotherapy was a negative factor if the patients developed stage III disease, as all stage II patients are at risk of doing. The impact of prior radiotherapy on the bone marrow is lasting. More persistent and profound leukopenia in patients treated earlier with radiotherapy (especially if the chest is included) limits the

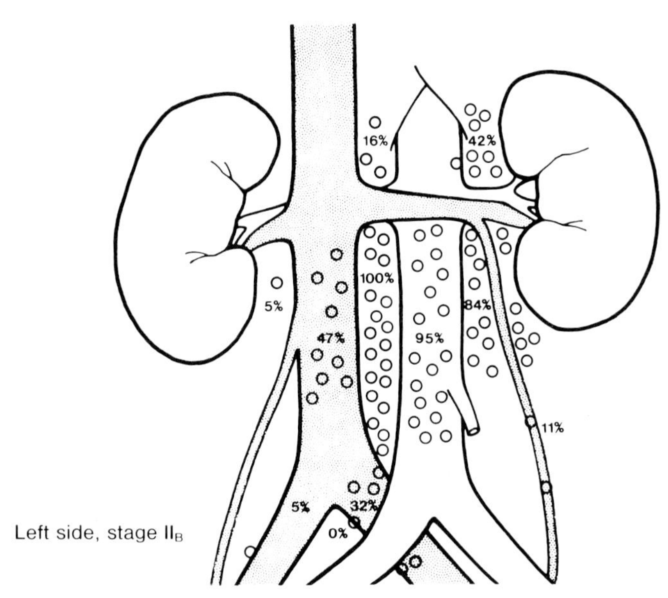

Figure 11.19. Left-sided stage II_B tumors have an impressive spread into the interaortocaval zone, precaval, and suprahilar zones.

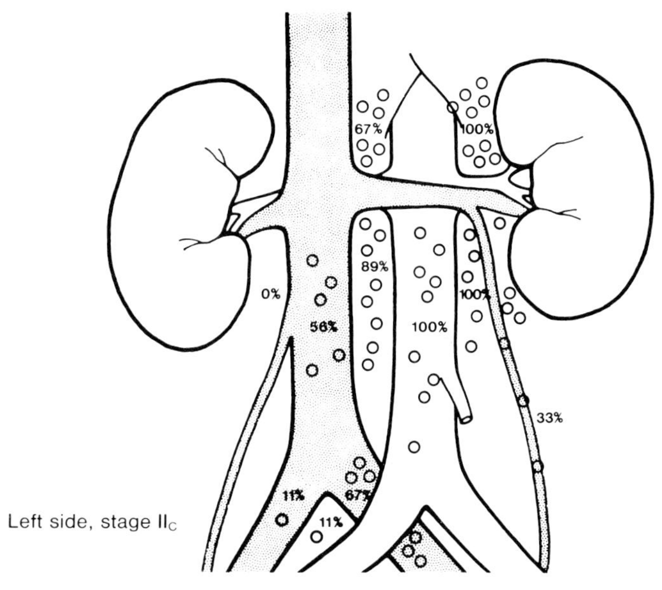

Figure 11.20. Left-sided stage II_C palpable masses involve the suprahilar zones by direct extension of tumor mass. Also, the iliac zones and precaval zones are frequently involved owing to tumor size.

Table 11.4.
Incidence of positive nodes related to zone and stage II_A, II_B, II_C; primary tumor right side

Zone	Stage			
	II_A	II_B	II_C[a]	Total
	(%)	(%)	(%)	(%)
1 (R. paracaval)	3/26 (12)	6/24 (25)	8/8 (100)	17/58 (29)
2 (Precaval)	12/26 (46)	23/24 (96)	8/8 (100)	43/58 (74)
3 (Interaortocaval)	23/26 (88)	23/24 (96)	8/8 (100)	54/58 (93)
4 (Preaortic)	6/26 (23)	21/24 (88)	8/8 (100)	35/58 (60)
5 (L. para-aortic)	1/26 (4)	3/24 (13)	2/8 (25)	6/58 (10)
6 (R. suprahilar)	0/26 (0)	8/24 (33)	5/8 (63)	13/58 (22)
7 (L. suprahilar)	0/26 (0)	3/24 (13)	3/8 (38)	6/58 (10)
8 (R. iliac)	1/26 (4)	4/24 (17)	6/8 (75)	11/58 (19)
9 (L. iliac)	1/26 (4)	2/24 (8)	2/8 (25)	5/58 (9)
10 (Interiliac)	0/26 (0)	2/24 (8)	2/8 (25)	4/58 (7)
11 (Gonadal)	2/26 (0)	3/24 (13)	3/8 (38)	8/58 (14)

[a] II_C, "B-3," or palpable bulky mass.

chemotherapist in his ability to deliver effective doses of chemotherapy. Still it must be said that radiotherapy is an effective alternative to RPLND in controlling low stage disease in areas where RPLND is not employed or available.[14]

Several comments are in order regarding tissue analysis of retroperitoneal tumors resected following chemotherapy (PVB).

CYTOREDUCTIVE SURGERY FOR METASTATIC TESTIS CANCER: CONSIDERATIONS OF TIMING AND EXTENT

Retroperitoneal surgery for extirpation of massive metastatic disease is greatly facilitated by preoperative treatment with four courses of PVB chemotherapy. We have done retroperitoneal lymphadenectomy for persistent tumor masses following PVB combination chemotherapy on over 120 patients. Fifty-one patients followed from 3–8 years have had their tissue reports analyzed relative to the integration of histologic findings. These include three major subsets: (1) persistent *malignancy*, (2) mature or immature *teratoma* and (3) nontumor tissue changes such as hemorrhage, inflammation, calcification, *fibrosis*, *necrosis*, *cystic change*. These changes were placed on a chart (see Table 11.6) so as to make readily visible the complex nature of these tumor masses and the multiplicity of tissue changes. (1) There were 19 patients with persistent *cancer* in at least some portion of the specimen resected. Eleven of these 19 also had mature teratoma and multiple areas of fibrotic and necrotic change as well.

Hence, it is clear that mere biopsy of one portion of this lesion could be misleading. It is apparent that these retroperitoneal spaces should be dissected completely owing to the vast diversity of these tumor masses histologically. Nine of these patients with cancer in their specimen have died. Two were never rendered NED after surgery despite aggressive efforts of salvage chemotherapy. Both continued with positive serotesting throughout their postoperative course. All but one death occurred within a year of surgery. Negative markers did not guarantee freedom of persistent cancer in these specimens as eight of these had negative serum markers following chemotherapy and yet were found to have cancer in their specimen. Fifteen of the 19 cancer patients had their tissues submitted in separate segments to allow for precise zonal analysis on the grid used to define distribution of nodal elements in the retroperitoneum. (2) Sixteen patients have been classified as *teratoma*, four of which also had elements of immature teratoma as well. Of these 16, there is 1 death from relapse with wide-spread angiosarcoma. (He had extensive radiotherapy in 1977 prior to retroperitoneal lymph node dissection). Also, another patient relapsed with pulmonary nodule resected as teratoma. Hence, 15 of 16 teratoma patients are alive and well. (3) There were 16 patients who had no evidence of tumor and were classified as basically *fibrosis-necrosis-cystic change*. All are living and well, but two patients developed recurrent disease, one in the true pelvis (anaplastic seminoma) and one in the chest with thoracotomy revealing active cancer. Both have responded to salvage chemotherapy after extirpative secondary surgery.

Table 11.5.
Incidence of positive nodes related to zone and stage II_A, II_B, II_C; primary tumor left side

Zone	Stage			
	II_A	II_B	II_C[a]	Total
	(%)	(%)	(%)	(%)
1 (R. paracaval)	0/14 (0)	1/19 (5)	0/9 (5)	1/42 (2)
2 (Precaval)	0/14 (0)	9/19 (47)	5/9 (56)	14/42 (33)
3 (Interaortocaval)	4/14 (19)	19/19 (100)	8/9 (89)	31/42 (74)
4 (Preaortic)	10/14 (71)	18/19 (95)	9/9 (100)	37/42 (88)
5 (L. para-aortic)	11/14 (79)	16/19 (84)	9/9 (100)	36/42 (86)
6 (R. suprahilar)	1/14 (7)	3/19 (16)	6/9 (67)	10/42 (24)
7 (L. suprahilar)	2/14 (14)	8/19 (42)	9/9 (100)	19/42 (45)
8 (R. iliac)	0/14 (0)	1/19 (5)	1/9 (11)	2/42 (5)
9 (L. iliac)	2/14 (14)	6/19 (32)	6/9 (67)	14/42 (33)
10 (Interiliac)	0/14 (0)	0/19 (0)	1/9 (11)	1/42 (2)
11 (Gonadal)	2/14 (14)	2/19 (11)	3/9 (33)	7/42 (17)

[a] II_C, "B-3," or palpable bulky mass.

It is quite clear that one cannot afford to biopsy a single area and expect it to be representative of the entire mass, as these tumor masses are variable in their composition. This lack of uniformity or homogeneity of the tissue requires its total removal and sectioning for accurate definition of all tissue elements.

Using preoperative PVB chemotherapy has allowed more effective local and systemic cytoreduction and provided an 80% overall survival (41/51) in this high risk group with advanced testis cancer.

TISSUE ANALYSIS OF RETROPERITONEAL TUMOR MASSES AFTER CHEMOTHERAPY

Survival of patients with massive retroperitoneal metastases from nonseminomatous germinal cell testis cancer has been enhanced dramatically by preoperative chemotherapy, consisting of cisplatinum, vinblastine, and bleomycin (PVB). Such chemical, systemic cytoreduction greatly reduces tumor bulk and facilitates retroperitoneal lymph node dissection (RPLND). There are no reliable pre- or intraoperative predictive criteria, however, to indicate the precise nature of this residual tissue. Even gross morphologic examination is unreliable in ascertaining the presence or absence of persistent cancer in these tissues which may assume a variety of gross appearances (cystic, solid, necrotic, fibrous). Fifty-one patients with advanced retroperitoneal disease and/or pulmonary metastases were operated (RPLND) for removal of persistent retroperitoneal mass lesions after three or four courses of PVB. These specimens were analyzed (Table 11.6) for the following gross and microscopic features: hemorrhage (30), inflammation (23), fat (7), calcification (5), fibrosis (36), necrosis (34),

Table 11.6.
Tissue analysis of specimens removed from 51 patients and step-sectioned.

		Histologic Findings												
Basic Histology	No. of Patients	Hemorrhage or Thrombus	Inflammation	Fat	Calcification	Fibrosis	Necrosis	Cystic	Immature Teratoma	Mature Teratoma	Embryonal Cancer	Teratocarcinoma	Choriocarcinoma	Seminoma
Fibrous-necrosis-cystic change	16	9	7	3	2	13	11	2	0	0	0	0	0	0
Teratoma	16	9	8	1	2	11	9	8	4	16	0	0	0	0
Cancer	19	12	8	3	1	12	14	3	9	4	19	6	4	1
Totals	51	30	23	7	5	36	34	13	13	20	19	6	4	1

[a] Please note the variety of specific, *i.e.* cancer or teratoma, and nonspecific changes in these specimens. Clearly, random biopsy of these tumors following chemotherapy is inadequate for completing accurate histopathologic study. Because subsequent management depends on accurate exclusion of malignant elements, which can be focal, total excision of these areas (full RPLND) is necessary.

Table 11.7.
Staging process for testicular cancer[a]

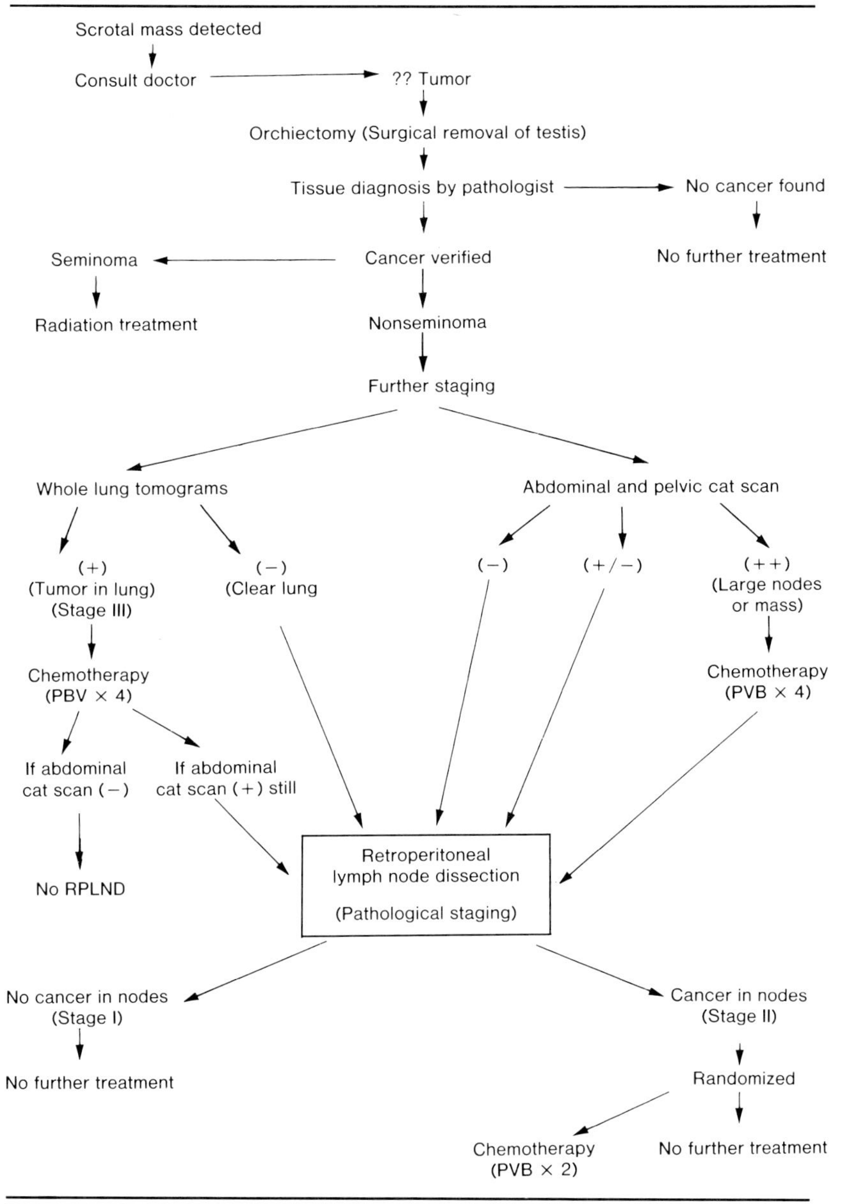

[a] The abbreviations used are: PVB, cisplatin, vinblastine, bleomycin, and RPLND, retroperitoneal lymphadenectomy.

cystic (13), immature teratoma (13), mature teratoma (20), and frank cancer: embryonal carcinoma (19), teratocarcinoma (6), choriocarcinoma (4) and seminoma (1). All patients had a combination of several of these features in widely varying gross and regional distributions. Nineteen patients (37%) had some focus of persistent malignancy, often small and seemingly distributed at random in a variety of gross presentations. Furthermore, the site of malignancy was often not in the central largest mass, which usually had necrotic or cystic features. It is concluded that mere gross examination and biopsy, or removal of the central portion of a residual tumor mass, is inadequate if persistent cancer is to be ruled out. Rather, as complete as RPLND as possible is recommended for this purpose.

SUMMARY

In summary, several conclusions can be drawn from our experience. Chemotherapy is opening new avenues in the management of these patients. It allows us to leave patients with proven histologic stage I disease untreated with close follow-up. Should stage III relapse occur, the patient can be salvaged with appropriate and aggressive combination chemotherapy, as our cases were. Patients with stage I disease should have a 100% survival rate if the retroperitoneum is dissected appropriately and the patient is followed closely postoperatively. Several options exist for the postoperative management of patients with stage II disease. Two courses are under cooperative study; (1) no treatment after lymphadenectomy, as in stage I; (2) combination chemotherapy after lymphadenec-

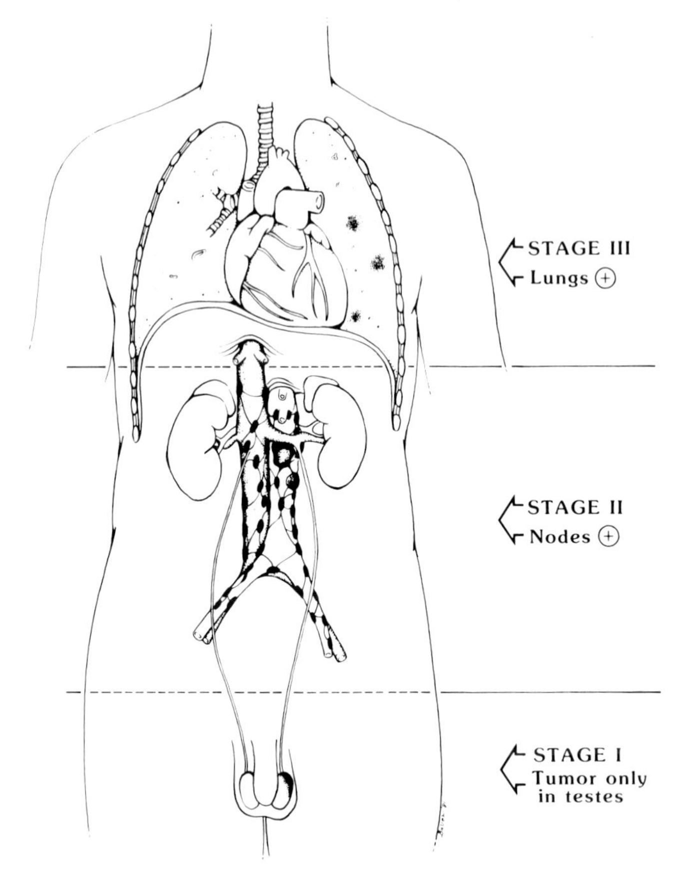

Figure 11.21. Schematic representation of the three basic stages of testis cancer. This is a helpful adjunct in aiding the patients to understand the principles of clinical and/or surgical staging.

tomy. (Table 11.3) Those patients in the no treatment group who develop stage III disease cross-over to combined chemotherapy with PVB. Since 1974, all but two of our patients with stage II disease who progressed to stage III have achieved complete remission with this three-drug combination. Another new horizon is the potential for chemical cytoreduction of disseminated stage III disease; persistent abdominal disease can now be resected more safely and completely. It is this author's opinion that chemotherapy provides a safer, more extensive initial cytoreduction than the contrary approach of primary surgical cytoreduction followed by postoperative chemotherapy[3] (Fig. 11.21, Table 11.7).

Serotesting for the β-subunit of human chorionic gonadotropin and for α-fetoprotein has been a helpful means of following patients with stage II disease and for detecting tumor before it can be seen by any of the conventional radiologic methods.

Although the role of retroperitoneal lymphadenectomy will doubtless change and improvements in noninvasive staging will certainly continue (serotesting for tumor-associated antigens, ultrasound, axial tomography, lymphangiography, and nuclear magnetic resonance), it would seem unlikely that completely accurate staging can be obtained without surgical dissection and histologic nodal examination. We have had recent experience with several patients in whom all these preoperative tests for metastases (including serotesting) were negative, yet they had evidence of multiple tumorous nodes on microscopic examination.[16] This suggests that the role of surgical staging with histologic nodal study will remain central to the accurate definition of the disease status and direction of therapy. Furthermore, in this disease, retroperitoneal surgery completely done seems to have positive influence on patient survival. But the question is: does retroperitoneal lymphadenectomy (for staging) need to be done at all? This decade will provide the answer. If not, the primary role for retroperitoneal lymphadenectomy in this disease will be for resection of residual tumor following chemotherapy for advanced disease.

REFERENCES

1. Cooper J. F., Leadbetter, W. F., Chute R. The thoracoabdominal approach for retroperitoneal gland dissection: its application to testis tumors. *Surg. Gynecol. Obstet. 90:*486, 1950.
2. Donohue, J. P., Einhorn, L. H., Williams, S. D. Is adjuvant chemotherapy necessary following retroperitoneal lymphadenectomy for nonseminomatous testis cancer? *Urol. Clin. N. Am. 7:*747, 1980.
3. Donohue, J. P., Einhorn, L. H., Williams, S. D. Cytoreductive surgery for metastatic testis cancer: considerations of timing and extent. *J. Urol. 123:*876, 1980.
4. Donohue, J. P., Maynard, B., Zachary, J. M. The distribution of nodal metastases in the retroperitoneum from nonseminomatous testis cancer. *J. Urol. 128:*315, 1982.
5. Donohue, J. P. Retroperitoneal lymphadenectomy, *Urol. Clin. N. Am.:* 517, 1977.
6. Donohue, J. P., and Rowland, R. G. Complications of retroperitoneal lymph node dissection. *J. Urol. 125:*338, 1981.
7. Donohue, J. P., Roth, L. M., Zachary, J. M., Rowland, R. G., Einhorn, L. H., Williams, S. G. Cytoreductive surgery for metastatic testis cancer: tissue analysis of retroperitoneal tumor masses after chemotherapy. *J. Urol. 127:*1111, 1982.
8. Einhorn, L. H., and Donohue, J. P. Improved chemotherapy in disseminated testicular cancer. *J. Urol. 117:*65, 1977.
9. Einhorn, L. H., and Donohue, J. P. Improved chemotherapy for germinal testis tumors. *Cancer 42:*293, 1978.

10. Ferguson, L. R. J., Bergan, J. J., Conn, J., Jr., *et al.* Spinal ischemia following abdominal aortic surgery. *Ann. Surg. 181:*267, 1975.
11. Fraley, E. E., Kedia, K., Markland, C. The role of radical operation in the management of nonseminomatous germinal tumors of the testicle in the adult. In *Controvery in Surgery,* p. 479, edited by R. L. Varco, and J. P. Delaney. W. B. Saunders, Philadelphia, 1976.
12. Goldinger, P. L., and Schweizer, O. The hazards of anesthesia and surgery in bleomycin-treated patients. *Semin. Oncol. 6:*121, 1979.
13. Patton, J. F., and Mallis, N. Tumors of the testis. *J. Urol. 81:*457, 1959.
14. Peckham, M. J. Combined management of malignant teratoma of the testis. *Lancet 2:*267, 1979; *Lancet 2:*678, 1982.
15. Ray, B., Hajdu, S. I., Whitmore, W. F., Jr. Distribution of retroperitoneal lymph node metastases in testicular germinal tumors. *Cancer 33:*340, 1974.
16. Rowland, R. G., Weisman, D., Williams, S. D., Einhorn, L. H., Donohue, J. P. Accuracy of preoperative staging in stage A and B nonseminomatous germ cell testis tumor. *J. Urol. 127:*718, 1982.
17. Scardino, P. T. Adjuvant chemotherapy is of value following retroperitoneal lymph node dissection for nonseminomatous testicular tumors. *Urol. Clin. N. Am. 7:*735, 1980.
18. Skinner, D. G. Nonseminomatous testis tumors: a plan of management based on 96 patients to improve survival in all stages by combined therapeutic modalities. *J. Urol. 115:*65, 1976.
19. Skinner, D. G., and Leadbetter, W. F. The surgical management of testis tumors. *J. Urol. 106:*84, 1971.
20. Staubitz, W. J., Early, K. S., Magoss, I. V., *et al.* Surgical treatment of nonseminomatous germinal testis tumors. *Cancer 32:*1206, 1973.
21. Van Buskirk, K. E., and Young, J. G. The evolution of the bilateral antegrade retroperitoneal lymph node dissection in the treatment of testicular tumors. *Milit. Med. 133:*575, 1968.
22. Vurgrin, D., Cvitkovic, E., Whitmore, W. F., Jr., *et al.* Adjuvant chemotherapy in resected nonseminomatous germ cell tumors of testis: stages I and II. *Semin. Oncol. 6:*94, 1979.
23. Whitmore, W. F., Jr. Treatment germinal tumors of the adult testes. *Cont. Surg. 6:*17, 1975.
24. Williams, S. D., Einhorn, L. H., Donohue, J. P. High cure rate of stage I or II testicular cancer with or without adjuvant chemotherapy. *Proc. Am. Soc. Clin. Surg. 21:*421, 1980.
25. Young, J. D., Jr. Retroperitoneal Surgery. In *Urologic Surgery,* Ed. 2, p. 848, edited by J. F. Glenn and W. H. Boyce. Harper & Row, New York, 1975.

12

A British Approach to the Management of Patients with Testicular Tumors

J. P. Blandy, M.A., D.M., M.Ch., F.R.C.S., F.A.C.S.
R. T. D. Oliver, M.D., M.R.C.P.
H. F. Hope-Stone, M.D., B.S., D.M.R.T., F.R.C.R.

Throughout the last 30 years there has been a considerable difference in the practice of surgeons on either side of the Atlantic in the management of retroperitoneal lymph nodes in nonseminomatous germinal cell tumors of the testis. Surgeons in North America have preferred to deal with the nodes by surgical removal: those in Britain have trusted to radiotherapy to sterilize them. Several attempts have been made to compare the two systems of management, though they have been invariably frustrated by differences in terminology, classification, and staging. On each occasion that an attempt has been made to compare the results, the comparison has been made invalid by the pace of the advances in other aspects of staging and treatment of the patients, and by authors attempting to compare the early results from their latest modification in treatment with those treated elsewhere some 5 or 10 years previously. Historically, on each occasion that such comparisons have been made, no significant difference could be found in the results of node dissection *versus* radiation, though until very recently the overall results of radiotherapy have been slightly better than those from lymph node dissection. (Table 12.1).

Since 1978, for the first time, the reported results of node dissection appeared to outstrip those of radiotherapy but these new comparisons coincided with the meteoric rise of chemotherapy, at first using one agent,[4] and in more recent years, using combinations such as those described by Samuels *et al.*[8] and Einhorn and Donohue[9]. So remarkable have been the effects of chemotherapy upon large and obvious metastases, that surgeons in both the lymph node dissection and radiotherapy camps have been obliged, if for different reasons, to reconsider their positions. The British, so long entrenched in defence of radiotherapy, have now to

Table 12.1.
Results of treatment of stage I and stage II testicular teratoma (historical data).[a]

Historical Period	Orchidectomy + Lymph Node Dissection		Orchidectomy + Paraaortic ± Mediastinal Radiation	
	N	Survival	N	Survival
		%		%
Pre-1970				
(5-year survival)	568[1]	51	421[1]	60
1970–1975				
(3-year survival)	185[2]	68	184[2, 3]	72
Post-1975				
(2-year survival)	117[4, 5]	94	71[6, 7]	90

[a] N, number of patients; superior numbers are References.

reconsider whether their use of radiotherapy is any longer justified for very early stages of the tumor, if this radiotherapy prejudices the possibility of using a full dose of chemotherapy at a later stage.[7, 9–11] Equally, the proponents of surgical resection of the lymph nodes have to ask themselves whether surgical removal of the nodes can add anything to what is already achievable by chemotherapy, particularly when the inevitable postsurgical adhesions will preclude the use of radiation should this be required later on for residual chemotherapy-resistant tumor. Both groups now find themselves arriving at a common position where they must consider most carefully whether or not any additional treatment is needed for the patient whose tumor appears to be confined to the testis (judged by all the most recent methods of investigation). Instead of routine node dissection or routine radiotherapy, it is possible to ask the question whether a judicious policy of watchful monitoring of tumor markers and CAT scan imaging with early treatment the moment metastases are detected might not be the better way of managing the patient. Such a question horrifies those of us who remember how dismal were the results of simple orchidectomy alone for tumors in the days before radiotherapy or node dissection. Nevertheless, as nearly 50% of patients diagnosed then as stage I can now be demonstrated to have metastases, it seems thoroughly justified to contemplate prospective surveillance studies of such stage I cases.

Many surgeons in the past asked the question why the dispute between lymphadenectomy and radiotherapy for nonseminomas was not long ago resolved by a prospective randomized trial such as that attempted by Maier and Lee.[6] However, a moment's consideration will show that there has never been sufficient time to recruit adequate numbers of patients for such a trial, at least during the last 20 years, without being overtaken by advances in treatment. The battleground has shifted year by year with such rapidity that there has never been an opportune moment to erect the cumbersome, if certain, apparatus of the controlled randomized prospective clinical trial. This is just as well, for testicular tumors are so uncommon, that the time needed to arrive at a significant difference between alternative modes of treatment would have been inordinately long. In Britain only about 300 nonseminomas occur *per annum* and, of these, less than 150 have no demonstrable hematogenous metastases; to recruit sufficient patients into a trial to demonstrate a 10% improvement in survival between two groups following different forms of therapy might need 10 years, allowing for a percentage of the patients not being entered. In that time, conventional 240 kv x-ray treatment was superceded by cobalt teletherapy, and cobalt by the linear accelerator; the operation of Chevassu was overtaken by that of Leadbetter; and that of Leadbetter by transabdominal retroperitoneal node dissection. In addition, in the last 5 years any slight differences between the two would have been completely obscured by the dramatic results of chemotherapy. In effect we might have actually held up progress had we all been too rigidly locked into clinical trials designed, with the best of motives, to examine questions, which, with benefit of hindsight can be seen to be irrelevant. The really outstanding advance in treatment of tumors of the testis owes nothing to clinical trial, everything to clinical acumen and imagination.

Today, we all expect that the young man who comes up with a testicular cancer will be cured, and it has been seriously suggested that any death from testicular cancer should be made the object of a confidential enquiry similar to that which today regularly follows the unexpected death of a mother in pregnancy. Such an inquisition would, of course, need to consider what type of treatment had been deployed at each stage, but it would find itself in grave difficulties, even today, to know which method ought to have been used, for step by step, ever since 1906 when Chevassu[12] first pleaded for earlier orchidectomy and more radical retroperitoneal node dissection, the benefit conferred by any form of treatment has always been only one element in a constantly advancing pattern of medical care. It is salutary to note that the results even of simple orchidectomy for nonseminoma showed almost as dramatic an improvement in the half-century between the reports of Chevassu[12] (1906) and Whitmore[13] (1970) as that which followed the use of one or other type of treatment of the retroperitoneal nodes (Tables 12.1 and 12.2). Indeed, the very gratifying improvement in the results of the therapy of known retroperitoneal node metastases has itself to be viewed against the steady improvement in the general health of the public, at least in Great Britain, which has followed the undoubted economic and nutritional changes of the last half-century. Comparisons of the results of treatment for one "clinical stage" *versus* another need to be viewed carefully against what is almost certainly a steady improvement in the standard of early diagnosis, the annual improvement in precision of diagnosis, and advances in hematology, antibiotics, anesthetics and all other aspects of medical care.

Table 12.2.
Natural history of clinical stage I testicular tumors after treatment by orchidectomy alone[a]

Era	N	Seminoma	Teratoma[a] TC	EC
		%	%	
Chevassu 1906[12]	128	22[b]	11	
Whitmore 1970[13]	106	50	40	17

[a] The abbreviations used are: N, number of patients; TC, teratocarcinoma, and EC, embryonal carcinoma.
[b] Percentage of survival.

Twenty years ago the results published by Patton and Mallis[14] led us to scrutinize the work at the London Hospital, and ask the questions whether and when we should be using radical node dissection (Hope-Stone et al. 1963[20]). We could not come to a clear answer then. The answer is even less clear today. Here we present our most recent attempt to audit the results of the treatment of germ cell tumors of the testis seen in the one institution over the last 30-year period from 1950–1980, the majority of whom have been treated by one group of surgeons and radiotherapists.

CLINICAL MATERIAL

Records of patients with testicular tumors have been kept in this Hospital since 1907[15] and were, before that time, the object of careful study by Curling,[16] and by Hutchinson.[17] From time to time they have been reviewed in the past[18] and there has never been a period when the condition was not a major interest of the surgeons of this institution. Few of the older records are, however, suitable for our purposes today. The present study is based predominantly on records of patients admitted between January 1960 and December 1977 whose histology has been reviewed and details extracted from case notes. Actuarial survival analyses of this information was performed using programs developed from the Vogelbach Computing Center statistical package for the social sciences (Northwestern University, Evanston, Ill.), transferred to computer data sheets and analyzed using the York package. Patients treated between 1950 and 1960 and those added since 1977 have been analyzed manually using the punch card method employed in previous analyses of this material.[3, 11, 19, 20]

Before 1977, all but two patients underwent orchidectomy: the exceptions had widespread tumor metastases which were biopsied. Since 1978, with the advent of effective chemotherapy for cases formerly thought to be hopelessly advanced, four additional cases were treated on the evidence of biopsy material from metastases and three on the evidence of metastases with markedly elevated HCG.

STAGING

Twenty years ago staging was on the basis of abdominal palpation, supplemented by excretion urography to show displacement of kidneys and ureters, plain radiography of the chest, and such crude measures of gonadotrophic activity as were in common use then for pregnancy testing. Year by year, these methods of investigation were progressively added to and made more precise with the introduction of whole lung tomography, lymphangiography, the more accurate biological assays of chorionic gonadotrophin and, later on, its measurement with radioimmunoassay techniques along with the radioimmunoassay of α-feto-protein and β-chain HCG. With the invention of computer-assisted tomography a new order of precision was added to the detection of metastases in the lung fields and permitted the identification of para-aortic metastases, often quite bulky, that had not displaced the ureters and certainly could not be felt by manual palpation of the abdomen even under anaesthesia in a fit and muscular young male. Because these staging investigations have been introduced gradually, it is impossible to compare the results of treatment at the end of the period under review with the results at the beginning except in the broadest of terms. For this reason, the results have been analyzed on the basis of two staging procedures: (1) Initial (preradiodiagnostic) clinical stage, and (2) final (postradiodiagnostic) clinical stage (Tables 12.3 and 12.4).

TREATMENT POLICY

Prior to 1963, patients were treated with 250 kv and seminoma without lung metastases received 2500–3000 rads in 3–4 weeks, and teratomas

Table 12.3.
Initial (preradiodiagnostic) clinical stage

Stage	Description
I.	No evidence of metastases in abdomen, neck, skin or central nervous system (CNS) on clinical examination.
II.	Clinical palpable lymph nodes in inguinal, common iliac or para-aortic region but no clinically detectable metastases in liver, neck, skin or central nervous system.
III.	As above, plus supraclavicular lymph node mass (or in the absence of testicular or para-aortic mass if biopsy of a mass in supra-clavicular region was indicative of a primary testicular tumor).
IV.	Obvious hard, enlarged and irregular clinically palpable liver, or clinical signs of CNS metastases in patient with biopsy-proven testicular tumor, or biopsy evidence of metastasis in another site, provided it had been biopsied on the basis of clinical symptoms or signs unsupported by radiological investigation.

Table 12.4.
Final (postradiodiagnostic) clinical stage[a]

Stage	Description
I.	Absence of metastases on chest x-ray (and/or whole lung tomography since 1970 and/or CT scan of lungs since 1978), lymphography (since 1968 and/or CAT scan of abdomen since 1978) and clinical examination.
IIA.	Para-aortic node less than 2 cm (common iliac or inguinal also considered in patients who have had previous inguinal or scrotal surgery).
IIB.	Para-aortic nodes ≥ 2 cm on lymphogram and/or CAT scan.
IIIA.	Para-aortic, mediastinal and/or supraclavicular lymph nodes but no tumor mass greater than 2 cm in diameter.
IIIB.	Mass ≥ 2 cm in any one or more of the above-mentioned sites.
IVA.	<3 lung metastases or multiple lung metastases <2 cm in diameter without clinically palpable abdominal mass.
IVB.	≥ 3 metastases, at least one of which was greater than 2 cm, or any lung metastases in patients with clinically palpable abdominal mass.
IVH.	Ultrasonic and/or isotopic and/or CAT scan and/or biochemical evidence of liver metastases. Any three of the four criteria had to be positive.

[a] Modified from Peckham *et al.*[7]

without lung metastases received 3500–4000 rads. From 1963–1972, patients were treated using a cobalt source. Seminomas received 3000 rads and teratomas 4000 rads. From 1973, patients have been treated over 4 weeks with an 8-Mev linear accelerator, using the same dosage schedule over 4 weeks given in 20 daily fractions. For all cases a simple technique using parallel opposed fields with an intravenous pyelogram (IVP) localization of the kidneys was used. Since 1972, a simulator has been used to improve the accuracy of treatment fields along with lymphography.

For stage I patients, treatment was to the para-aortics and pelvic lymph nodes only. For stage II patients, the para-aortics and pelvis were first treated to the standard dose and then, 1 month later, prophylactic treatment was given to the mediastinum and supraclavicular fossa using a T-shaped field. For stage III, treatment was given to chest and abdomen but the site of the largest volume of disease was treated first. In the early years, patients with lung metastases received either whole lung irradiation (2000 rads) or one of several single agents or combinations of drugs currently under investigation at that time, but there were no large series of patients receiving a single standard treatment until 1978 when use of bleomycin, vinblastine and cisplatinum according to the Einhorn and Donohue[9] regime was introduced. Since then, with increasing experience with the combination and encouraging results from other workers, it has been used for patients with earlier stage lymph node metastases as well, but so far only for patients with proven metastasis.

RESULTS

Four hundred and fifty-nine cases have been reviewed (Table 12.5) of whom 238 treated from 1960–1977 are the object of detailed computerized survival analyses.

Actuarial survival of patients treated from 1960–1977 are analyzed according to preradiodiagnostic clinical stage (Figs. 12.1 and 12.2). The histological classification of the tumors is that described by Pugh and Cameron.[21] Survival of men with clinically detectable metastases (*i.e.* stages II and III) is much worse than those in stage I, whatever the histological type of the tumor, and as reported previously from this institution,[3] there is a suggestion that survival of teratomas plateaus after the 4th year. For seminomas there is a continuing decline in survival even after 10 years—a factor that must be viewed against the incidence of nontumor deaths in this relatively older group of men, many of whom were older than 50 at the time of diagnosis (Table 12.6). Late relapse of nonseminoma is rare, but in this series there was one man, presenting with an MTU (malignant teratoma undifferentiated (embryonal carci-

Table 12.5.
The London Hospital testicular tumour series

Year of Diagnosis	Number of Cases
<1960	160
1960–1977	238
1978–1980	61

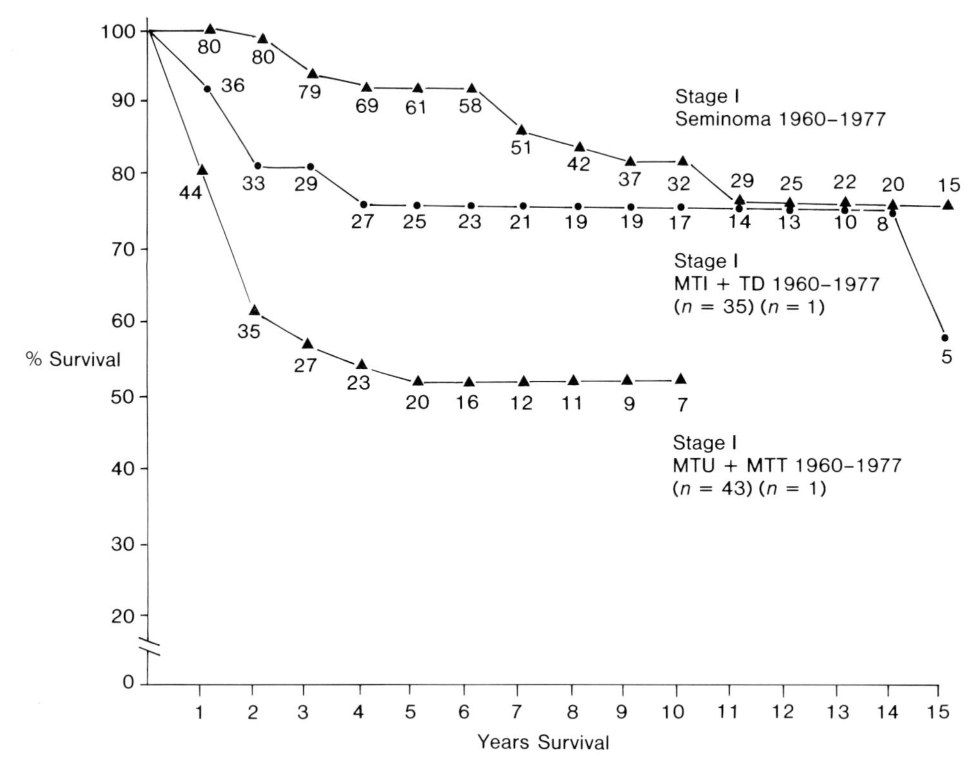

Figure 12.1. Actuarial survival of patients with initial clinical stage I seminoma, MTI + TD and MTU + MTT, 1960–1977. (*MTI*, malignant teratoma intermediate; *TD*, teratoma differentiated; *MTU*, malignant teratoma undifferentiated; and *MTT*, malignant teratoma, trophoblastic.)

noma)), treated by orchidectomy and abdominal radiation, who remained well for 16 years only to develop widespread metastases which, at autopsy, were found to be of the same histological type as his original tumor. Examination of his remaining testicle failed to demonstrate any evidence of a second primary.

Considering these results by the year of diagnosis and comparing them with the previously reported cases treated prior to 1960 show that irrespective of stage there has been a gradual improvement in survival over the last 30 years (Table 12.7). At the same time there has been a reduction in the proportion of men diagnosed as seminoma, and those in whom the diagnosis was only made when there were bulky retroperitoneal metastases (Tables 12.8 and 12.9).

Analyzed according to the criteria of the final (postradiodiagnostic) stage, there is an improvement in the survival of men with stage I tumors (Table 12.9). But there has been very little advance in the survival of the stage II cases when one allows for the larger proportion who had less advanced small-volume node metastases. It is hard to escape the conclusion that the overall improvement in survival seen in Table 12.7 may be merely a reflection of treating patients with less advanced disease and a more precise detection of early metastases.

CAT scanning, introduced in 1978, further increased the sensitivity of the detection of small lymph node and lung metastases and −65% of

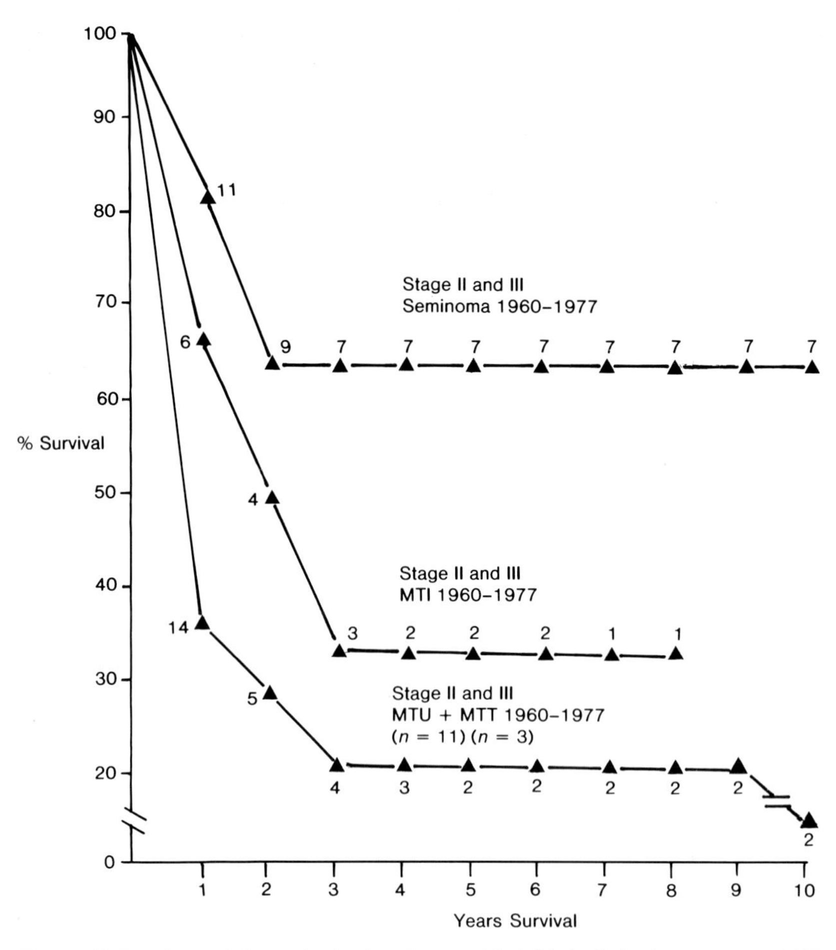

Figure 12.2. Actuarial survival of patients with initial clinical stage II and III seminoma, MTI + TD and MTU + MTT 1960–1977. (*MTI*, malignant teratoma intermediate; *TD*, teratoma differentiated; *MTU*, malignant teratoma undifferentiated; and *MTT*, malignant teratoma trophoblastic.)

Table 12.6.
Mean age[a] *versus* histological type (patients treated between 1960 and 1977)[b]

	N	Mean Age ± SD	Range
Seminoma	115	41 ± 13[c]	16–81
MTU	65	33 ± 11[d]	16–79
MTI	49*	29 ± 11[e]	15–71
TD	1	36	
MTT	4	30 ± 6	23–37
Unclassified germ cell	3		31–48

[a] One patient with no age recorded in notes, excluded.
[b] The abbreviations used are: N, number of patients; MTU, malignant teratoma undifferentiated; MTI, malignant teratoma intermediate; TD, teratoma differentiated; and MTT, malignant teratoma trophoblastic.
[c] *versus*[d], $p < 0.001$.
[c] *versus*[e], $p < 0.001$.
[d] *versus*[e], probability not significant.

teratomas with initial clinical Stage I presentation were thus "upstaged" (Table 12.10). (The staging error seems to be less important for seminomas, where only 3/21 (14%) were upstaged: one of these, a patient with large abdominal mass and three small lung metastases on CAT scan, had a spontaneous disappearance of the latter while his para-aortic nodes were undergoing radiotherapy).

IMPACT OF INTENSIVE PLATINUM COMBINATION THERAPY ON OVERALL SURVIVAL

As mentioned, earlier treatment policy has evolved during the past 3 years. Initially, use of platinum combination therapy was restricted to all patients, whatever the histological type, with proven lung metastases but more recently with increasing confidence it has been used to treat earlier stages of disease. This policy was accelerated by the death from chemotherapy-induced leucopenic sepsis with no residual disease of a patient with seminoma who presented initially with bulky clinical stage II disease,

Table 12.7.
Influence of initial clinical stage and year of diagnosis on survival of patients with testicular tumors at the London Hospital (all histologies)

Year of diagnosis	Overall		Stage I		Stage II or III	
	Number of Patients	% of Survival at 5 Years	Number of Patients	% of Survival at 5 Years	Number of Patients	% of Survival at 5 Years
		%		%		%
<1960	160	58 (93)[a]	NA[b]	NA[b]	NA[b]	
1960–1969	113	64 (70)	70[c]	79 (54)	23	30 (7)
1970–1977	125	71 (48)	92[d]	76 (38)	10	40 (4)

[a] Number of patients exposed to risk in determining the 5-year survival point on curve.
[b] Notes not reviewed. See Table 12.9 for data on final (postradiological) stage and survival taken from previously compiled punch cards.
[c] Twenty patients (13 alive) no data on initial clinical stage available. Notes lost; data from punch cards used.
[d] Twenty-three patients (17 alive) no data on initial clinical stage available. Notes lost; data from punch cards used.

Table 12.8.
Influence of histology and year of diagnosis on survival of patients with testicular tumors at the London Hospital[a]

N	Year of Diagnosis	Seminoma		MTI		MTU	
		N	% of Survival at 5 Years	N	% of Survival at 5 Years	N	% of Survival at 5 Years
			%		%		%
160 (93)[b]	<1960	101	65 (66)	32	63 (20)	27	22 (7)
111[c] (68)	1960–1969	61	82 (46)	23	74 (17)	27	19 (5)
124[c] (47)	1970–1977	54	92 (26)	28	64 (10)	42	49 (11)

[a] The abbreviations used are: MTI, malignant teratoma intermediate; MTU, malignant teratoma undifferentiated; and N, number of patients.
[b] Number of patients exposed to risk in determining the 5-year survival point on curve.
[c] Three patients with inadequate tissue to define type of tumor excluded.

Table 12.9.
Influence of final clinical stage and year of diagnosis on survival of patients with testicular tumors at the London Hospital (all histologies)[a]

N	Year of Diagnosis	Stage I			Stage II A and B (Combined)						Stages III and IV (Combined)					
		N	% of Survival at 5 Years		N	% of Survival at 5 Years					N	% of Survival at 5 Years				
160 (93)	<1960	110	74	(81)	26	42	(11)				24	4	(1)			
					Stage II A			Stage II B			Stage III A and IV A			Stage III B and IV B		
					N	% of Survival at 5 Years		N	% of Survival at 5 Years		N	% of Survival at 5 Years		N	% of Survival at 5 Years	
113 (70)	1960–1969	72	83	(58)	6	67	(4)	19	42	(8)	7	0	(0)	9	0	(0)
125 (48)	1970–1977	72	86	(32)	25	75	(11)	8	40	(2)	7	26	(1)	13	23	(2)

[a] Conventions as in Table 12.8.

Table 12.10.
Contribution of modern radiology to changing stage of previously untreated patients with testicular tumors (1978–1980).[a]

	Seminoma		Teratoma	
	N	Upstaged	N	Upstaged
Initial Clinical Stage I	13	1 (1)[b]	20	13 (11)
Initial Clinical Stage II and III	8	2 (1)	20	7 (2)

[a] N, number of patients.
[b] Number of patients upstaged excluding patients with metastases on chest x-ray.

Table 12.11.
Postradiodiagnostic stage and survival in the pre- and postcisplatinum era (all histologies).[a]

	Stage I			Stage II			Stage III and IV			
	N	% Alive 1 Year	% Alive 2 Years	N	% Alive 1 Year	% Alive 2 Years	N	% Alive 1 Year	% Alive 2 Years	
1960–1977	144	97 (144)[b]	90 (140)	58	83 (58)	70 (46)	36	44 (36)	22 (16)	$n = 238$
1978–1980	19	100 (16)	94 (7)	12	83 (10)	71 (6)	23	85 (18)	55 (5)	$n = 53$

[a] N, number of patients.
[b] Number at risk

Table 12.12.
Histology and response to cisplatinum combination chemotherapy of previously untreated patients with metastatic testicular tumors.[a]

	N	Complete Response	Current Status		
			Alive 6 Months	Disease Free >6 Months Off Treatment	Dead
Seminoma	4	3	4	3	
MTI	6	3(+2)[b]	5	5	1
MTU	15	12[c]	8	8	7
MTT[d]	7	2(+1)[b]	3	3	4
Total	32				

[a] The abbreviations used are: N, number of patients; MTI, malignant teratoma intermediate; MTU, malignant teratoma undifferentiated, and MTT, malignant teratoma trophoblastic.
[b] Patients rendered disease free by surgical excision of differentiated teratoma.
[c] One patient died from fulminating influenzal pneumonia and had no tumor at autopsy.
[d] Three patients diagnosed on the basis of bulky metastases with grossly elevated HCG (210 mg/l, 12 mg/l and 3.5 mg/l) and normal α-fetoprotein. At completion of treatment histology of testis revealed necrotic tissue in the first patient, differentiated teratoma in the second patient, and viable tumor in the third.

relapsed after radiotherapy and then died during a course of chemotherapy; and the death from uncontrolled tumor of two patients with small volume postradiological stage IIA disease who relapsed after radiotherapy and were unable to tolerate full dosages of combination therapy because of profound hematological toxicity.

When analyzed on the basis of final (postradiodiagnostic) clinical stage (Table 12.11) there is already a clear indication that patients with advanced disease are doing better than patients treated prior to 1978 but the numbers are as yet too small and follow-up too short to be certain that there will be an increase in long-term cure. For patients with early Stage I and II tumors there is as yet no clear indication of impact of the new chemotherapy but it must be remembered that three of the four deaths which occurred in this group of patients were among those who relapsed after radiotherapy and then received chemotherapy.

RESPONSE OF PATIENTS TO PLATINUM, BLEOMYCIN AND VINBLASTINE

Of 61 patients with newly diagnosed testicular tumors referred for staging 24 patients (12 in final stage I and 4 in stage IIB seminomas; 5 in stage I MTI (malignant teratoma); 2 in stage IIA MTU; and 1 in stage I MTT (malignant teratoma trophoblastic) received radiotherapy to para-aortic region as primary treatment and 37 received chemotherapy as primary treatment. There are 5 patients currently on treatment and showing evidence of response and 32 patients (Table 12.12) have been evaluated for response to chemotherapy. In addition, five patients who received radiotherapy (two in stage IIB seminomas, one in stage I MTI, and two in stage IIA MTU) subsequently relapsed and were referred for chemotherapy; the response of these patients and a further nine patients who had also relapsed after previous radiotherapy are recorded in Table 12.13. Complete response is based on results of clinical examination, tumor markers and CAT scan. Only patients with previously irradiated seminoma have done as well as unirradiated patients.

INFLUENCE OF TUMOR VOLUME AT START OF TREATMENT ON SURVIVAL AFTER CHEMOTHERAPY

The number of patients treated with chemotherapy is inadequate to make a formal survival analysis on the basis of stage and histology.

Table 12.13.
Histology and response to cisplatinum combination chemotherapy of previously irradiated patients with metastatic testicular tumors.[a]

		Complete Response	Current Status		
			Alive >6 Months	Disease Free >6 Months Off Treatment	Dead
Seminoma	3	3	2[b]	2	1
MTI	6	0(+1)[c]	2	0	4
MTU	5	0	2	0	3
Total	14				

[a] The abbreviations used are: MTI, malignant teratoma intermediate; and MTU, malignant teratoma undifferentiated.

[b] One patient died disease free in leucopenic phase of fourth course of chemotherapy.

[c] One death due to hemorrhage from duodenal ulcer (mesenteric artery with irradiation arteritis was eroded by duodenal ulcer). Autopsy showed no viable malignancy, but one small focus of cartilage.

Table 12.14.
Influence of tumor volume on survival of patients with MTU and MTT tumors.[a]

	N	Number of Deaths	Actuarial Survival at 18 Months
			%
Patient with abdominal nodes or lung metastases, ≤2 cm	5	0	100 (2)[b]
Patients with abdominal nodes or lung metastases, >2 cm	14	7	54 (9)
Patient with clinically palpable liver	3	3	0

[a] The abbreviations used are: MTU, malignant teratoma undifferentiated; MTT, malignant teratoma trophoblastic; and N, number of patients.
[b] Number at risk

However, there is already a suggestion for patients with MTU and MTT tumors, which is the largest group, that tumor volume is an important determinant of survival (Table 12.14).

DISCUSSION

Results reported in the literature show a steady improvement in survival for stage I and II nonseminomatous germ cell tumors with either radiotherapy or node dissection.[1-7] During this period, it seemed at first that men did slightly better with radiotherapy than with node dissection: 60% *versus* 51% before 1970, 72% *versus* 68% up to 1976. Since 1976 the results seem to have been better after node dissection (94% *versus* 90%) though it has to be asked whether this difference did not arise because centers with the best results from node dissection were the same centers where the best results were being obtained and some of them were using adjuvant chemotherapy.[4, 5]

As for the patient, it is impossible to quantify the relative acceptability of one course of treatment *versus* the other. When there is so little to choose between either form of therapy, the decision ought to take into account the morbidity of treatment. Lymphadenectomy entails a big abdominal incision, intestinal adhesions, loss of ejaculation,[22] and, even in the best hands, some morbidity from wound infection, lower limb edema, and pulmonary embolism.[23, 24] It is true that these are relatively slight in the best centers,[25] but the operative and postoperative hazards of skeletonizing the cava and the aorta and the ureters in less-than-optimal centers may well be under-reported.

No less necessary is it to take note of the morbidity of radiation therapy in less than optimal hands: it is true that centers reporting their results regularly find negligible incidences of bowel damage, of radiation nephritis and of spinal cord lesions. [2, 3, 20, 26] But they do occur elsewhere and cannot be ignored. Doctors are not all equal in their expertise and radiotherapy is no less a field for skill and judgement than is lymphadenectomy.

A good deal of the controversy has centered upon the matter of sexual function. After bilateral node dissection, men are seldom able to ejaculate and only rarely produce children probably from the necessary removal of the presacral nerves.[22] Ejaculation, with the maintenance of fertility after radiotherapy if it is possible to shield the contralateral testicle, is well established.[26]

Our own long-term follow-up, which would appear to be unique in centers expressing an interest in these cancers, seems to suggest that there may be another, perhaps more important, difference between the results of radiotherapy and of node dissection. In our experience, there continued to be a small but definite risk of late relapse, even 16 years after otherwise successful treatment by radiotherapy. Unfortunately, we cannot find any similar very long-term follow-up in the literature of men in comparable groups who have been treated by node dissection. When we have arrived at the situation where we are comparing cure-rates that approach 100% this risk of late relapse assumes increasing importance.

Equally important in the very long run may be the question of late hazards of radiation therapy in terms of carcinogenesis or ischemic damage to the kidney. In our own series there have been cases of known second nontesticular cancers and deaths from cardiovascular disease. It is possible that following lymphadenectomy, and without adjuvant radiotherapy or chemotherapy, these late deaths might not occur so often: but the evidence is wanting, since no such long-term follow-up has been carried out in any of the reported surgical series. It is, on the contrary, well-known that there is an increased risk of a second cancer in any patient who has had a first one, and cardiovascular disease is the most frequent cause of death in this country. It is therefore not by any means necessary to attribute these deaths to the radiation, but they do emphasize the importance of long term (10–20 year) follow-up of patients.

The results from this one institution mirror those in the literature, which also show a gradual improvement in survival over the last 30 years. Since this improvement occurs irrespective of technical advances in staging, *i.e.* according to initial clinical stage, it is quite possible that there has been a change in the natural history of the disease during this same period of time. This is suggested by the reduction in the proportion of men presenting with seminomas and of those with large-volume abdominal disease (Tables 12.8 and 12.9).

Because of this, and the fact that modern staging techniques can demonstrate metastases in nearly 50% of patients who would previously have been diagnosed as stage I, it is necessary to look again at the need for treatment in men in whom all the modern panoply of diagnostic tests fails to discover any metastases. It is possible that cases regarded as stage I by modern criteria, *i.e.* where markers, CAT scan and lymphangiogram are all negative, might well expect an 80% chance of cure by orchidectomy alone. We know that in men with "small volume" disease, chemotherapy can achieve a survival of 95%[7, 27] to 100% (this series). While it is true that giving routine radiotherapy to all the men in this group can also achieve close to 100% survival, if by mischance the initial staging is wrong, and they need chemotherapy at a later date, this initial dose of radiation may limit their subsequent tolerance to chemotherapy.[7, 11–13]

Today, we do not know what is the likelihood of relapse occurring in men thought, by all modern tests, to be in stage I. But if it were (as seems likely) to be of the order of 20%, and even if no more than 90% of them could be cured by chemotherapy if their metastases were detected at an early stage, then the overall survival for the group would be 98%, and 80% of the patients would have been let off a highly unpleasant course of chemotherapy, the long term risks of which have yet to be quantified or a dose of radiation that is not without its own hazards.

Proponents of node dissection may at this stage argue that examination of the operation specimen would make the issue clear by providing precise evidence as to the surgical stage: but a node dissection is a formidable procedure if its only value is to add a further 20% accuracy to an already very accurate barrage of preoperative investigations, and all this at the cost of ejaculatory infertility.

Today 90–94% of men thought to be in stage I can be cured either by lymph node dissection or radiation, and it is hard for those of us who have been using either form of treatment to give it up lightly when the results are so good. Nevertheless, we feel that the time has now come when the question must be put to the test. It is essential that nobody goes away with the notion that there is no need for any routine adjuvant treatment. Men with nonseminomatous tumors must not be deprived of adjuvant therapy unless they can be meticulously followed up. In this context because of the need for detailed staging procedures only available in specialist centers, such patients should continue to be referred to centers with a special interest in germ cell tumors.

At the other end of the spectrum, a new question has been raised in recent years concerning the correct management of the man who presents with very advanced disease, the man who until recently was thought to be inoperable, and fit only for palliative management. Today his enormous metastases melt away with chemotherapy, and we are left with the problem of what to do about residual radiological abnormality detected at the completion of treatment when it is known that two-thirds of such lesions do not have viable malignancy on histological section.[27] It is tempting to attempt to remove it. The operation—often referred to as a "debulking" operation—is frequently difficult and not a little dangerous, since the walls of the aorta and cava are often severely damaged by the necrosis of the adjacent tumor. It remains to be seen whether the attempt is justified by the results, that is to say we need to know what is the benefit to the minority from removal of a small nest of dormant tumor that has demonstrated its resistance to chemotherapy, compared to the risks for the majority in undergoing a major operation to remove only dead tissue. It is possible that the addition of radiotherapy to sites of residual disease may reduce the need for surgery and this will need to be tested by trial in the future. Even so, it will be necessary to continue to get precise pathological information on the effect of our treatment.

One fact which continues to emerge from study of patients with testicular tumors is that far too many young men are still being referred only when their disease is far advanced. The tragedy is that they could, in nearly every case, have been saved by earlier diagnosis and more vigorous treatment. Of 21 patients coming up in the last 2 years with bulky metastases, no fewer than 7 had a lump in the testicle that could and should have been diagnosed earlier. However clever we may have become with our surgery or our radiotherapy or our chemotherapy, we still have a major task of education to accomplish.

Looking back over this experience of 20 years it seems that the wheel has come full circle. No longer is there any interest in the protracted argument of lymph node dissection *versus* radiation: the war has moved on, and the old entrenched positions need no longer to be defended. Now we must ask ourselves whether radiotherapy or node dissection need to be given to men who come up in the earliest stages of nonseminoma. Both protagonists now have to look ahead, to try to define how best to offer their patients the benefits of chemotherapy, of surgical debulking, and of radiation. New questions replace the old ones. For very different reasons, and by very different routes, we seem to have come to the same position.

Acknowledgments—We are grateful to our colleagues in the North East Metropolitan Region for referring patients for treatment; and to colleagues in the London Hospital, A. Paris, B. Mantell and G. Mair, for permission to study patients treated by them, and to Steven Evans for performing the computer analysis.

REFERENCES

1. Caldwell, W. L. *South. Med. J. 62:*1232, 1969.
2. Peckham, M. J., and McElwain, T. J. In *Recent Advances in Urology*, Vol. 2, p. 324, edited by W. F. Hendry Churchill-Livingstone, Edinburgh, 1976.
3. Blandy, J. P. *et al.* Tumours of the Testicle William Heinemann Medical Books, London, 1970.
4. Skinner, D. G. *J. Urol. 115:*65, 1976.
5. Donohue, J. P. *et al. Cancer 42:*2903, 1978.
6. Maier, J. G., and Lee, S. N. *Urol. Clin. N. Amer. 4:*477, 1977.
7. Peckham, M. J., Barrett, A., McElwain, T. J., and Hendry, W. F. Combined management of malignant teratoma of the testis *Lancet 1:*267–270, 1979.
8. Samuels, M. L., Lanzotti, V. J., Holoye, P. Y., Eamonn, B. L., Smith, T. and Johnson, D. E. *Cancer Treat. Rev. 3:*185, 1976.
9. Einhorn, L. H., and Donohue, J. *Ann. Int. Med. 87:*293, 1977.
10. Stoter, G., *et al.* Combination chemotherapy comprising *cis*-dichloroplatinum, vinblastine and bleomycin, in a highly compromised group of patients with disseminated testicular nonseminomas. *Lancet 1:*941–945, 1979.
11. Oliver, R. T. D., *et al.* Chemotherapy of metastatic testicular tumors. *Br. J. Urol. 52:*34–37, 1980.
12. Chevassu, M. Tumeurs du testicule Thèse de Paris No 193 G Steinheil, 1906.
13. Whitmore, W. F. In *Proceedings of the Sixth National Cancer Conference*, p. 219. J. B. Lippincott, Philadelphia, 1970.
14. Patton, J. F., and Mallis, N. Tumors of the testis *J. Urol. 81:*457–481, 1959.
15. Howard, R. J. Malignant disease of the testis *Practitioner 79:*794, 1907.
16. Curling, T. B. *A Practical Treatise on the Diseases of the Testis* Longman, Brown, Green & Longmans, London, 1843.
17. Hutchinson, J. *An Atlas of Illustrations of Pathology Fasc X Diseases of the Testis*, edited by H. K. Lewis. New Sydenham Society, London, 1894.
18. Cairns, H. W. B. *Lancet 1:*845, 1926.
19. Blandy, J. P. *Urology*, p. 1203. Blackwell Scientific Publications, Oxford, 1976.
20. Hope-Stone, H. F., Blandy, J. P., and Dayan, A. D. *Br. Med. J. 1:*984, 1963.
21. Pugh, R. C. B., and Cameron, K. M. In *Pathology of the Testis*, Blackwell Scientific Publications, London, 1976.
22. Kedia, K. R., Markland, C., and Fraley, E. E. Sexual function after high retroperitoneal lymphadenectomy *Urol. Clin. North Am. 4:*523–527, 523–527, 1977.
23. Sago, A. L., Ball, T. P., and Novicki, D. E. Complications of retroperitoneal lymphadenectomy *Urology, 13:* 241–243, 1979.

24. Beck, P. H., and Stutzman, R. E. Complications of retroperitoneal lymphadenectomy for nonseminomatous tumors of the testis *Urology 13:* 244–247, 1979.
25. McLorie, G. A., and Skinner, D. G. Metastatic nonseminomatous testis tumors: morbidity of treatment *J. Urol. 124:*479–481, 479–481, 1980.
26. Werf-Messing, B., van der *Int. J. Radiat. Oncol. Biol. Phys. 1:*235, 1976.
27. Einhorn, L., and Donohue, J. *Semin. Oncol. 6:*87, 1979.

13

Radiation Therapy for Patients with Testicular and Extragonadal Seminoma

William U. Shipley, M.D.

TESTICULAR SEMINOMAS

Introduction

Pure seminoma is the most common subtype*[1] of testicular cancer.[2] Pure seminoma is the most radiosensitive malignancy managed in radiotherapy clinics, although solid deposits of leukemia are of almost equal radiosensitivity. These tumors can usually be sterilized by doses of 2000–3000 rads of external beam irradiation.[3] Because of the exquisite (but as yet radiobiologically poorly understood) radiation sensitivity of seminomatous deposits, radiation therapy rather than surgical resection is the treatment choice for the retroperitoneal lymph nodes in patients presenting with this germ cell tumor. For instance, the 3- and 5-year survivals for patients treated with radiation therapy following radical orchiectomy for stage I seminoma are 97% (Table 13.1). This extraordinarily high success rate, reported from most clinics, makes the seminoma to date surpassed only by skin cancer as the most successfully managed group of tumors in all of clinical oncologic practice.

Surgery by radical orchiectomy is the appropriate diagnostic step and the treatment of choice for control for the primary tumor in a patient presenting with a testicular tumor.[9-11] The rationale for the use of external beam radiation therapy, or possibly surgery, to treat the regional (retroperitoneal) lymph node metastases in the curative management of patients with testicular seminoma is that, at presentation, a substantial (15%–30%)

* Dixon and Moore classification[1] of germ cell testicular tumors. Group I, pure seminoma; group II, embryonal carcinoma, pure or with seminoma; group III, teratoma, pure or with seminoma; group IV, teratoma with embryonal and/or choricocarcinoma, with or without seminoma; group V, Choriocarcinoma, pure or with embryonal carcinoma and/or seminoma.

Table 13.1.
Radiation therapy in testicular seminoma: clinical stage I

Institution	Number	% of 3-year Disease-Free Survival
		%
Walter Reed[4]	284	97
Royal Marsden Hospital[5]	78	98
M. D. Anderson Hospital[3]	79	94
Stanford University[6]	71	100
Rotterdam Institute[7]	91	100
Massachusetts General Hospital[8]	135	98
Total	738	97

number of patients will have metastases to only the retroperitoneal lymph nodes. Thus, the control of the disease at this first sight of metastases by local treatment will lead to cure in well over 90% of patients in this group.

The clinical staging* for the evaluation of possible extragonadal metastatic disease in patients with testicular seminoma should include lung tomograms, bipedal lymphangiogram, and quantitative pre- and postorchiectomy HCG and α-fetoprotein (AFP). An elevated AFP indicates with near certainty that nonseminomatous malignant germ cell elements are present and treatment decisions should be so modified.[17] Lymphangiography has an accuracy of 70%–80% when compared to pathological staging as reported from many large centers[11, 18–21] In patients with negative or minimally positive lymphangiograms, the retroperitoneal CT scan has not added accuracy to a clinical staging. If the lymph nodes are shown to be substantially involved with bulky deposits on lymphangiogram, then retroperitoneal CT scan will often add helpful information of possible extranodal extension of the tumor as well as of possible involvement of lymph nodes above the level of L2 or in the renal hila where metastases are not usually demonstrated by lymphangiography.

Clinical Evaluation

Several important postorchiectomy evaluations are necessary prior to the formulation of the final treatment recommendations. The slides from the radical orchiectomy specimens must be reviewed by an experienced pathologist. In our experience, this had led to a change in diagnosis with regard to the subtype of germinal tumor in 10–20% of the patients referred. I believe that this is understandable due to the infrequency with which a general pathologist within a community hospital, where often radical orchiectomy is carried out, is called upon to diagnose these relatively uncommon tumors. Because of the unique radiosensitivity, pure

* Clinical staging of testicular carcinoma, presented both by Maier and Lee[14] and Peckham[15] based on their experience and that of the M.D. Anderson Hospital.[16] Clinical stage I, lymphangiogram negative, no evidence of metastases; clinical stage IIA, lymphangiogram positive with maximum diameter of metastases less than 2 cm, evidence of metastases confined to retroperitoneal nodes; clinical stage IIB, lymphangiogram positive with maximum diameter of metastases 2 cm or greater, evidence of metastases confined to retroperitoneal nodes; clinical stage III, involvement of supra- and infradiaphragmatic lymph nodes, no evidence of extralymphatic metastases; and clinical stage IV, extralymphatic metastasis.

seminoma is important to distinguish from nonseminomatous germ cell tumors. For example, the control of bulky retroperitoneal nodal metastases by external beam irradiation for patients with seminoma (usually with doses of 4000 rads or less) is <90%.[3] While the local control of similar-stage patients treated with radiation therapy with nonseminomatous testicular carcinoma is only 31%.[12]

Often patients are referred with the histologic diagnosis of an "anaplastic" seminoma with the implication that this may have important treatment implications. However, recent review of anaplastic seminoma of the testes, by the same institution that originated this subcategory, has revealed this has a similar presentation, response to radiation, and prognosis as compared to typical seminoma when evaluated by stage.[13] This review and difficulty of defining this entity histopathologically has led to the committee pathologists at the recent International Symposium of Human Testes Cancer to conclude that the term anaplastic seminoma should be abandoned (R. E. Scully, personal communication).

Radiation Treatment Techniques

Lymphangiographic visualization of the retroperitoneal nodes is essential in the careful design of appropriate retroperitoneal treatment fields with radiation therapy. The exact definition of the field depends on the unique characteristics of a given patient and the type of megavoltage equipment available. Figure 13.1 demonstrates radiotherapeutic fields that we have employed in the patients with clinical stage I or IIA testicular seminoma. The lymphatic drainage differs for the left and right testicles and, therefore, so should the field in the region of the ipsilateral renal hilum. The fields are contoured with individually cut cerroband blocking. These paired anterior and posterior fields are both treated daily on our 10-mv linear accelerator. The boundaries of the fields usually are: *superiorally* to include the origin or the thoracic duct or the entire anterior surface of the T11 veterbral body; *inferiorally* to include the internal inguinal ring and (not shown on the diagram) the linguinal incision; *laterally* to include the ipsilateral renal hilum, usually more generous on the left than on the right; and the contralateral retroperitoneal lymph nodes of the para-aortic, or paracaval and common illiac groups. These should be expanded to include additional areas in the following two, not uncommon, situations: (1) in patients who have a prior history of inguinal or scrotal surgery, that may predispose to atypical lymphatic drainage, the inferior portion of the field should be extended to include the contralateral inguinal region; and (2) if there has been histological evidence of epididymal invasion by the tumor, the fields should be enlarged to include the ipsilateral hypogastric lymph nodes as a potential site of metastatic drainage. The excretory urogram must be carefully evaluated at the time of simulation with the patient in the treatment position to assure the exact localization of the kidneys with respect to radiation fields. When such care is taken to localize the kidneys properly, the risk of radiation-induced injury is essentially limited. A gonadal shield protecting the contralateral testicle should be used during simulation and treatment of the retroperitoneal fields. With the use of gonadal shielding (usually clam shell-like devices),

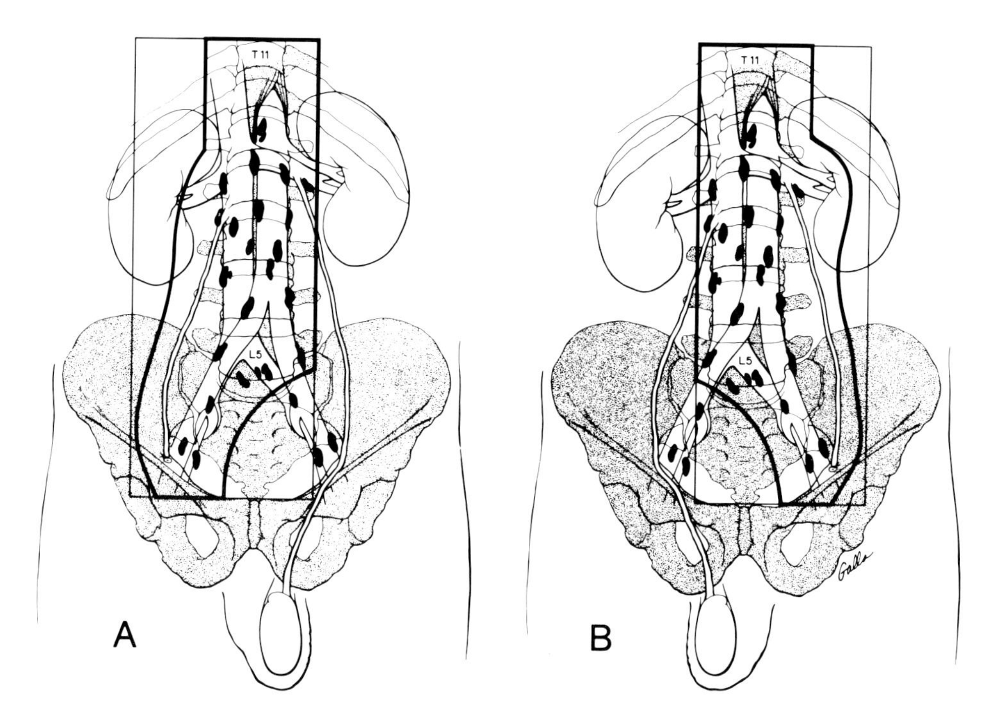

Figure 13.1. Contoured anterior and posterior radiation treatment fields for patients *with* clinical Stage I or IIA testicular seminoma, but *without* epididymal involvement or prior inguinal surgery. (The lead scrotal chamber or shield to protect the contralateral testis is not shown.) *A*, right testicular tumor; *B*, left testicular tumor.

the radiation dose to the contralateral testis is approximately 1.5%–2.0% of the prescribed dose. This is the result of both externally and internally scattered protons.[22] Recently we have used additional lead shields outside the primary beam 10 cm above the contralateral testicle to shield high energy protons scattered from the machine treatment head. This technique and the use of a more comprehensive gonadal shield preventing the majority of internally scattered protons from hitting the testicle has lowered the dose to the contralateral testicle to approximately 0.1% of the treatment dose (Kubo and Shipley, in preparation).

The treatment of patients with clinical stage II seminoma should include radiation of the mediastinum and left supraclavicular regions as elective treatment following retroperitoneal irradiation. Care should be taken to match these supradiaphragmatic fields with the retroperitoneal portals using appropriate gap, moving junction, or junctional wedge techniques to assure neither underdosing nor an area of high dose overlap in the region of spinal cord.[23]

Treatment Results

Friedman[24] reported more than three decades ago on the exquisite sensitivity of the retroperitoneal lymph nodes metastases from pure seminoma to external irradiation. More recent analyses of the doses of megavoltage therapy necessary to sterilize such metastatic deposits from pure seminoma confirm his original observations that 3000 rads given with conventional fractionation (150–200 rad/day; 5 sessions/week) using megavoltage beams is nearly certain of sterilizing these metastases (Tables 13.1 and 13.2). Only 1 of 132 patients developed an in-field local failure when a range of doses, varying with clinical settings, from 2000–4500 rads were given by the M.D. Anderson Hospital group.[3] Of course, local control of seminoma like other tumors and normal tissue tolerance depend on the time-dose relationships determined by the radiation fractionation scheme rather than on only total dose.[25] On review of our seminoma experience since 1950, only one stage I patient of 135 irradiated (with megavoltage doses of 2300–3000 rads) has recurred in the treated field. However, that patient was given an uncommonly protracted irradiation course of more than 5 weeks.[8] The cure rate for patients with this early stage of seminoma who were initially designated as having an anaplastic subtype by the genito-urinary branch of the Armed Forces Institute of Pathology, and who were treated by orchiectomy and retroperitoneal lymphatic irradiation, is not lower than those men with the other histologic subtypes. Specifically, for 77 patients with a median follow-up of 97 months, the 10-year survival was 96% and 87% for stage I and II patients, respectively, with the anaplastic form of pure seminoma.[13]

The treatment results of patients with clinical stage I seminoma treated with the external beam irradiation following orchiectomy are shown in Figure 13.2 and Table 13.1. The combined 3-year survival of 738 patients reported from six major treatment centers is 97% with a range of 94%–100%. Generally, these outstanding results were achieved without the elective irradiation of the mediastinal and supraclavicular lymph nodal regions. Patterns of failure have been analyzed both by the M. D. Anderson group and ourselves. In this combined group, only one of 194 patients treated without elective irradiation of the supradiaphragmatic regions failed in the supraclavicular lymph nodes.[3, 8] Peckham and McElwain[5] have reported that patients with seminoma who in their series did receive elective mediastinal irradiation had a higher incidence of intercurrent death due to myocardial infarction than in the much larger group of patients who did not receive irradiation to this area. Although this latter report was not a statistically significant difference, the general consensus and this author's preference is that elective treatment of mediastinum and the left supraclavicular region in the clinical stage I patients is not indicated.

The results of treating patients with stage II seminoma by external beam irradiation therapy is shown in Table 13.2. For 190 patients, the average 3-year disease-free survival was 86% with a range of 74%–93%. The radiation in nearly all instances included elective irradiation of the mediastinum and supraclavicular regions, usually doses of 2000–3000 rads following retroperitoneal treatment. Doornbos *et al.*[3] reported two of five patients failing in the supraclavicular lymph nodes in those stage II seminoma patients who were not treated electively to this area. These results and the 15%–20% incidence of proven histologic involvement of the supraclavicular lymph nodes in patients with clinical stage II testicular cancer by left supraclavicular nodal biopsy make elective supradiaphragmatic treatment essential in the management of patients with this stage disease.[25, 26] In patients with bulky retroperitoneal lymph node disease

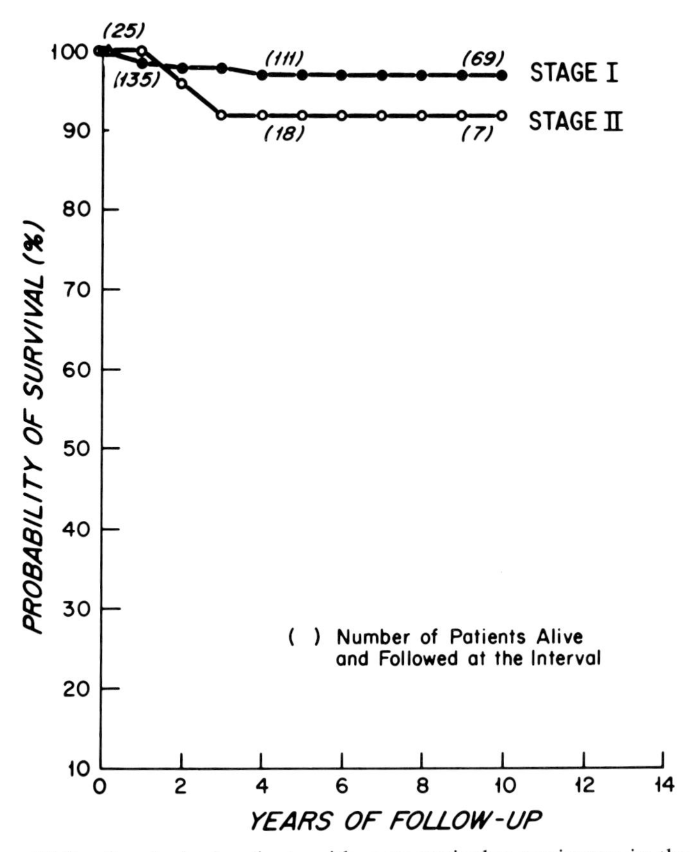

Figure 13.2. Survival of patients with pure testicular seminoma in the Massachusetts General Hospital Series, 1950–1976.[8]

Table 13.2.
Radiation therapy in testicular seminoma: clinical stage II

Institution	Number	% of 3-year Disease-Free Survival
		%
Walter Reed[4]	34	76
Royal Marsden Hospital[5]	27	93
M.D. Anderson Hospital[3]	30	74
Stanford University[6]	27	89
Rotterdam Institute[7]	46	91
Mass. General Hospital[8]	26	88
Total	190	86

(clinical stage IIB), modifications of the usual treatment techniques for retroperitoneum are necessary. The whole abdominal cavity should initially be treated to doses in the range of 2000 rads to prevent marginal recurrence in those tumors that may extensively infiltrate beyond the lymph nodes. The boost dose to the bulk disease should be raised to levels of 4000 rads with careful shaping of the cone-down retroperitoneal fields to exclude 50%–70% of the renal parenchyma from receiving doses in excess of 2400 rads. Retroperitoneal exploration following radiation should be considered when radiologic regression has not occurred.

A small minority of patients, probably less than 5%, present with clinical stage III and IV seminoma. The success rate in these patients treated with radiation therapy is less certain because of the small number of patients reported. The composite experience suggests that about one-half the patients with these advanced stages treated with radiation alone can be cured.[3–8] However, now multidrug chemotherapy, which has shown to be effective in disseminated seminoma, should be considered for advanced stages. Our present treatment policy with stage III or IV patients is irradiation to the involved and potentially involved lymph nodal regions usually supplemented with 1500 rads with full lung irradiation and followed by 1 year of cyclophosphamide.

PURE TESTICULAR SEMINOMA WITH ELEVATED HCG

In the 5 of 83 patients treated with seminoma at the Walter Reed Hospital, 10–30 years ago, presence of a positive HCG by the relatively insensitive urinary bioassay technique predicted a lethal outcome in all 5.[4] However, these five patients all presented with very advanced disease. No effective chemotherapy was available and the metastatic seminoma masses did show the usual radiation sensitivity to local therapy (Maier, personal communication). Over the last decade, the much more sensitive and specific (no interference with LH) radioimmunoassay to the β-subunit of HCG has been developed.[28] A small minority of patients with pure seminoma present with an elevated serum HCG by antibody assay to this β-subunit.[17, 29] Javapour and associates[17] found an elevated HCG in 5%, or in 3 of 60 patients, presenting with a primary tumor confirmed to be pure seminoma on review of serial histologic sectioning. Immunoperoxidase staining of the primary tumor identified HCG within benign cytiotrophoblastic giant cells associated with the seminoma. Patients with an elevated AFP should be managed as having nonseminomatous tumor. An elevated AFP occurs only in the presence of embryonal carcinoma or yolk sac tumor.[17] Our experience[8] and that reported by others[30] has been that patients with pure seminoma and an elevated HCG have metastatic masses with the usual excellent radiosensitivity and all 10 remain in complete remission following the usual treatment with radiation therapy. We have irradiated five patients (stage I (3), stage IIB (1), stage IV (1) with pure seminoma (on review of histologic step-sections) and an elevated HCG. All are in complete remission both clinically and serologically with a follow-up of 2, 3, 4, 8, and 13 years. The Stage IIB patient had a 9 × 5 × 5-cm retroperitoneal mass completely obstructing the right illiac vein. He was treated with 2000 rads to the whole abdomen and a boost to 4000 rads to the original bulky disease in the retroperitoneum. He was subsequently given a course of radiation of 2600 rads to the mediastinum and left supraclavicular region. At the completion of the retroperitoneal irradiation, the serum HCG was negative, and the repeat ultrasound showed clearance of the obstructing mass. Two months later a retroperitoneal exploration revealed no mass, and all resected tissue was fibrotic and free of tumor. He remains free of disease now, 4 years following diagnosis. The stage IV patient, who had even more massive retroperitoneal disease and a 5-cm pulmonary mass that was cytologically seminoma on needle biopsy, is in complete remission following similar treatment plus whole lung irradiation and cyclophosphamide chemotherapy for 1 year.

Our present treatment strategy is similar to that recommended by Whitmore[11] with pure seminoma and an elevated HCG: step-sectioning of the primary tumor to demonstrate any nonseminomatous tumor elements, if present; otherwise, the treatment is by radiation therapy with doses that are usual for the patient's clinical stage. If the HCG remains elevated following irradiation, then additional treatment by surgery or chemotherapy is essential, as is suggested by a compilation of complicated cases recently published in the urologic literature.[31]

SECOND TESTICULAR TUMORS

In our series, 4 patients, or approximately 2% of 171 seminoma patients, developed a second testicular tumor. In addition, two other patients had developed a seminoma following successful treatment of an initial nonseminomatous testicular tumor. The mean interval between the diagnosis of the two consecutive tumors was 11 years with a range of 6–18 years. Three of the four tumors that developed after initial seminoma were pure testicular seminomas occurring 6, 7, and 12 years following treatment of the initial tumor. All three of these patients were successfully retreated after orchiectomy and retroperitoneal irradiation by similar treatment and all are alive without evidence of disease at 4, 6, 19 years of follow-up since the diagnosis of the second primary tumor. This increased incidence of second testicular tumors has been previously described.[3, 32, 33]

VARIATIONS IN TUMOR HISTOLOGIC TYPE IN METASTATIC SITES

In our review, 15 of the 17 patients that failed initial treatment had pathological material evaluated from the metastatic site. In two instances, a different pattern (embryonal carcinoma) was found in the metastatic tumor from the primary seminoma. In a clinical stage IIB patient, the widespread abdominal disease recurred which proved to be embryonal carcinoma. A stage I patient failed in an isolated rib that was treated successfully by high dose irradiation. Others have reported that pure testicular seminoma can metastasize with different histologic patterns[3, 4, 34] although this is a rare (less than 3% of treated patients) event.

Radiation Tolerance and Complications

Retroperitoneal irradiation is well tolerated by the young men undergoing this treatment. They nearly always continue their work or education during treatment with little, if any, interruption. Approximately half the patients treated experienced mild nausea which is usually controlled with antiemetic medication. Weekly hemograms should be checked during treatment because 10% of the patients require treatment interruption from moderate, but never severe, leukopenia or thrombocytopenia. Acute radiation colitis or enteritis is uncommon in this dose range of 3000–4000 rads when given with conventional fractionation (150–200 rads, 5 sessions/week). Should such symptoms occur, they are usually controlled with an antispasmotic medication and subside shortly following completion of treatment. Delayed late or gastrointestinal reactions such as radiation enteritis or bowel obstruction are not seen following treatment with doses at this level if they are not combined with retroperitoneal lymph node resection.[6]

Patients undergoing retroperitoneal irradiation with conventional gonadal shielding receive to the contralateral testicle 1.5%–2% of the treatment dose (45–60 rads) which causes a transient oligospermia. The oligospermia persists for 12–18 months following radiation therapy, but in nearly all instances, returns to pretreatment levels in 18–24 months.[35, 36] Recently, with our improved gonadal shielding mechanisms, which allow only 0.1% of the given dose to the contralateral testicle, we have not observed any reduction in sperm count following radiation therapy. However, patients should be instructed that it would be wise to wait a full year following radiation therapy prior to insemination to maximize the opportunity for repair from any genetic damage from this low level (~3 rads) of radiation.

Treatment Recommendations

Patients found on radical inguinal orchiectomy to have a pure testicular seminoma should be treated with external beam irradiation as outlined below.

CLINICAL STAGE I

Retroperitoneal irradiation to the first echelon lymph node region as outlined in Figure 13.1. The dose should be in the range of 3000 rads with megavoltage equipment given in 150- to 200-rad fractions over 3–4 weeks. Elective mediastinal or left supraclavicular irradiation is not indicated.

CLINICAL STAGE IIA

Retroperitoneal fields similar to those shown in Figure 13.1 should be treated to 3000 rads in 4 weeks followed by an additional boost of 600 rads given to the areas of lymphangiographically involved lymph nodes. The mediastinal and left supraclavicular regions should be treated electively with doses in the range of 2600 rads over 2-1/2 weeks following completion of the retroperitoneal irradiation.

CLINICAL STAGE IIB

The whole abdominal cavity should be treated to a dose of 2000 rads. A boost dose to the retroperitoneal masses and the para-aortic and ipsilateral iliac lymph nodes should be given to raise the total dose level to 4000 rads in 5–6 weeks. Subsequently, the mediastinum and left supraclavicular fossa should receive 2600 rads as in stage IIA.

CLINICAL STAGES III–IV

Treat with radiation to all involved or potentially involved lymph nodal regions to 2600 rads and boost areas of bulk disease in the retroperitoneum to 4000 rads and solitary pulmonary nodules to 3600 rads. Patients with pulmonary or pleural disease should also be treated with full lung irradiation to 1500 rads. In patients who have had bulky abdominal disease, as in stage IIB, the whole abdominal cavity should receive 2000 rads. Following irradiation, patients should be treated with a year of cyclophosphamide.

PATIENT FOLLOW-UP

Recurrences following radiation therapy for patients with seminoma almost all occur within the first 2 years of presentation. Accordingly, patients should be followed closely for 2 years by physical exam, chest x-ray and, if they were originally positive, serum HCG every 3 months for 2 years. Follow-up after this should be annually for 5 years. The high (>50%) cure rate even if metastases develop, occasionally of nonseminomatous histology, justifies this close surveillance.

Conclusions

1. Pure testicular seminoma is a highly curable disease when treated by conventional external beam radiation therapy to the involved or potentially involved regional-draining lymph nodes.
2. Despite high success rates, close follow-up for the first 2–3 years is necessary. Appropriate salvage treatment for the minority of patients who develop a recurrence often is curative.
3. Further improvement in overall survival may be achieved by aggressively treating those patients with lesions who have had a poor prognosis, *i.e.* stages IIB, III, and IV. This should be done by combining comprehensive external beam with irradiation and chemotherapy that emphasizes the alkylating agent, cyclophosphamide.
4. HCG and "anaplastic" seminomas are as curable by radiation therapy as are all seminomas.
5. Two percent of patients with testicular tumor will develop a tumor in the contralateral testicle in the next 5–20 years.

EXTRAGONADAL SEMINOMAS

Extragonadal germ cell tumors occur *with very low frequency* and are histologically identical with those of malignant neoplasms of testicular origin; they have been recently thoroughly reviewed by Einhorn.[37] They occur most commonly in the anterior mediastinum,[38–43] the retroperitoneum[41–47], and the pineal as well as other midline cerebral and cerebellar locations.[42, 43, 48, 49] These germ cell tumors are similar in at least three ways to their malignant counterparts arising in the testes. First, they occur in the same age distribution as the primary testicular tumors. Second, they have roughly the same frequency in distribution of pathologic subtypes with 50% or more being seminomas. Thirdly, the response of these rare tumors to radiation therapy and chemotherapy can be reasonably inferred to be similar to their histologic counterpart arising in the testes.[37, 40, 49] Cox[40] recently reviewed over 100 documented cases of mediastinal seminoma. He concluded that doses of 3000 rads over 3 weeks gave excellent local control which is similar to the radiocurability for metastatic deposits from testicular seminoma at any site. Likewise, the radiocurability of the suprasellar germinomas separate these rare tumors from most other brain tumors.[49]

It is important to alert our colleagues in general, thoracic and brain surgery that these tumors exist as clinical entities because, for the seminomatous subtypes, there is a reasonably good prospect of cure with radiotherapy and now, with advances in multidrug chemotherapy, the potential for cure in the nonseminomatous tumors. If the surgeon is aware of the possible diagnosis of an extragonadal seminoma, and this is possible to confirm on frozen section, then the surgeon need not take undue risks to compromise normal structures by a "complete" resection. There is no indication for orchiectomy in these patients if the testes are normal to palpitation. Finally, there is no role for retroperitoneal lymph node resection in a patient with a mediastinal seminoma. The published information on cure rate and patterns of failure following localized radiation therapy for patients with mediastinal and retroperitoneal seminomas indicate elective irradiation to uninvolved fields above or below the diaphragm seems unnecessary.[38, 46]

The clinical evaluation of the patient with mediastinal or retroperitoneal seminoma should include whole lung tomograms and a lymphangiogram. A computed body tomograph will likely assist in radiation treatment planning. The radiation dose given by conventional fractionation should be 4000–4500 rads for extragonadal seminomas in the mediastinum, the retroperitoneum, and the brain. At the present time, there does not appear to be an initial role for chemotherapy in the extragonadal seminomas.[37]

Conclusions

1. Extragonadal seminomas of the anterior mediastinum, retroperitoneum and brain are definite clinical entities.
2. These tumors should be treated in a similar fashion to their testicular counterpart.
3. The extragonadal seminomas have a high cure rate with definitive external beam radiation therapy using doses of 4000–4500 rads.
4. There is no need to perform an orchiectomy on such patients.

REFERENCES

1. Dixon, F. J., and Moore, R. A. Tumors of the male sex organs. Atlas of Tumor Pathology. Section VIII, FAS 31b and 32. Armed Forces Institute of Pathology, Washington, D.C., 1952.
2. Culp, D. A., Boatman, D. L., and Wilson, V. B. Testicular tumors: 40 years experience. *J. Urol. 110*:548–553, 1964.
3. Doornbos, J. F. Hussey, D. H., and Johnson, D. E. Radiotherapy for pure seminoma of the testis. *Radiology 116*:401–404, 1975.
4. Maier, J. G., and Sulak, M. H. Radiation therapy in malignant testis tumors, Part I, Seminoma. *Cancer 32*:1212–1216, 1973.
5. Peckham, M. J., and McElwain, T. J. Radiotherapy of testicular tumors. *Proc. R. Soc. Med. 67*:300–303, 1974.
6. Earle, J. D., Bagshaw, M. A., and Kaplan, H. S. Supervoltage radiation therapy of testicular tumors. *AJR 117*:653–661, 1973.
7. van der Werf-Messing, B. Radiotherapeutic treatment of testicular tumors. *Int. J. Radiat. Oncol. 1*:235–248, 1976.
8. Dosoretz, D. E., Shipley, W. U., Blitzer, P. H., Gilbert, S., Prat, J., Parkhurst, E. C., and

Wang, C. C. Megavoltage irradiation for pure testicular seminoma: results and patterns of failure. *Cancer 48:*2184–2190, 1981.
9. Whitmore, W. F., Jr. Germinal tumors of the testis. *Proceedings of the 6th National Cancer Conference.* J. B. Lippincott, Philadelphia, 1970.
10. Prout, G. R., Jr. Germinal tumors of the testis. *Cancer Medicine Holland,* pp. 1696–1708, edited by F. James and E. Frei, III. Lee & Febiger, Philadelphia, 1973.
11. Whitmore, W. F., Jr. Surgical treatment of adult germinal testis tumors. *Semin. Oncol. 6:*85–102, 1979.
12. Tyrrell, C. J., and Peckham, M. J. The response of lymph node metastases of testicular teratoma to radiation therapy. *Br. J. Urol. 48:*363–370, 1976.
13. Percarpio, B., Clemants, J. C., McLeod, D. G., *et al.* Anaplastic seminoma: an analysis of 77 patients. *Cancer 43:*2510–2513, 1979.
14. Maier, J. G., and Lee, S. N. Radiation therapy for nonseminomatous germ cell testicular cancer in adults. *Urol. Clin. North Am. 4:*477–493, 1977.
15. Peckham, M. J. An appraisal of the role of radiation therapy in the management of nonseminomatous germ cell tumors of the testis in the era of effective chemotherapy. *Cancer Treat. Rep. 63:*1653–1658, 1979.
16. Hussey, D. H., Luk, K. H., and Johnson, D. E. The role of radiation therapy in the treatment of germinal cell tumors of the testis other than pure seminoma. *Radiology 123:*175–180, 1977.
17. Javadpour, N., McIntire, K. R., Waldmann, T. A., and Bergman, S. M. Role of alphafetoprotein and human chorionic gonadotrophin in seminoma. *J. Urol. 120:*687–690, 1978.
18. Wallace, S., and Jing, B. S. Lymphangiography: diagnosis of lymph node metastases from testicular malignancies. *JAMA 213:*94–97, 1970.
19. Maier, J. G., and Schamber, D. T. The role of lymphangiography in the diagnosis and treatment of malignant testicular tumors. *AJR 114:*482–491, 1972.
20. Ray, B., Hajdu, S. I., and Whitmore, W. F., Jr. Distribution of retroperitoneal lymph node metastases in testicular germinal tumors. *Cancer 32:*340–348, 1974.
21. Safer, M. L., Green, J. P., Crews, Q. E., Jr., and Hill, D. R. Lymphangiographic accuracy in staging of testicular tumors. *Cancer 25:*1603–1605, 1975.
22. Shipley, W. U. The role of radiation therapy in the management of adult germinal testis tumors. In *Testicular Tumors,* pp. 47–67, edited by L. H. Einhorn. Mason Publishing, New York, 1980.
23. Boyer, A. L., Doppke, K. P., Linggood, R. M., *et al.* Treatment of large irregular advanced fields using a 10 mv X-ray Beams., *Int. J. Radiat. Oncol. Biol. Phys.* (In press) 1983.
24. Friedman, M. Tumors of the testis and their treatment. In *Clinical Therapeutic Radiology,* edited by U. V. Portmann. Thomas Nelson & Sons, New York, 1950.
25. Donohue, R. E., Pfister, R. R., Weigel, J. W., and Stonington, O. G. Supraclavicular node biopsy in testicular tumors. *J. Urol. 9:*546–548, 1977.
26. Buck, A. S., Schramber, C. T., Maier, J. G., and Lewis, E. L. Supraclavicular node biopsy and malignant testicular tumors. *J. Urol. 107:*619–621, 1972.
28. Vaitukaitis, J. L., Braunstein, G. D., and Ross, G. T. The radioimmunoassay which specifically measures human chorionic gonadotrophin in the presence of human luteinizing hormone. *Am. J. Obstet. Gynecol. 113:*751–758, 1972.
29. Lang, P. H., and Fraley, E. E. Serum alpha-fetoprotein and human chorionic gonadotrophin in the treatment of patients with testicular tumors. *Urol. Clin. North Am. 4:*393–406, 1977.
30. Mauch, P., Weichselbaum, R., and Botnick, L. The significance of positive chorionic gonadotrophins in apparently pure seminoma of the testis. *Int. J. Radiat. Oncol. Biol. Phys. 5:*887–889, 1979.
31. Lange, P. H., Nochomovity, L. E., Rosai, J., *et al.* Serum Alpha-Fetoprotein and Human Chorionic Gonadotropin in Patients with Seminoma. *J. Urol. 124:*472–478, 1980.
32. Patton, J. F., Hewitt, C. B., and Mallis, N. Diagnosis and treatment of tumors of the testis. *JAMA 171:*219A–2201, 1959.
33. Stephen, R. A. The clinical presentation of testicular tumors. *Br. J. Urol. 34:*448–451, 1962.
34. Maier, J. G., Sulak, M. H., and Mittemeyer, B. T. Seminoma of the testis: analysis of treatment success and failure. *AJR 102:*596–602, 1968.

35. Smithers, D. W., Wallace, D. M., and Austin, D. E. Fertility after unilateral orchiectomy and radiotherapy for patients with malignant tumours of the testis. *Br. Med. J. 4:*77–79, 1973.
36. Orecklin, J. R., Kaufman, J. J., and Thompson, R. W. Fertility in patients for malignant testicular tumors. *J. Urol. 109:*293–295, 1973.
37. Einhorn, L. H. Extragonadal germ cell tumors. In *Testicular Tumors*, pp. 185–204, edited by L. H. Einhorn, Masson Publishing, New York, 1980.
38. Schantz, A., Sewall, W., and Castleman, B. Mediastinal germinoma. *Cancer 30:*1189–1194, 1972.
39. Martini, N., Golbey, R. B., Hajdu, S. I., Whitmore, W. F., and Beattie, E. J. Primary mediastinal germ cell tumors. *Cancer 33:*763–769, 1974.
40. Cox, J. D. Primary malignant germinal tumors of the mediastinum. *Cancer 36:*1162–1168, 1975.
41. Johnson, D. E., Laneiri, J. P., Mountain, C. F., and Luna, M. Extra-gonadal germ cell tumors. *Surgery 73:*85–90, 1973.
42. Cha, E. M. Ectopic seminoma in the retroperitoneum and mediastinum. *J. Urol. 110:*47–53, 1973.
43. Utz, D. C., and Buscemi, M. F. Extragonadal testicular tumors. *J. Urol 105:*271–274, 1971.
44. Das, S., Bochetto, J. R., and Alpert, L. I. Primary retroperitoneal seminoma. *Cancer 36:*595–598, 1975.
45. Montague, D. K. Retroperitoneal germ cell tumors with no apparent testicular involvement. *J. Urol. 113:*505–508, 1975.
46. Abell, M. R., Fayos, J. V., and Lampe, I. Retroperitoneal germinomas (seminomas) without evidence of testicular involvement. *Cancer 18:*273–290, 1965.
47. Friedman, N. B. Comparative morphogenesis of extragenital and gonadal teratoid tumors. *Cancer 4:*265–276, 1951.
48. Simson, R. L., Lampe, I., and Abell, M. R. Suprasellar germinomas. *Cancer 22:*533–544, 1968.
49. Rubin, P., and Kramer, S. Ectopic pinealoma: a radiocurable neuroendocrinologic entity. *Radiology 85:*512–523, 1965.

14

Adjuvant Chemotherapy

Part A

The Negative View*

Stephen D. Williams, M.D.
Lawrence H. Einhorn, M.D.

BACKGROUND

Theoretic considerations and abundant clinical experience in other tumor types make attractive the use of adjuvant chemotherapy in nonseminomatous germ cell tumors (NSGCT). A small number of patients with pathologic stage A tumors and a substantial number of stage B patients are destined to relapse after retroperitoneal lymphadenectomy (RPLND) even under the best of circumstances. Presumably, these patients fail because of undetected micrometastases present at the time of surgery.

It is quite likely that patients with minimal tumor burden respond better to chemotherapy and that small undetected tumor foci may be totally obliterated by drugs. There is compelling clinical evidence in such diseases as breast cancer, certain sarcomas, etc., that the risk of recurrence is reduced when chemotherapy is given immediately after therapy directed at the primary tumor in patients with no evidence of disease.

Unfortunately, there is only minimal data available regarding the utility of adjuvant therapy in NSGCT, none of which has been done in a random prospective fashion. The ultimate worth of adjuvant therapy awaits the completion of well designed prospective trials; nonetheless, a few conclusions can be drawn.

INDIANA EXPERIENCE

The results of the chemotherapy protocols at our institution for disseminated disease are outlined in Chapter 15. As the full curative potential of platinum-based combination chemotherapy for disseminated disease was appreciated, our approach to the management of "early" stage disease underwent modification.

* Supported in part by PHS MO1 RROO 750-06 and Southeastern Cancer Study Group #CA-19657.

From 1974–1979, we had opportunity to care for 116 consecutive unselected patients with pathologic stage A or B NSGCT. All had orchiectomy, usually prior to referral, followed by RPLND done at our hospital. The surgical technique is described in another chapter. In addition, 20 patients were referred to us for follow-up care after having all of their surgery elsewhere. RPLNDs on these patients were done by several different urologists and varied in technique. All had stage B disease.

All patients had all gross tumor removed and had no pathologic evidence of microscopic residual disease. All had normal whole lung tomograms, and serum markers (β-HCG and α-fetoprotein (AFP)) were allowed to return to normal if elevated preoperatively. Intraoperative actinomycin-D was not used.

Regardless of postoperative treatment, every attempt was made to obtain monthly chest radiographs and markers for the first postoperative year and every-other-month studies for the second year. Many of these studies were done under the supervision of the referring physician. A few patients were briefly lost to follow-up, but the vast majority of these studies were done as planned. At the time of this analysis, follow-up on all patients was complete, and none have been followed less than 2 years.

Sixty-three patients had pathologic stage A disease. None received adjuvant treatment of any sort. Five (7.9%) relapsed and received chemotherapy with cisplatin + vinblastine + bleomycin ± adriamycin (PVB ± A). All attained complete remission and remain free of disease at a minimum of 18 months following initiation of chemotherapy.

Our approach to patients with stage B disease changed over the period of this study. Initially actinomycin-D was given to 30 patients monthly for 1 year and every other month for the second year. This drug was chosen because of its known activity in metastatic disease and its relative lack of serious toxicity. Subsequently, 13 unselected patients received PVB, 7 initially in a feasibility study and 6 more recent patients as part of a random prospective trial. They received the lowered dose (0.3 mg/kg) of vinblastine and only two courses of cisplatin (total treatment, 6 weeks).

More recently, 30 consecutive patients received no adjuvant treatment. By this time, it had become apparent that in excess of 95% of patients with "minimal" metastatic disease will attain complete remission with chemotherapy. It was thought that relapsing patients, after RPLND, would be diagnosed early at a time when systemic therapy would have an extremely high probability of cure.

Table 14A. 1 shows the results of treatment of the stage B patients. Of

Table 14A.1.
Stage B results of different treatments

	Actinomycin D	PVB[a]	Observation
Number	30	13	30
Relapse	14	0	11
Presently NED	29[b]	13	29[c]

[a] The abbreviations used are: PVB, cisplatin, vinblastine, bleomycin; and NED, no evidence of disease.

[b] One cancer death.

[c] One death from unrelated causes.

note, the risk of relapse of the actinomycin-D and "no therapy" patients was quite similar, and none of the PVB patients has recurred. Two of these patients have died, one of cancer and one of unrelated causes.

Four of these patients had pathologic stage B_3 disease and three patients relapsed. The risk of relapse of stage B_1 *versus* B_2, was quite similar, and although the numbers are fairly small, no other obvious risk factor has been identified.

Table 14A. 2 shows the extent of disease of relapsing patients. As can be seen, the majority had "minimal" metastatic disease at diagnosis, and marker determination was quite helpful in the early diagnosis of relapse. Abdominal ultrasonography and/or computerized tomography was routinely done at the time of relapse, and only 3/116 Indiana patients recurred below the diaphragm.

Overall, 134/136 patients are presently disease free, and length of observation is such that virtually all are beyond risk of relapse.

DISCUSSION

Our experience in consecutive unselected patients with NSGCT provides convincing evidence for the effectiveness of modern treatment strategies in this disease. Meticulous lymphadenectomy, with or without adjuvant treatment but with effective systemic therapy, should relapse occur, has yielded a survival rate approaching 100%.

Thus, at this time, one can legitimately evaluate various avenues of treatment not only in terms of effectiveness but also in cost to the patient in terms of acute and chronic treatment sequelae. Unfortunately, at this time, there is a paucity of data but some tentative conclusions, in our opinion, can be made.

Some investigators have routinely used actinomycin-D postoperatively for stage A patients pointing to an observed recurrence rate of 3.6% in such patients has compared to their previous historical experience.[1] The relapse rate in our 63 stage A patients was 7.9% which is not significantly inferior. More importantly, all 5 relapsing patients were salvaged with subsequent chemotherapy. Admittedly, actinomycin-D is a relatively safe drug, but it does cause substantial subjective toxicity. We believe that the minimal, if any, benefit seen from treatment is not warranted, and in

Table 14A.2.
Extent of metastatic disease at relapse[a]

	Number (%)
Minimal pulmonary	13 (43.3)
Advanced pulmonary	4 (13.3)
Minimal abdominal	4 (13.3)
Advanced abdominal	2 (6.7)
Elevated marker only	5 (16.7)
Other	2 (6.7)
Total	30

[a] Total "minimal" relapse = 24/30 (80%); 9/30 relapses (30.0%) detected initially by an elevated marker only.

excess of 90% of such patients would be receiving unnecessary chemotherapy.

The situation for stage B disease is more complex. Table 14A. 3 outlines available data regarding the use of adjuvant therapy in this situation. Various treatment regimens have been used, but all basically employ vinblastine + bleomycin with or without cisplatin. Of note, nonplatinum-containing regimens appear to have a small but finite risk of recurrence after chemotherapy. This small group of patients is of great concern, as they would be at least relatively refractory to vinblastine and bleomycin, two of the most active drugs. It is quite likely that many of these patients could not be salvaged with subsequent chemotherapy.

On the other hand, the reported patients receiving platinum-based regimens have, with one exception, remained disease-free. As the major toxicity of these regimens is myelosuppression from vinblastine, we can see little justification for using a form of treatment not containing this agent, which is the single most active drug in this disease.

There is, however, a more fundamental question. The regimens used as surgical adjuvant therapy are intensive and will have a small potential for causing drug-related death and an, as of yet, unknown risk of late sequelae. In our experience, around 65% of patients with resected stage B_1 and B_2 disease will be cured by RPLND. Patients receiving no therapy and subsequently relapsing, in our experience, have universally been cured by chemotherapy for metastatic disease. It could well be that an expectant approach for all such patients will ultimately yield as high a cure rate as the use of adjuvant therapy but avoid systemic therapy in many. The answer at present is unknown but a large multicenter trial is currently in progress. In this study, patients are randomly allocated from RPLND to either observation or a brief but intensive platinum-containing adjuvant regimen. The results are eagerly awaited.

For the present, however, we believe delayed chemotherapy is a valid treatment option provided the following conditions are met:

Table 14A.3.
Adjuvant chemotherapy in resected stage B testicular cancer

Institution	Treatment	Number	Results	Ref.
UCLA	B_1: Actinomycin-D	11	2 relapses 1 death	1
	B_2: VBL[a] + Bleo	16	2 relapses 0 deaths	1
M. D. Anderson	VBL + Bleo or Bleo-COMF	32	4 deaths	2
Memorial	"Mini-VAB"	62	10 relapses 6 deaths	3
Memorial	VAB	29	0 relapses	4
Memorial	VAB-6	43	1 relapse	5
Instituto Nationale Tumori, Milano	PVB	24	0 relapses	6
Indiana	PVB	13	0 relapses	

[a] The abbreviations used are: VBL, vinblastine; Bleo, bleomycin; COMF, cytoxan-oncovin-methotrexate-5 Fu, VAB, vinblastine + actinomycin-D + bleomycin; PVB, cisplatin, vinblastine, bleomycin.

1. Completely resected stage B NSGCT by a surgeon experienced in the management of such patients.
2. Normal whole lung tomograms (or chest computerized tomography) and radioimmunoassay AFP and HCG that normalize after surgery.
3. Postoperative follow-up monthly for 1 year and every other month for the second year with chest x-ray, HCG and AFP.
4. Institution of PVB or a comparable regimen immediately at relapse, should it occur, by physician experienced in the use of such regimens.

Data from our institution strongly supports the worth of this approach and until completion of the appropriate random prospective clinical trials, we believe this is a valid treatment option.

REFERENCES

1. Skinner, D. G., and Scardino, P. T. Relevance of biochemical tumor markers and lymphadenectomy in management of nonseminomatous testes tumor: current perspective. *J. Urol. 123:*378–382, 1980.
2. Samuels, M. L., and Johnson, D. E. Adjuvant therapy of testis cancer: the role of vinblastine and bleomycin. *J. Urol 124:*369–371, 1980.
3. Vugrin, D., Whitmore, W. F., Cvitkovic, E., *et al.* Adjuvant chemotherapy combination of vinblastine, actinomycin-D, bleomycin, and chlorambucil following retroperitoneal lymph node dissection for stage II testis tumor. *Cancer 47:*840–844, 1981.
4. Vugrin, D., Whitmore, W., Cvitkovic, E., *et al.* Adjuvant chemotherapy with VAB-3 of stage II-B testicular cancer. *Cancer 48:*233–237, 1981.
5. Sogani, P., Vugrin, D., Herr, H., Whitmore, W., and Golbey, R. VAB-6 with or without maintenance in resected nonseminomatous germ cell tumors of the testes stage II-B (Abstract). *Proc. Am. Soc. Clin. Oncol. 22:*433, 1981.
6. Monfardini, S. Unpublished data.

Part B

Adjuvant Chemotherapy is of Value Following Retroperitoneal Lymph Node Dissection for Nonseminomatous Testicular Tumors

Peter T. Scardino, M.D.

INTRODUCTION

The purpose of adjuvant chemotherapy following radical surgery for cancer is to eradicate well-established but clinically undetectable micrometastases. The efficacy of adjuvant chemotherapy is based on firm experiments and clinical evidence, including the kinetics of drug cell interactions, experimental studies in laboratory animals, and controlled clinical trials in patients.

Experimental tumors consistently demonstrated the phenomenon of gompertzian growth: the growth of a tumor is always exponential but the growth rate decreases exponentially as the tumor enlarges.[1] Consequently, the smaller the mass (or tumor burden) present, the greater the percentage of cells actively dividing. Rapidly dividing tumor cells are more susceptible to chemotherapy. In addition, the drugs act by first order kinetics. A given effective dose of drug kills a constant percentage of the total tumor cell population irrespective of the size of the population.[2] Consequently the chances of curing a tumor with drugs is inversely proportional to the mass or burden of tumor present when treatment is started.

Studies in laboratory animals have unequivocally demonstrated the efficacy of adjuvant chemotherapy.[3-6] Both transplanted and spontaneous murine tumors have a higher cure rate when treated with surgery plus adjuvant chemotherapy than with either modality alone.

In premenopausal breast cancer[7, 8] and in Wilms' tumor,[9] randomized controlled clinical trials have demonstrated a statistically significant decrease in recurrence rate and increase in survival in patients treated with adjuvant chemotherapy following surgery. Improved cure rates have also been achieved with adjuvant chemotherapy after surgery for embryonal rhabdomycosarcoma and ovarian cancer and probably for osteogenic sarcoma as well.[10]

Adjuvant Therapy in Testicular Cancer

However, in testicular cancer the argument for adjuvant chemotherapy is complicated by the superb results of intensive chemotherapy, with or without adjuvant *surgery*, for advanced metastatic disease.[11] Consequently, one must assess the *relative* risks and benefits of two alternative methods of treatment—adjuvant chemotherapy in all patients *versus* intensive chemotherapy in those who relapse—which, in the final analysis, may be equally curative. The decision for or against adjuvant chemotherapy should be based on the probability of recurrence after retroperitoneal lymph node dissection, the prognosis associated with recurrence, and the relative risks and efficacy of the adjuvant chemotherapy regimens used *versus* the intensive (or "rescue") regimen to be used.

The use of adjuvant chemotherapy is only appropriate in patients who have already received *optimal surgical therapy*: radical orchiectomy and complete retroperitoneal lymphadenectomy. This paper will not address the ability of clinical staging studies to detect retroperitoneal nodal metastases. Nor will it debate the necessity for a *complete* retroperitoneal lymph nodes dissection in the primary and secondary areas at risk, an operation which elimates retroperitoneal recurrence, makes radiotherapy unnecessary, and which can be performed with a low mortality ($< 0.5\%$) and with minimal morbidity.[12-15] The only long-term ill effect of retroperitoneal lymphadenectomy is loss of ejaculation in the majority of patients.

Our experience with chemotherapy was recently reported in detail.[12] A total of 122 consecutive patients were treated by Staubitx and by Skinner *et al.* Initial staging studies included physical examination, chest film, excretory urogram, serum HCG and α-fetoprotein (AFP), and in some cases whole lung tomograms. All patients received 4 mg of actinomycin-

D intravenously over 5 days beginning on the day of the operation. Subsequent adjuvant chemotherapy was based on the pathologic stage.

Of 78 patients with negative nodes, only 2 (3%) relapsed, and both were salvaged with chemotherapy. No patient with negative nodes has died of testis tumor. Of 44 patients with positive nodes (stages B_1 and B_2), 6 (14%) relapsed. Four of these 6 (67%) responded to intensive chemotherapy; two died of tumor. The adjuvant therapy regimen resulted in only two deaths due to tumor in 122 patients followed at least 24 months. The relapse rate was reduced from 18% to 3% in stage A and from 33% to 14% in stage B_1 and B_2 patients. Only 8% of the patients required intensive chemotherapy rather than 24% if no adjuvant had been given.

The relapse rate for stage B_1 alone was 18%, which can be reduced further by a more intensive regimen incorporating vinblastine plus bleomycin rather than actinomycin-D alone for such patients, as we are now doing.[16] Although Whitmore (Vugrin *et al.*[16]) has not advocated adjuvant therapy, the data from Memorial Sloan-Kittering Cancer Center demonstrate its effectiveness quite well; there were no relapses among 33 stage B_1 patients treated with "mini-VAB" (vinblastine-actinomycin D and bleomycin) following lymphadenectomy.[16]

Therefore, to demonstrate the value of adjuvant chemotherapy following retroperitoneal lymph node dissection for early stage (A, B_1, B_2—see Table 14.B1)[17] nonseminomatous testicular cancer we must consider the following questions:

1. Risk and prognosis of recurrence after retroperitoneal lymph node dissection
   a. What is the risk of developing metastases following retroperitoneal lymph node dissection?
   b. Can we predict which patients are most likely to develop recurrent disease?
   c. What is the prognosis for those patients whose disease recurs?
   d. Can such recurrence be detected early, when the tumor burden is small?
2. Safety and efficacy of adjuvant chemotherapy
   a. Are the drugs used in the adjuvant regimen effective for metastatic disease in the dosage used?
   b. What is the acute and chronic toxicity of these drugs?
   c. If the tumor recurs despite adjuvant chemotherapy, is the recurrent tumor less responsive to standard intensive chemotherapy?

Table 14B.1.
Pathological staging system for testicular cancer

Stage	Description
A	Limited to testis
B	Metastases to retroperitoneum
	B_1 Microscopic metastases to ≤5 lymph nodes
	B_2 Metastases to >5 nodes, or any node >2 cm, or any extracapsular spread
	B_3 Massive, palpable retroperitoneal metastases
C	Metastases beyond retroperitoneum, positive markers after lymphadenectomy

3. Safety and efficacy of intensive chemotherapy
   a. How effective is high dose intensive chemotherapy?
   b. How toxic is it, both short and long-term?
4. Adjuvant *versus* intensive chemotherapy
   a. Which is more expensive, adjuvant chemotherapy for all patients or intensive chemotherapy for those who recur?
   b. What other factors justify the use of adjuvant chemotherapy?

RISK AND PROGNOSIS OF RECURRENCE AFTER RETROPERITONEAL LYMPH NODE DISSECTION

What is the Risk of Developing Metastases Following Retroperitoneal Lymph Node Dissection?

Whitmore[14] had compiled the results of retroperitoneal lymph node dissection for nonseminomatous tumors in seven series reported between 1968 and 1976. Surgical treatment alone resulted in a 5-year survival of 87% for all patients with pathological stage A and 63% for pathological stage B disease. Almost all patients with massive retroperitoneal metastases are excluded from these series of patients who were treated surgically for cure and received no radiation therapy or chemotherapy. Hence, the risk of developing metastases following retroperitoneal lymph node dissection alone in approximately 13% of the lymph nodes are negative (stage A) and 37% if the lymph nodes are positive (stages B_1 and B_2), but massive disease is not present.

Can We Predict Which Patients Are Most Likely to Develop Recurrent Disease?

Our ability to predict which patients will ultimately develop systemic metastases following retroperitoneal lymph node dissection is poor. Preoperative staging studies done before the retroperitoneal node dissection may identify patients with systemic disease, who should be treated initially with chemotherapy rather than lymphadenectomy. We have utilized only the chest film and excretory urogram in all patients, and abdominal sonography and whole lung tomograms in some patients to identify pulmonary metastases and bulky abdominal disease. Although testicular cancers occasionally metastasize to the liver, brain, bone and other sites, it has not been cost-effective to perform routine radionucleide or radiographic studies of these organs before lymphadenectomy. If the staging studies are negative and lymphadenectomy is performed, the risk of recurrence correlates most closely with the status of the lymph nodes.[12] The extent of the primary tumor, the finding of a focus of choriocarcinoma within the primary tumor or the nodal metastases,[18] and the prelymphadenectomy level of human chorionic gonadotropin (HCG) or AFP[19] (Tables 14B.2 and 14.B3) have not been shown to alter the prognosis substantially when modern therapeutic modalities are used. Consequently it has not been possible to estimate the risk of recurrence based on prelymphadenectomy prognosis factors, and we have relied upon pathologic staging as the best prognostic indicator.[12]

Table 14B.2.
Prognostic significance of serum α-fetoprotein (AFP) determined after orchiectomy but before retroperitoneal lymph node dissection in 24 patients with positive retroperitoneal nodes, pathologic stage B_1 and B_2. The frequency of elevated AFP and the absolute value of AFP were not statistically significantly different in the patients with recurrence compared to those without, nor in the patients who died compared to those who survived. The wide range of values precludes the use of prelymphadenectomy AFP levels to determine the risk of recurrence or death from disease.

	Recurrence	No Recurrence	Death	Survival
Frequency[a]	5/8 (63%)	5/16 (31%)	3/3 (100%)	8/21 (38%)
Mean[b]	122	872	172	689
±SD	±132	±3236	±2823	±223
Range	0–330	0–13,000	14–330	0–13,000

[a] Number of positive/total patients
[b] ng/ml

Table 14B.3.
Prognostic significance of serum HCG in 37 patients (see title, Table 14B.2). There were no statistically significant differences in the frequency of elevated levels or in the absolute values of HCG between patients with tumor recurrence and those without, nor between patients who died of cancer and those who survived.

	Recurrence	No Recurrence	Death	Survival
Frequency[a]	7/11 (64%)	9/26 (35%)	4/4 (100%)	12/33 (36%)
Mean[b]	99	47	240	30
±S.D.	±225	±143	±349	±115
Range	0–760	0–653	0–760	0–653

[a] No. positive/total patients.
[b] nanograms per milliliter.

What is the Prognosis for Those Patients Whose Disease Recurs?

The prognosis for patients whose tumor recurs after lymphadenectomy depends upon the tumor burden present when metastases are discovered and treatment is initiated. The complete response rate with intensive chemotherapy is quite good (88–100%) for those patients who are treated when the tumor burden is minimal, but the results are much less satisfactory (45–67%) if there is advanced pulmonary or abdominal disease, or both.[20] Brain and liver metastases are almost uniformly fatal.

Can Such Recurrence be Detected Early, When the Tumor Burden is Small?

Although an occasional patient will develop hepatic or cerebral metastases as the first evidence of recurrence, in the majority of patients evaluations every month for the first year and 2 months for the second year after lymphadenectomy should detect early recurrence. A physical examination, chest film, and serum HCG and AFP determinations would be the minimum required at each visit. The tumor markers are capable of identifying recurrence weeks or months before any other clinical studies in some patients,[19, 21] but in a recent series only 3 of 7 patients who developed recurrence had elevated marker levels *before* any other clinical evidence of recurrence.[12] Furthermore, since testicular tumors have one of the most rapid doubling times of any solid tumor in man, widespread metastases can appear and progress dramatically in a matter of weeks. To detect recurrent disease early requires not only sensitive radiographic studies and tumor markers, but responsible patients who can be relied upon to keep each appointment. Reports of severe psychological and emotional problems, including heavy multiple drug use in these young men, must be a source of concern to the physician who depends upon frequent follow-up visits to detect early recurrence.[22]

SAFETY AND EFFICACY OF ADJUVANT CHEMOTHERAPY

Is the Adjuvant Regimen Effective for Metastatic Disease in the Doses Used?

A well-established principle of adjuvant chemotherapy is that drugs must be able to induce complete clinical remission in patients with advanced disseminated tumor. Actinomycin-D has an 18–23% complete response rate and a 33–36% overall response rate when used as a single agent.[20] Vinblastine and bleomycin, whether in combination with actinomycin-D or not, have achieved complete responses in 19–45% and overall responses in 60–88% of patients with advanced disease.[20] There is no doubt that these drugs are effective for advanced disease and are suitable as adjuvant agents.

What is the Acute and Chronic Toxicity of these Drugs?

In the adjuvant program we have reported,[12] actinomycin-D has been used alone as an adjuvant for patients with negative nodes in a total dose of 4 mg over 5 days beginning the day of the operation and repeated again in 2 months. Acute toxicity, occasional stomatitis and skin rash, have been minimal. The extensive use of this drug in children with Wilms' tumor has been monitored over many years and no long-term complications have been noted. Vinblastine and bleomycin have been used as adjuvant therapy for patients with positive retroperitoneal nodes in a variety of regimens.[12, 16, 24] Vinblastine can cause severe myalgia, peripheral neuropathy and myleosuppression in doses of 0.4 mg/kg given over 2 days. Samuels *et al.*[24] have noted the necessity to discontinue the full course of prophylactic chemotherapy in one patient with peripheral neuropathy of 32 patients treated with adjuvant vinblastine-bleomycin. The acute toxicity associated with bleomycin, particularly when given as a continuous infusion, included stomatitis, alopecia, and pneumonitis. Samuels had to abort adjuvant chemotherapy in one patient who developed pneumonitis. There was one duodenal ulcer and one episode of retroperitoneal fibrosis with ureteral obstruction. Two patients developed sepsis and one died of *Candida* septicemia.[24] On the other hand, Skinner and Scardino[12] and Vugrin *et al.*[16] reported no major complications or mortality from their adjuvant therapy programs, which was less intensive than that of Samuels. Although these is no evidence of long-term toxicity of either vinblastine, bleomycin or the combination, sufficiently long follow-up and adequate numbers of patients are not yet available.[25]

Does Prior Adjuvant Chemotherapy Lessen the Response to Intensive Chemotherapy if the Tumor Recurs?

In our series,[12] six patients treated with adjuvant actinomycin-D or vinblastine and bleomycin developed metastatic disease. Five of these six patients were subsequently cured with intensive combination chemotherapy, even though the intensive therapy included the same drugs used as adjuvant agents. Einhorn and Donohue[11] have also reported that prior "chemoprophylaxis" does not decrease the response rate to intensive chemotherapy when compared to patients who relapse after surgery alone.

SAFETY AND EFFICACY OF INTENSIVE CHEMOTHERAPY

How Effective is High Dose Intensive Chemotherapy?

The most widely used intensive chemotherapy regimens include cisplatin vinblastine, and bleomycin (PVB)[11] along with the other agents (Vab-III, VAB-IV).[26] The complete response rate with PVB was 61–70% with an additional 13–17% of patients rendered complete responders after surgical resection of residual disease for an overall complete response rate of 74–87%. Of these patients, 4–12% have subsequently relapsed and 65–83% are alive and free of disease. The complete response rate is inversely proportional to the extent of disease.[11] Using the VAB-III and VAB-IV programs, Golby *et al.*[26] have reported 62–73% complete response rates with chemotherapy plus surgical resection of residual disease. However, 13–27% of the patients have subsequently relapsed and only 45–60% are alive and free of disease. We can conclude that the long-term "cure" rate of patients with metastatic testicular cancer treated with intensive combination chemotherapy is in the range of 60–70%, although the prognosis for any one individual is most closely related to the extent of disease at the time of treatment. While patients treated with minimal disease may have a 90–100% complete response rate and a high probability of ultimate cure, those who relapse with advanced pulmonary metastases or with hepatic or cerebral metastases will have a much lower chance of cure even with the most intensive chemotherapy available.

Acute and Chronic Toxicity of Intensive Chemotherapy?

The acute toxicity of the PVB regimen has been moderately severe in all reports. Acute gastrointestinal reaction including nausea and vomiting has been universal. Almost all patients experience fever and chills related to the bleomycin. All have alopecia and a weight loss which averaged 20 pounds.[11] Myalgia secondary to vinblastine is a common problem and occasionally is severe enough to require narcotic analgesics and dosage modification. Vinblastine caused profound leukopenia associated in 25% of the patients with sepsis requiring hospital admission and administration of intravenous antibiotics. Almost 10% of the patients in the Einhorn and

Donahue[12] series had documented Gram-negative septicemia. Among 66 patients there were two drug-related deaths, one due to bleomycin pulmonary fibrosis and the other to vinblastine-induced leukopenia with septicemia. The mortality rate for intensive combination chemotherapy has ranged from 1–8%.[11, 27, 28] The VAB regimens have not been reported to cause drug-related deaths, but the acute reversible toxicity is comparable to that with PVB and the rate of complete responders and long-term disease-free patients appear to be less with the VAB regimens than with PVB.[20]

ADJUVANT *VERSUS* INTENSIVE CHEMOTHERAPY

Cost Comparison

The cost in dollars of an adjuvant chemotherapy program for all patients *versus* an intensive chemotherapy program for those who recur after surgery is only of secondary importance. But it is interesting to note that the adjuvant chemotherapy program would result in a 5–10% reduction in the overall cost of care for these patients. The costs can be estimated by determining the cost of each drug and calculating the combined costs for each drug regimen for each patient. Based on the proportion of stage A and B patients and on the recurrence rate for each stage,[12] one can calculate that the cost of the drug alone for stage A patients is approximately $133 and for stage B patients would be approximately $1905, or $930/patient overall. This figure includes the cost of the adjuvant chemotherapy given to all patients and of the intensive chemotherapy given to the patients whose disease recurs in spite of the adjuvant therapy. The cost of the intensive chemotherapy regimen is based on the average of four cycles of PVB per patient given only to those patients who relapse after lymph node dissection, and assumes a 6-day hospital stay for each cycle. In the "no adjuvant" group, the average cost per patient with negative nodes would be $732, and for those with positive nodes the cost would be $1348, or a combined cost of $1009/patient. The cost of the intensive chemotherapy program assumed a 6-day hospitalization for each of the four cycles of the drug.

Such calculations are only a rough estimation since they do not reflect the relative cost of more frequent, intensive follow-up examinations for those patients receiving no adjuvant therapy nor the increased cost associated with the morbidity of the intensive chemotherapeutic regimen. Of course, a more effective adjuvant chemotherapy program would result in a proportionately decreased cost for each patient in the adjuvant therapy group.

Are There Other Factors Which Justify the Use of Adjuvant Chemotherapy?

The young age of patients with testicular cancer and the frequent finding of patients with serious psychological and emotional problems[18] suggests that patients should be treated with effective therapy at the time of initial presentation, when their relationship with the physician is optimal and their concern for their future is at its peak. These factors work to motivate a relatively immature patient to stick with his therapy, at least for a period of time. Such patients cannot always be relied upon to return to the doctor for frequent check-ups when they are feeling well. Some of these young men who are transients in the community cannot be relied upon to return to the same physician in the same community consistently. Often times patients with this rare disease are referred from long distances away or from foreign countries where frequent follow-up visits would be difficult if not impossible. Patients who would be considered appropriate candidates for a prospective randomized trial of adjuvant therapy are not comparable in a socioeconomic sense to the general population of testicular tumor patients. Mentally retarded, psychologically disturbed, transient, or foreign individuals would generally be excluded from such protocols, though they make up a significant proportion of testicular tumor patients seen in any major medical center.

CONCLUSION

Adjuvant chemotherapy is indicated in all patients after retroperitoneal lymph node dissection for nonseminomatous testicular cancer unless there is a specific contraindication to the use of these drugs in the individual patient. Adjuvant therapy markedly reduces or even eliminates systemic recurrence.[12, 16, 24] The risk of relapse after retroperitoneal lymph node dissection is high enough (13–37%) to justify graded adjuvant chemotherapy regimens based on the specific risk of recurrence at each stage. At this time the most accurate guide to prognosis following retroperitoneal lymph node dissection is the pathologic stage of the tumor and the levels of postoperative tumor markers.[12, 19] There is no evidence of long-term deleterious side effects of the drugs and dosages used for adjuvant chemotherapy, especially with PVB, have not been well documented and may include permanent high frequency hearing loss and impaired renal and gonadal function. The increased risk of later development of second cancers, well documented following the administration of alkylating agents.[25] to which cisplatin is most closely akin, can only be determined with long-term observation of these patients.

It is debatable whether a randomized prospective controlled trial of adjuvant chemotherapy using the intensive PVB regimen, as in the current intergroup stage II adjuvant chemotherapy protocol sponsored by the National Cancer Institute, will be able to settle the debate regarding the value of adjuvant chemotherapy in testicular cancer. This study actually addresses the question of how two cycles of intensive PVB used as an adjuvant following retroperitoneal lymph node dissection in all patients with positive nodes compares to three or four cycles of PVB used therapeutically in patients carefully monitored for recurrence under the rigors of a planned protocol. Although acute toxicity may vary somewhat depending upon the number of cycles of PVB, chronic toxicity—long-term effects on hearing, renal function, fertility, and the development of late second cancers—may not. Based on current experience, the results of either arm of this study can be expected to approach 100% survival, so that statistically significant differences in survival are unlikely to be found even with very large numbers of patients in each treatment arm. It would seem more appropriate to address the question of whether *low-dose, graded,* adjuvant chemotherapy regimens, appropriate to the risk of recurrence within each pathologic stage, is superior to observation alone, with intensive chemotherapy at relapse. Such a study would allow meaningful comparisons of recurrence rate, survival data, and acute and chronic toxicity between these distinctly different approaches to management. Until such a study is completed, the weight of evidence favors the use of low dose, graded, adjuvant chemotherapy in all patients following retroperitoneal lymph node dissection for nonseminomatous testicular cancer.

REFERENCES

1. Laster, W. R., Jr., Mayo, J. G., Simpson-Herren, L., *et al.* Success and failure in the treatment of solid tumors—II. Kinetic parameters and "cell cure" of moderately advanced carcinoma 755. *Cancer Chemother. Rep. 53:*169–188, 1969.
2. Wilcox, W. S. The last surviving cancer cell—the chances of killing it. *Cancer Chemother. Rep. 50:*541–542, 1966.
3. Martin, D. S., Fugmann, R. A., and Hayworth, P. Surgery, cancer chemotherapy, host defenses, and tumor size. *J. Natl. Cancer Inst. 29:*817–834, 1962.
4. Schnabel, F. M., Jr. Concepts for systemic treatment of micrometastases. *Cancer 35:*15–24, 1975.
5. Schnabel, F. M., Jr. Surgical adjuvant chemotherapy of metastatic murine tumors. *Cancer 40:*558–568, 1977.
6. Simpson-Herren, L., Sanford, A. H., and Holmquist, J. P. Cell population kinetics of transplanted and metastatic Lewis lung cancer. *Cell Tissue Kinet. 7:*349–361, 1974.
7. Shimkin, M. D., and Moore, G. E. Adjuvant use of therapy in the surgical treatment of cancer. *JAMA 167:*1710–1714. 1958.
8. Bonadonna, G., Valagusa, P., Rossi, A., *et al.* Are surgical adjuvant trials altering the course of breast cancer? *Semin. Oncol. 5:*450–464, 1978.
9. Burgert, E. O., and Glidewell, O. Dactinomycin in Wilms' tumor. *JAMA 199:*464–468, 1967.
10. Zubrod, G. C. Historic milestones in curative chemotherapy. *Semin. Oncol. 6:*490–505, 1979.
11. Einhorn, L. H., and Donohue, J. P. Combination chemotherapy in disseminated testicular cancer: the Indiana University experience. *Semin. Oncol. 6:*87–93, 1979.
12. Skinner, D. G., and Scardino, P. T. Relevance of biochemical tumor markers and lymphadenectomy in the management of nonseminomatous testis tumors: current perspective. *J. Urol. 123:*378–382, 1980.
13. Donohue, J. P., Einhorn, L. H., and Perez, I. M. Improved management of nonseminomatous testis tumors. *Cancer 42:*2903–2908, 1978.
14. Whitmore, W. F., Jr. Surgical treatment of adult germinal testis tumors. *Semin. Oncol. 6:*55–68, 1979.
15. Babaian, R. J., and Johnson, D. E. Management of stages I and II nonseminomatous germ cell tumors of the testis. *Cancer 45:*1775–1781, 1980.
16. Vugrin D., Cvitkovic, E., Whitmore, W. F. Jr., and Golbey, R. B. Adjuvant chemotherapy in resected nonseminomatous germ cell tumors of testis: stages I and II. *Semin. Oncol. 6:*94–98, 1979.
17. Scardino, P. T., and Skinner, D. G. Germ cell tumors of the testis: improved results in a prospective study using combined modality therapy and biochemical tumor markers. *Surgery 86:*86–93, 1979.
18. Skinner, D. G. Advances in the management of nonseminomatous germinal tumors of the testis. *Br. J. Urol. 49:*553–560, 1977.
19. Scardino, P. T., Cox, H. D., Waldmann, T. A., *et al.* The value of serum tumor markers in the staging and prognosis of germ cell tumors of the testis. *J Urol. 118:*994–999, 1977.
20. Jacobs, E. M., and Muggia, F. M. Testicular cancer: risk factors and the role of adjuvant chemotherapy. *Cancer 45:*1782–1790, 1980.
21. Lange, P. H., McIntire, K. R., Waldmann, T. A., *et al.* Serum alpha-fetoprotein and

human chorionic gonadotrophin in the diagnosis and management of nonseminomatous germ cell testicular cancer. *N. Engl. J. Med. 295:*1237–1240, 1976.
22. Gorzinsky, J. G., and Holland, J. C. Psychological aspects of testicular cancer. *Semin. Oncol. 6:*125–129, 1979.
23. Jaffe, N., McNeese, M., Mayfield, J. K., *et al.* Childhood urologic cancer therapy related sequelae and their impact on management. *Cancer 45:*1815–1822, 1980.
24. Samuels, M. L., Johnson, D. E., and Bracken, R. B. Adjuvant chemotherapy in metastatic testicular neoplasia: results with vinblastine-bleomycin. In *Cancer of the Genitourinary Tract*, pp. 173–180, edited by D. E. Johnson and M. L. Samuels. Raven Press, New York, 1979.
25. Meyer, W., and Leventhal, B. Late effects of cancer therapy. In *Complications of Cancer*, pp. 397–416, edited by M. D. Abeloff. Johns Hopkins University Press, Baltimore, 1979.
26. Golbey, R. B., Reynolds, T. F., and Vugrin, D. Chemotherapy of metastatic germ cell tumors. *Semin. Oncol. 6:*82–86, 1979.
27. Anderson, T., Javadpour, N., Schilsky, R., *et al.* Chemotherapy for testicular cancer: current status of the National Cancer Institute combined modality trial. *Cancer Treat. Rep. 63:*1687–1692, 1979.
28. Sampson, M. D., Stephens, R. L., Rivkin, S., *et al.* Vinblastin, bleomycin, and cis-dichlorodiammineplatinum (II) in disseminated testicular cancer: preliminary report of a Southwest Oncology Group Study. *Cancer Treat. Rep. 63:*1663–1669, 1979.
29. Krikorian, J. G., Daniels, J. R., Brown, B. W., Jr., *et al.* Variables for predicting serious toxicity (vinblastin dose, performance status, prior therapeutic experience): chemotherapy for metastatic testicular cancer with cis-dichlorodiammineplatinum (II), vinblastine, and bleomycin. *Cancer Treat. Rep. 62:*1455–1463, 1978.

15

Chemotherapy of Disseminated Testicular Cancer*

Stephen D. Williams, M.D.
Lawrence H. Einhorn, M.D.

HISTORICAL PERSPECTIVE

Testicular cancer was a chemosensitive tumor even in the earlier era of single-agent chemotherapy. Actinomycin-D with or without chlorambucil and methotrexate became the standard treatment for disseminated testicular cancer throughout the decade of the 1960s and would induce a 50% objective response rate including 10–20% complete remissions. During the latter part of the 1960s and the early part of the 1970s, several other agents became available that demonstrated activity in testicular cancer including vinblastine, mithramycin, and bleomycin. The major significance of these pioneering studies in addition to demonstrating single agent activity was the fact that 10–20% of these patients achieved a complete remission and that, furthermore, approximately half of those who achieved a complete remission were ultimately cured. It also became evident in these earlier studies that testicular cancer is not a disease associated with late relapse. If a patient was destined to relapse after achieving a complete remission, virtually all relapses would occur within 2 years from the initiation of chemotherapy and the majority within 1 year. This has continued to be true, in our experience with cisplatin combination chemotherapy, in which approximately 99% of patients who are continuously disease free for 1 year are cured of their disease.

Although it was encouraging that approximately 50% of those early complete remissions with actinomycin-D, mithramycin, or vinblastine were cures, one does have to realize the implication that the cure rate was only 5–10% for the total patient population since the overall complete remission rate was only 10–20%. In addition to having a higher complete response rate it is also expected that modern combination chemotherapy

* Supported in part by U.S. Public Health Service Grant MO1 RR00 750-06 and Southeastern Cancer Study Group Grant CA19657

will have a considerably lower relapse rate. The reduction in relapse rate is likely due to both more effective induction chemotherapy and also an increased capability to define complete remission.

A final point of interest in these earlier studies was the durability of complete remission in the absence of maintenance therapy. Kennedy utilized mithramycin for 6 months and then discontinued therapy. Thus, there was already evidence that maintenance therapy may be unnecessary. Certainly, similar situations exist in other chemosensitive tumors such as Hodgkin's disease, where no benefit ensues from long-term chemotherapy. Combination chemotherapy with vinblastine plus bleomycin was pioneered by Samuels and represented a major advance in the disease. This two-drug regimen is synergistic as it produced a higher complete remission rate than one would predict from the single agent activity of each component. Actinomycin-D, as a single agent, is as active as vinblastine as a single agent, but one does not see this apparent synergism when the latter two are combined, as one gets merely the expected additive result.

Initial studies with vinblastine plus bleomycin (VB-I) was started by Samuels in 1970, using dosages of 0.4–0.6 mg/kg of vinblastine plus bleomycin 15 mg/m^2 twice weekly.[1] There were 17 of 51 (33%) complete remissions with VB-I with a relapse rate of 23%.

In 1973, Samuels[2] changed his method of administration of bleomycin therapy from intermittent to continuous infusion (VB-III). The bleomycin in this study was given in a dosage of 30 units in 1000 ml of 5% glucose and water over a 24-hour period of 5 consecutive days starting on day 2 of the treatment program. The vinblastine was given in a total dosage of 0.4 mg/kg split into two fractions on days 1 and 2, but a minimum dosage of 30 mg was required as the initial dosage. Therapy was repeated every 4–5 weeks as toxicity permitted. There was a 53% complete remission rate (47 complete remissions in 89 patients) with this regimen. The toxicity with vinblastine plus bleomycin has been described by Samuels.[2] Essentially, bacteriologically proven septicemia occurred in 13% of these patients and was responsible for four drug-related deaths. Bleomycin pulmonary fibrosis was seen in 7% of this patient population and half of the patients developing this complication died as a result.

Although Samuels[2] demonstrated a superiority with VB-III utilizing continuous infusion bleomycin as opposed to his earlier data with VB-I, this nevertheless represents historical control data rather than a random prospective study. It certainly is possible (as is true of all historical control studies) that there are other factors involved such as increased physician familiarity with the drugs involved as well as a different referral pattern. It is also interesting to note that the possible superiority for continuous infusion bleomycin was apparent only for embryonal carcinoma. When cisplatin is added to vinblastine plus bleomycin, approximately 90% of patients with embryonal carcinoma will achieve a disease-free status, and therefore, it seems unlikely, if not impossible, to ever demonstrate superiority for continuous infusion of bleomycin in cisplatin-containing regimens. Another major advance in the treatment of testicular cancer was the discovery of the activity of *cis*-diamminedichloroplatinum in germinal neoplasms. Cisplatin is one of a group of coordination compounds that strongly inhibit bacterial replication. This drug has significant single-agent activity in patients with refractory testicular cancer and, furthermore, in its earlier studies, had relatively minimal myelosuppression.[3]

VAB PROGRAMS

The Memorial Group in New York evaluated combination chemotherapy with vinblastine plus actinomycin-D plus bleomycin (VAB-I) from June 1972–April 1974.[4] Unfortunately, this treatment regimen produced only 14% complete and 22% partial remissions in 71 evaluable patients.[5] Although the dosages and method of administration were markedly different from those of Samuels vinblastine plus bleomycin program, a rather low complete remission rate with VAB-I raised a serious question as to the role, if any, of actinomycin-D in modern day remission induction chemotherapy.

VAB-II incorporated cisplatin and gave bleomycin by continuous infusion. This protocol was utilized from June 1974–January 1976, and produced an overall 50% complete remission rate; however, only 24% are presently disease free.[6]

The Memorial Group next evaluated a complicated seven-drug regimen (VAB-III) from July 1975–January, 1977. Adriamycin, cyclophosphamide, and chlorambucil were added to the above mentioned drugs. There was a 54% complete remission rate in 74 patients and an additional 7% were rendered disease free with surgical resection of residual disease. Forty-five percent are presently disease free with a minimum followup of 2 years.[7]

From September 1976–July 1978, patients were treated with a similar regimen called VAB-IV. There was a 61% complete remission rate in 41 patients who had no prior chemotherapy, and an additional 19 patients were rendered disease free with surgical resection of residual disease for an overall disease-free status of 80%. Sixty-eight percent of these patients are disease free in the most recent publication with a minimum followup of 12 months.[8] A modification of the VAB-IV regimen has recently been completed by the Eastern Cooperative Oncology Group and, unfortunately, their results were quite inferior to those published by the Memorial Group, as only 30% of the patients are currently disease free. The reasons for this discrepancy are not readily apparent.

From December 1978–December 1979, 29 patients were treated with VAB-VI. VAB-VI was a major departure from the previous VAB programs; in this regimen, cisplatin was given every 3–4 weeks rather than every 3–4 months in the previous VAB regimens, and the duration of therapy decreased from 2–2½ years to 12 months. Sixty-four percent of 25 evaluable patients achieved a complete remission with chemotherapy, and an additional 28% were rendered disease free with resection of residual disease for an overall disease-free status of 92%. With a minimum followup of 8 months, 84% of these patients are currently disease free.[9]

CISPLATIN PLUS VINBLASTINE PLUS BLEOMYCIN (PVB)

In August 1974, we began studies utilizing cisplatin plus vinblastine plus bleomycin in disseminated testicular cancer.[10] In our initial study, 50 patients with disseminated germ cell tumors of the testis were treated with PVB. Three patients died within 2 weeks of initiation of chemotherapy and were considered inevaluable. We no longer use the term "inevaluable" and all subsequent studies included all patients entered on chemotherapy trials. The treatment regimen in this initial study is shown in Table 15.1. Most patients received three courses of cisplatin. However, if a complete remission was not achieved after three courses, a fourth course was given. After completion of the 12 weeks of remission induction, maintenance therapy was given with vinblastine 0.3 mg/kg every 4 weeks for a total of 2 years of chemotherapy.

The primary goal was to increase the complete remission rate and potential for cure. Partial remission was not considered a worthwhile goal unless the patient was left with localized disease that could be surgically removed.

Thirty-three of 47 evaluable patients (70%) achieved complete remission (defined as a complete disappearance of all clinical, radiographic, and biochemical evidence of disease, including normal whole lung tomograms, serum β-HCG, and α-fetoprotein). The remaining 14 patients achieved partial remission (greater than 50% decrease in measurable disease). Furthermore, 5 of these 14 patients were rendered disease free following surgical removal of residual localized disease after significant reduction of tumor volume with chemotherapy. The therapeutic results are outlined in Table 15.2.

Table 15.1.
Treatment regimen for using platinum plus vinblastine plus bleomycin (PVB)

Platinum	20 mg/m^2 I.V. × 5 days every 3 weeks for 3–4 courses[a]
Vinblastine	0.2 mg/kg I.V. days 1 and 2[b] every 3 weeks for 3–4 courses[a]
Bleomycin	30 units I.V. weekly × 12

[a] In more recent experiences, all patients receive 4 courses.
[b] Total dose vinblastine = 0.3 mg/kg for subsequent studies.

Table 15.2
Therapeutic results from cisplatin plus vinblastine plus bleomycin plus or minus adriamycin (PVB ± A)

Program	No.	C.R.[a]	NED Surgery	Overall C.R.	Presently NED[+]
		%	%	%	%
1974–1976					
PVB	47	70	11	81	57
1976–1978					
PVB 0.3[b]	27	59	19	78	70
PVB 0.4[b]	26	65	23	88	77
PVBA	24	72	8	80	72
Total	78	68	14	82	73
1978–1980					
PVB	87	64	11	75	68
PVBA	84	68	11	79	74
Total	171	66	11	77	71

[a] The abbreviations used are: C.R., complete remission; NED, no evidence of disease.
[b] See text.

These patients now have been followed for a minimum of 5½ years and all are off chemotherapy. Four patients died in complete remission in the early part of this study. Two of these deaths were due to Gram-negative sepsis, one from bleomycin-induced pulmonary fibrosis, and one from multiple small bowel fistulae and obstruction secondary to previous surgery. One of the septicemia deaths was from *Klebsiella pneumoniae* in a chronic alcoholic who had no evidence of granulocytopenia during this fatal pneumonia. Thus, this regimen was directly responsible for two drug-related fatalities.

Only 6 of these 33 complete remissions have relapsed. Five of these relapses occurred within 9 months of initiation of therapy and the sixth relapse occurred at 17 months.

Although our original PVB regimen produced very respectable therapeutic results, the toxicity was of concern. Although cisplatin is potentially nephrotoxic, this has not been a clinical problem since the routine utilization of saline hydration. The most important factors are felt to be hydration and the ensuring of adequate urinary volume. This is usually accomplished by continuous intravenous hydration with normal saline beginning the night before the first day of cisplatin and continuing at a rate of 100 ml/h during the 5-day course. Outpatient cisplatin can be given by prehydrating the patient with 500 ml normal saline over 2 hours before and after each dosage. Mannitol diuresis or furosemide has not been felt necessary. The safety of this method of administration of cisplatin has also demonstrated in 171 patients entered in a Southeastern Cancer Study Group protocol evaluating maintenance vinblastine therapy.[11] Nephrotoxicity was negligible in this large patient population, and in our experience the majority of patients will complete treatment with creatinine clearances greater than 100 ml.

Clinically significant bleomycin pulmonary fibrosis, likewise, has been an uncommon complication, although, in patients with prior mediastinal irradiation or who are above age 50, more caution is necessary. Diffusion capacity, with correction for anemia, is the most valuable pulmonary function test, but basically, the bleomycin is usually continued unless there are inspiratory basilar rales or a respiratory lag on physical examination or radiologic evidence of pulmonary fibrosis.

The major serious toxicity had been related to high dose (0.4 mg/kg) vinblastine. Myalgias, constipation, and paralytic ileus were all troublesome side effects, but severe granulocytopenia and potential sepsis was the most worrisome toxicity. Thirty-eight percent of the original PVB patients required hospitalization for granulocytopenia and fever and 15% had documented infection. This toxicity was limited to induction and was not seen during maintenance.

In an attempt to reduce hematologic toxicity, a random prospective trial was initiated in 1976 comparing our standard PVB with the same regimen using a 25% dosage reduction (0.3 mg/kg) for vinbastine during remission induction.[12] It was felt that the reduced vinblastine dosage would reduce the hematologic toxicity, but the critical question was whether it would maintain the same therapeutic results. The third arm investigated the worth of the addition of adriamycin (A) (50 mg/m^2) to the PVB regimen (vinblastine = 0.2 mg/kg).

Seventy-eight patients were entered on this study, and all have been followed for a minimum of 3½ years. The degree of myelosuppression for high dose vinblastine (0.4 mg/kg) was similar to our original PVB study. The 25% reduction in the vinblastine dosage resulted in the expected decrease in hematological toxicity, as only 15% developed granulocytopenic fever and there were no documented infections.

The results of therapy are illustrated in Table 15.2. The overall complete remission (C.R.) rate (68%) and surgical resection rate for localized residual disease (14%) were remarkably similar to our original PVB study. The therapeutic results are almost identical for the three separate induction regimens. The relapse rate remained low, with all relapses occurring within 1 year of initiation of therapy.

The most important determinant to achieving complete remission was extent of disease. Thirty of 31 patients with minimal metastatic disease achieved C.R.; the only patient not achieving a C.R. had a median sternotomy with removal of small residual bilateral pulmonary nodules that were mature teratoma pathologically.

Fifty-three of these 78 patients (68%) remain continuously free of disease. In addition, five other patients are currently disease free with salvage chemotherapy with cisplatin plus VP-16 combination chemotherapy (see below). Thus, 58 patients (74%) are currently alive and disease free.

The role of maintenance therapy in disseminated testicular cancer has never been clearly established. It is quite possible that in a disease where remission induction therapy is so effective and C.R. can be defined so accurately, maintenance therapy may be unnecessary. To test this hypothesis, a third generation study was begun in June 1978, randomizing patients achieving C.R. to standard maintenance vinblastine (0.3 mg/kg monthly for 21 months) *versus* no maintenance therapy after the 12 weeks of remission induction therapy.[11] This study was done by the Southeastern Cancer Study Group. All patients received four courses of cisplatin combination chemotherapy to insure uniformity in the remission induction.

Patients were initially randomized to receive four courses of PVB (vinblastine = 0.3 mg/kg) or PVB + A as outlined above. Those patients achieving chemotherapy-complete remissions and those disease free by resection of mature teratoma were eligible for the maintenance randomization. Patients having surgical resection of residual carcinoma were not placed on the maintenance program; they received two "adjuvant" courses of PVB.

One hundred and seventy-one evaluable patients were the subjects of this study, with a minimum follow-up of 18 months. There was no obvious difference in the ability of either regimen to produce a complete remission or a disease-free status with the addition of surgical resection of persistent disease (Table 15.2).

One hundred and thirteen patients were eligible for the maintenance phase. The results of the maintenance randomization are shown in Table 15.3. Eighteen of the 58 patients randomized to vinblastine refused maintenance; all have remained without evidence of disease. The relapse rate was only 7% (4 of 55) among patients randomized to no maintenance,

Table 15.3.
Results of 1978–1980 maintenance study

	Vinblastine[a]	Observation	Total
Total	58	55	113
Relapse	5	4	9
Presently NED[b]	56[c]	52[c]	108

[a] Eighteen patients refused vinblastine after randomization; none of these patients relapsed *versus* 5/40 relapses in patients actually receiving the drug.
[b] NED, no evidence of disease.
[c] Four patients NED with salvage therapy.

and these patients have been on no therapy for a minimum of 15 months. One hundred and eight patients (96% of the 113 randomized) are currently free of disease since 4 of these 9 patients with relapses achieved a sccond durable complete remission with cisplatin plus VP-16 salvage chemotherapy. We feel that this is a large enough patient population followed for an adequate period of time to show conclusively that maintenance therapy is not required in well staged complete responders.

These data from our institution and numerous other institutions and cooperative groups prove quite convincingly that around 80% of patients with nonseminomatous testicular cancer will achieve disease-free status and the relapse rate is relatively low with or without maintenance therapy. One would have a very difficult time statistically demonstrating that any changes in remission-induction chemotherapy in the entire patient population could improve upon these results. Accordingly, future endeavors will have two potential goals in this disease. One goal will be to reduce toxicity of induction treatment and to find patient populations who have a high complete remission rate and need less therapy. On the other hand, a poor risk group can be defined who might potentially benefit from innovative strategies. Our next study in the Southeastern Cancer Study Group will compare induction chemotherapy with platinum, vinblastine, and bleomycin to that with platinum plus VP-16 plus bleomycin. It is thought that the short- and long-term toxicity with the latter regimen would be less and, hopefully, it will be proved to be at least therapeutically equal.

CHEMOTHERAPY OF SEMINOMA

The discussion on the chemotherapy of metastatic seminoma must begin with the realization that what appears to be metastatic seminoma may in reality be nonseminomatous disease. Patients who are initially treated with orchiectomy with a diagnosis of pure seminoma may have a different cell type than their original presentation. In 1980, the results of the first 19 consecutive patients with disseminated seminoma treated with PVB ± adriamycin were published.[13] All patients have a minimum follow-up of 2½ years. Twelve of these 19 patients (63%) achieved a complete remission, and none of these patients relapsed. Five of the six patients with no prior radiotherapy achieved complete remission.

A more recent analysis was conducted combining our results at Indiana University with those of Dr. Cortes-Funes in Madrid, Spain, and those of the Dutch Multi-Center Group.[14] Of 54 patients treated, 37 or 69% achieved a complete remission. Thirty of these 37 complete responders have been followed for a minimum of 1 year. There have been only three relapses, and furthermore, 18 of 19 patients who received no previous radiotherapy achieved complete remission. As might be expected, there is considerably more severe and prolonged myelosuppression in patients with prior radiotherapy despite the fact that the vinblastine dosage is reduced 25% in such patients. The results of chemotherapy with PVB in metastatic seminoma are comparable to those achieved in nonseminomatous germ cell tumors.

Although alkylating agents have been recommended in the treatment of metastatic seminoma, there is little hard data to justify their inclusion as part of a chemotherapy protocol in the 1980s and certainly no justification for using single alkylating agent therapy. The largest series of metastatic seminoma published using alkylating agent therapy was the Russian experience with the drug sarcolysin.[15, 16] This study has been widely quoted and is a primary reason for the widespread use of alkylating agents in metastatic seminoma. The authors noted "good clinical effect" in the treatment of seminoma with "38 remissions in 42 cases" and further noted that "19 out of 42 were alive and fit for work 2–6 years after the treatment was instituted."

It is possible that many of these patients had stage II or even stage I disease. None of the articles mention how many of the 42 patients had prior radiotherapy. Therefore, the preference for alkylating agents in metastatic seminoma may have been based upon mistaken interpretation of data. The American experience is considerably more sparse. MacKenzie[17] reported the initial Memorial Group experience with chlorambucil. Four patients with metastatic seminoma were treated, and two partial and two complete remissions were obtained; however, one of the complete remissions relapsed, and the other one remained disease free for 20 months at the time of the original publication. This latter patient did not have prior radiotherapy. MacKenzie also observed two of three partial remissions of pulmonary metastases with actinomycin-D and two of four partial remissions with actinomycin-D plus chlorambucil plus methotrexate.

The Memorial Group experience in metastatic seminoma has been updated.[18] This series included 18 patients with seminoma. Only three of these patients had no prior radiotherapy, and two of these three patients achieved complete remission and remained disease free with chemotherapy. Only five patients achieved complete remission: two with chlorambucil alone out of nine patients for a complete remission rate with this drug of 22%; one with nitrogen mustard plus radiotherapy; and two patients with chlorambucil plus actinomycin-D (although one of these two patients also received radiotherapy). On the basis of these data, it appears that alkylating agents clearly have activity in seminoma, but the overall complete remission rate appears to be between 20 and 30%. Alkylating agents were also considered to be radiomimetic and, therefore, a logical foundation for the chemotherapy of a disease that is exquisitely radiosensitive. However, some of these early studies include patients relapsing in irradiated fields, and the concept of a radiomimetic drug in such a clinical setting seems illogical. Therefore, it seems there is no basis for alkylating agent therapy in the treatment of metastatic seminoma or metastatic testicular cancer in general, especially when one considers the potential for long term toxicity, such as second neoplasm, with prolonged courses of alkylating agents.

Therefore, the results in metastatic seminoma with PVB are quite comparable to the results with the same chemotherapy regimen in nonseminomatous tumors. There is no data to indicate a difference in response rate or potential curability of metastatic seminoma compared to nonseminomatous tumors. Chemotherapeutic strategy for disseminated seminoma should parallel that employed for nonseminomatous germ cell tumors.

EXTRAGONADAL GERM CELL TUMORS

Extragonadal germ cell tumors account for about 1–2% of all germ cell tumors and, indeed, are probably more common than were previously realized. They are histologically identical to those of malignant germ cell tumors of testicular origin and can arise from the anterior mediastinum, retroperitoneum, or the pineal. They may rarely also occur at other miscellaneous sites.

Patients with primary retroperitoneal or primary mediastinal seminomas are usually best treated with radiation therapy with an expected 75% cure rate. However, patients with extragonadal germ cell tumors which are not pure seminomas should never be treated with radiation therapy as primary treatment. The results of PVB for extragonadal germ cell tumors are identical to the results obtained with the same treatment regimen for primary testicular cancer taking into account that these patients present with large volume disease. In a combined series from Indiana and Vanderbilt Universities, there are presently 16 out of 30 patients with primary extragonadal germ cell tumors treated with PVB who are presently alive and disease free and presumably cured. Almost all of these patients have a minimum followup of at least 1 year. Again, these results are almost indistinguishable from that which can be obtained with large volume disease of a similar quantity for testicular cancers.

There are several important concepts in the diagnosis and management of extragonadal tumors. First, these tumors should be treated in the same manner as their testicular counterparts, that is retroperitoneal or mediastinal seminoma should be treated primarily with radiotherapy, and extragonadal embryonal, teratocarcinoma, and choriocarcinoma should be treated with chemotherapy. Second, there is no indication for orchiectomy in these patients unless the testis is abnormal to palpation. However, especially in retroperitoneal germ cell tumors, it is also worthwhile to obtain a testicular ultrasound to see if there is a primary tumor in the testis. This is more than academic interest because there is evidence that there may be a relative blood-testicular barrier for chemotherapy. This phenomenon has been recognized for years in acute lymphoblastic leukemia. Also, we have had nine patients with disseminated testicular cancer with a primary tumor in the testis where the testis was not initially removed. Although large bulky metastatic disease disappeared with chemotherapy (or was found to be merely necrotic tissue at the time of surgical removal), subsequent orchiectomy in these nine patients revealed that two of them still had microscopic evidence of embryonal carcinoma. Third, the diagnosis of germ cell tumor must be considered in any young adult with an anterior mediastinal mass or retroperitoneal tumor that is pathologically interpreted as "malignant neoplasm" or undifferentiated carcinoma.[19] At the very least, serum β-HCG and α-fetoprotein should be obtained, and it may not be unreasonable to give one provocative course of PVB in such patients. If it truly is a germ cell tumor, one should see rapid regression of measurable disease with one course of therapy.

SALVAGE THERAPY

Although 80% of patients with disseminated testicular cancer will achieve a disease-free status with PVB (either with chemotherapy alone or surgical resection of residual disease), there still remains a patient population who ultimately will require salvage therapy. These, of course, are those patients who fail to ever achieve a disease-free status (about 20%) or those patients who relapse after complete remission (about 10%).

Prior to the introduction of VP-16 in 1978, secondary chemotherapy consisted of a variety of treatment programs including cisplatin plus adriamycin, cisplatin plus adriamycin plus vincristine plus bleomycin or, if the patient was refractory to platinum, actinomycin-D-based chemotherapy, adriamycin plus cyclophosphamide, or other regimens. Prior to 1978, we never achieved a 1-year disease-free survival with any treatment program in such patients. Furthermore, in 31 drug trials in 22 patients, we failed to ever achieve a partial remission or complete remission in any patient with noncisplatin therapy.

The investigational epipodophyllotoxin, VP-16, has definite single agent activity in germinal neoplasms and is the only drug we have ever seen that would induce response in platinum-refractory patients. We began using VP-16 salvage therapy in 1978. Forty-five heavily pretreated patients received platinum plus VP-16 with or without bleomycin and adriamycin, depending upon prior therapy.[20, 21] Forty-two had prior platinum-based chemotherapy, but none were refractory to this drug. A number had received various other drug combinations. Mininum follow-up is 15 months. Complete remission was attained in 24% and an additional 30% were rendered disease free with surgical resection of residual disease, for an overall no evidence of disease (NED) status of 54%. There are 40% currently disease free with a 15-month minimum follow-up. We feel this is a significant achievement considering the previous poor results in this patient population.

Our present salvage program is illustrated in Table 15.2. Adriamycin has been deleted from our current programs because of no good evidence of its benefit and its contribution to the mucositis and myelosuppression of this regimen. This therapy is applicable for any patient who is not refractory to any of the three study drugs (*i.e.* no progression within 4 weeks of the last cisplatin or bleomycin therapy). This salvage program can produce formidable myelosuppression because it is employed in a heavily pretreated patient population. However, the 40% apparent cure rate in a patient population that previously had a zero cure rate is significant testimony to its activity. At the present time, as mentioned previously, we are conducting our fourth generation study randomizing patients with testicular cancer to receive cisplatin plus vinblastine plus bleomycin *versus* cisplatin plus VP-16 plus bleomycin as first line therapy.

In a patient who has unresectable partial remission following PVB, it has been our policy to continue vinblastine maintenance therapy until disease progression. At the time of progression, they are refractory only to vinblastine, and such patients are treated with salvage chemotherapy with cisplatin plus VP-16 plus bleomycin at that time. We prefer that approach in contrast to the immediate introduction of salvage therapy because there are occasional patients who are serologically negative and have an "unresectable partial remission" who, in reality, have only residual necrotic, fibrous tissue. Also, it is very difficult to give a patient seven or eight consecutive courses of cisplatin combination chemotherapy; the period of maintenance vinblastine therapy allows mental and physical recovery from the effects of the previous chemotherapy.

LONG-TERM COMPLICATIONS OF THERAPY

The reproductive effects of cisplatin-based combination chemotherapy are unknown. A prospective study of this problem is currently underway at our institution, and the results are premature, but the effects are likely to be substantial with a high incidence of azoospermia and oligospermia with, as of yet, an unknown chance for recovery. However, a few of our patients have fathered children several years after completion of treatment. There does not appear to be any significant long-term problems with nephrotoxicity or pulmonary toxicity. The risk of second neoplasms is unknown and none, as of yet, are directly attributable to cisplatin-based chemotherapy. Cisplatin is associated with a positive Ames test, a predictor of carcinogenicity, and the risk of this complication is of real concern.

As others have observed, Raynaud's phenomenon is not infrequently seen. It appears that ultimately this is reversible but months or years may be required. The risk of premature coronary disease is unknown.

SUMMARY AND CONCLUSIONS

Cisplatin-based chemotherapy will, with or without subsequent surgical excision of residual disease, produce disease-free status in around 80% of patients so treated. The relapse rate from complete remission is around 10% or slightly less and does not appear to be affected by maintenance chemotherapy. Thus, around 70% of patients with disseminated testicular cancer will be cured. In the cohort of patients not cured by initial therapy, salvage chemotherapy with cisplatin plus VP-16 will allow a few more patients to be long-term disease-free survivors.

By manipulation of initial drug dosages and more experience with this regimen, acute toxicity has been reduced and, in experienced hands, the drug-related mortality should be quite low. The spectrum and frequency of long-term toxicity has not totally been defined. There has been no chronic renal disease or lung disease and normal reproductive function will return in some patients. Neurotoxicity can be a long-term problem but appears to diminish with time. Premature coronary artery disease and the induction of second neoplasms continues to be a potential problem with little data available regarding their frequency.

In addition to the evaluation of VP-16-containing therapy as first line, there are several other potentially fruitful areas of investigation. Highly desirable would be a reliable method initially to select which patients are destined not to be cured with standard therapy so they may be placed on trials of innovative treatment at the time of diagnosis of metastatic disease. Potential regimens include modification of dose, schedule of the drugs used in induction therapy, or the addition of other active agents. It is conceivable that high dose chemotherapy with autologous marrow rescue might also improve therapeutic results.

The fate of patients with disseminated testicular cancer is vastly improved from that of 10 years ago and it is likely that in the next decade the cure rate will be even higher with more precisely defined and lesser toxicity.

REFERENCES

1. Samuels, M. L., Lanzotti, V. J., Holoye, P. Y., Boyle, L. E., Smith, T. L., and Johnson, D. E. Combination chemotherapy in germinal cell tumors. *Cancer Treat. Rev. 3:*185–204, 1976.
2. Samuels, M. L., Johnson, D. E., and Holoye, P. Y. Continuous intravenous bleomycin (NSC-125066) therapy with vinblastine (NSC-49842) in stage III testicular neoplasia. *Cancer Chemother. Rep. 59:*563–570, 1975.
3. Higby, D. J., Wallace, H. J., Albert, D. J., and Holland, J. F. Diaminodichloroplatinum: a phase I study showing responses in testicular and other tumors. *Cancer 37:*1219–1225, 1974.
4. Wittes, R. E., Yagoda, A., Silvay, O., Magill, G. B., Whitmore, W., Krakoff, I. H., and Golbey, R. B. Chemotherapy of germ cell tumors of the testis. *Cancer 37:*637–645, 1976.
5. Cvitkovic, E., Cheng, E., Whitmore, W. F., and Golbey, R. M. Germ cell tumor chemotherapy update. *Proc. Am. Soc. Clin. Oncol. 18:*324, 1977.
6. Cheng, E., Cvitkovic, E., Wittes, R. E., and Golbey, R. B. Germ cell tumors: VAB II in metastatic testicular cancer. *Cancer 42:*2162–2168, 1978.
7. Reynolds, T., Vugrin, D., Cvitkovic, E., Chang, E., Braun, D., O'Hehir, M., Dukeman, M., Whitmore, W., Golbey, R. VAB-3 combination chemotherapy of metastatic testicular cancer. *Cancer 48:*888–898, 1981.
8. Vugrin, D., Cvitkovic, E., Whitmore, W. F., Jr., Cheng, E., and Golbey, R. B. VAB-4 combination chemotherapy in the treatment of metastatic testis tumors. *Cancer 47:*833–839, 1981.
9. Vugrin, D., Herr, H., Whitmore, W. F., Jr., Sogani, P., Golbey, R. VAB-6 combination chemotherapy in disseminated cancer of the testis. *Ann. Intern. Med. 95:*59–61, 1981.
10. Einhorn, L. H., and Donohue, J. *Cis*-diamminedichloroplatinum, vinbastine, and bleomycin combination chemotherapy in disseminated testicular cancer. *Ann. Intern. Med. 87:*293–298, 1977.
11. Einhorn, L. H., Williams, S. D., Turner, S., Troner, M., Greco, F. A. The role of maintenance therapy in disseminated testicular cancer: a Southeastern Cancer Study Group protocol. *Proc. Am. Soc. Clin. Oncol. 22:*474, 1981.
12. Einhorn, L. H., and Williams, S. D. Chemotherapy of disseminated testicular cancer. *Cancer 46:*1339–1344, 1980.
13. Einhorn, L. H., and Williams, S. D. Chemotherapy of disseminated seminoma. *Cancer Clin. Trials 3:*307–313, 1980.
14. VanOosterom, A. T., Williams, S. D., Funes, H. C., Vendrik, C. P., Huinink, W. W. The treatment of advanced seminomas with cisplatin, velban, and bleomycin. *Abstracts of UICC Conference on Clinical Oncology,* October 28–31, 1981.
15. Blokin, N., Larionou, L., Perevodchekova, N., Chebotareva, L., and Merkalove, N.

Clinical experience with sarcolysin in neoplastic disease. *Ann. NY Acad. Sci. 68:*1128–1132, 1958.
16. Chebotarva, L. I. Late results of sarcolysen therapy in tumors of the testis. Acta UN Int. Cong. Cancer. *20:*390–391, 1964.
17. MacKenzie, A. R. The chemotherapy of metastatic seminoma. *J. Urol. 96:*790, 1966.
18. Whitmore, W. F., Smith, A., Yagoda, A., Cvitkovic, E., and Golbey, R. Chemotherapy of seminoma. *Recent Results Cancer Res. 60:*244–249, 1977.
19. Richardson, R. L., Schaumacher, R. A., Fer, M. F., Hande, K. R., Forbes, J. T., Oldham, F. K., and Greco, F. A. The unrecognized extragonadal germ cell cancer syndrome. *Ann. Int. Med. 94:*181–186, 1981.
20. Williams, S. D., Einhorn, L. H., Greco, F. A., Oldham, R., and Fletcher, R. VP-16-213 salvage therapy for refractory germinal neoplasms. *Cancer 46:*2154–2158, 1980.
21. Williams, S. D. (Unpublished data).

16

Management of Nonseminomatous Germ Cell Tumors of the Testis: the Royal Marsden Hospital Experience

M. J. Peckham, M.D.

The management of nonseminomatous germ cell tumors of the testis can be considered under two headings: the management of patients with no clinical evidence of residual disease following orchiectomy (stage I), and the management of patients with clinical evidence of metastatic disease (stages II, III and IV). It is convenient to consider the management of patients with metastases in two broad subgroups, those where metastatic disease is small in volume and those who have bulky disease. The first group have an extremely high probability of cure with currently available chemotherapy and the main effort in this area is to reduce the toxicity of treatment without loss of efficacy. Conversely, in patients with bulky metastatic disease, treatment failures still occur and efforts are being directed towards the precise definition of the high risk group of patients and the development of more effective treatment. The treatment philosophy in testicular nonseminoma at the Royal Marsden Hospital has differed radically in concept from that employed in most American centers. Surgery (other than orchiectomy), is not employed as the initial form of management in any stage group. The main role of surgery is to resect residual masses after chemotherapy. In the latter group, efforts are being made to develop methods capable of identifying patients who need surgery and to distinguish patients with a high chance of residual malignancy from those in whom the residual mass is either differentiated teratoma or necrotic and fibrotic tissue.

A further major difference in management has been the abandonment of any form of immediate treatment following orchiectomy in patients with clinical stage I disease in whom serum markers are either negative or revert rapidly to normal levels after orchiectomy and who do not have tumor in the cut end of the spermatic cord. The background and preliminary results of this study are discussed below.

STAGING METHODOLOGY

The following investigations were performed: lymphography, chest radiography and whole lung tomography, intravenous urography, renal and hepatic function tests and full blood count. The liver and retroperitoneum were ultrasonically scanned until CAT scanning became available in mid-1977. Since then all patients have had CAT scans of the liver, retroperitoneum and lungs unless obvious metastatic disease rendered this unnecessary.

All patients had sequential serum sampling for α-fetoprotein (AFP) and β-HCG levels from the time of presentation.

STAGING CLASSIFICATION

This describes the extent of the tumor, the site(s) of involvement and the tumor volume.

I. Lymphogram negative, no evidence of metastases
II. Lymphogram positive, metastases confined to abdominal nodes, 3 subgroups are recognized:
  A. Maximum diameter of metastases <2 cm
  B. Maximum diameter of metastases 2–5 cm
  C. Maximum diameter of metastases >5 cm
III. Involvement of supradiaphragmatic and infradiaphragmatic lymph nodes. No extralymphatic metastases
  Abdominal status:
    A, B, C as for stage II
IV. Extralymphatic metastases
  Suffixes as follows:
    O, lymphogram negative
    A, B, C as for stage II
  Lung status:
    L_1, <3 metastases
    L_2, multiple metastases, none exceeding 2 cm maximum diameter
    L_3, multiple metastases, one or more exceeding 2 cm diameter
  Liver-status*:
    H_+, liver involvement

---

* Criteria for liver involvement:
of the four following parameters, three should be positive before liver involvement is diagnosed
1. Abnormal liver function tests
2. Positive CT scan
3. Positive ultrasonic or isotopic scan
4. Clinical enlargement

SURVEILLANCE STUDY IN CLINICAL STAGE I NONSEMINOMA

As has been argued elsewhere,[10] an analysis of historical data strongly suggests that at least 80% of men with clinical stage I disease are likely to be cured by orchiectomy alone. Furthermore, given the effectiveness of chemotherapy in small volume metastases, the detection of relapsing stage I patients with a minimal tumor load means that the probability of cure is extremely high.

Before undertaking such a study it was recognized that excellent treatment results in stage I disease have been reported with radical node dissection and deferred chemotherapy,[3] radical node dissection and routine chemotherapy[14] and radiotherapy with deferred chemotherapy.[12] The issue under investigation is not curability but curability with avoidance of unnecessary therapy. Before embarking on the study, a detailed analysis was carried out on stage I patients receiving lymph node irradiation after orchiectomy between 1974 and 1979.[13] The objective was to examine factors predisposing to relapse. As shown in Table 16.1, two factors with prognostic significance were identified: the behavior of serum markers following orchiectomy and involvement by tumor of the spermatic cord. The data were inadequate to evaluate the significance of intratumor vascular invasion or lymphatic permeation. In this study histology was not a significant factor, although in previous studies the relapse rate had been significantly higher in embryonal carcinoma than in teratocarcinoma.[11] Tissue staining for HCG did not significantly influence the outcome.

In 1979 routine lymph node irradiation following orchiectomy was discontinued in stage I nonseminoma regardless of histology or serum marker status. Entry criteria included negative serum markers or rapid normalization of serum markers following orchiectomy. If tumor was demonstrated in the cut end of the spermatic cord the patient was excluded from the surveillance study. In practice, no example of this was encountered. Patients who showed persistent elevation of serum AFP and/or β-HCG levels after orchiectomy were designated stage Im. Since

Table 16.1.
Prognostic factors in patients with stage I nonseminomatous germ cell tumors of the testis receiving lymph node irradiation

Factor	Of Prognostic Significance	Comment
Histology[a]	Yes	Relapse rate embryonal carcinoma > teratocarcinoma ($p < 0.05$)
Periorchiectomy serum AFP and/or HCG levels raised[b]	(No)	Delay between orchiectomy and first sample complicates interpretation of results
Rate fall of serum marker levels after orchiectomy[b]	Yes	Rapid fall: relapse rate—15% Slow/incomplete fall: relapse rate—64% ($p < 0.05$)
Tissue staining for HCG[b]	No	
Involvement of spermatic cord by tumor[b]	Yes	Positive: relapse rate—60% Negative: relapse rate—18% ($p < 0.05$)

[a] Data from Peckham *et al.*, 1977.[11]
[b] Data from Raghaven *et al.*, 1982.[13]

they obviously had metastatic disease, despite a failure of clinical staging procedures to demonstrate it, these patients received chemotherapy. Preorchiectomy serum marker levels were obtained wherever possible and attempts made to obtain at least twice-weekly measurements during the postorchiectomy period to allow the regression rate to be measured. The histology of the primary tumor was reviewed in all cases and the material processed for the presence of tissue HCG and AFP, using the immunoperoxidase method.[7] The primary tumor was examined histologically for evidence of vascular invasion and lymphatic permeation and the local extent of the tumor in terms of the involvement of the spermatic cord, epididymis and tunica were described.

The major objective of the surveillance study is to establish the cure potential of orchiectomy alone in patients staged by lymphography, intravenous urography, ultrasonic scanning of the liver and retroperitoneum and CT scanning of the thorax and abdomen. Patients in the study are seen at monthly intervals for the first year with CT scans performed at alternate visits, the follow-up interval is extended to 2 months in the second year and to 3 months in the third year. A second objective of the study is to see whether a group of patients can be defined where the relapse probability following orchiectomy alone is high enough to warrant immediate chemotherapy. The results of the surveillance study, particularly the tempo of relapse will determine future follow-up intervals and the clinical investigations needed to monitor patients on follow-up. It is possible that a group of patients may be defined where the cure rate by orchiectomy alone will approach 100%.

Results

Table 16.2 summarizes the number of patients who have been entered into the study since 1979 and, over the same period, the number who proved ineligible by virtue of persistently elevated serum markers. Table 16.3 shows patients followed for a minimum of 1 year after orchiectomy and the relapse rate in relation to histology of the primary tumor. The relapse rate has been strongly influenced by histology of the primary tumor with no relapses having occurred so far in patients with teratocarcinoma. It was thought initially that this might reflect a slower tempo of relapse in patients with teratocarcinoma compared with embryonal carcinoma. However, a retrospective analysis of the time to relapse in patients treated with radiotherapy between 1963 and 1979 (Fig. 16.1) shows an identical pattern for embryonal carcinoma and teratocarcinoma, suggesting that the preliminary observations of the surveillance study reflect a

Table 16.2.
Clinical stage I testicular nonseminoma: number of patients entered into surveillance study after orchiectomy requiring immediate chemotherapy (the Royal Marsden Hospital, 1979–1981.)

Entered into surveillance study	57
Excluded because of persistently elevated markers	2
Excluded because of tumor in the cut end of the spermatic cord	0
Total patients	59

low incidence of occult metastases in teratocarcinoma patients. As shown in Table 16.4, all relapses have occurred within 1 year of orchiectomy and most within 6 months. All patients who have relapsed are disease free following chemotherapy.

Table 16.3.
Clinical stage I nonseminoma testis: relapse rate according to histology after orchiectomy alone (the Royal Marsden Hospital, 1979–1981)

Histology	Total Patients	Number Relapsing	Percentage	Observation Time Since Orchiectomy
				(months)
Embryonal carcinoma	13	6	46.1	12–34
Teratocarcinoma	16	0	0	12–38
Trophoblastic malignant teratoma	2	0	0	12, 28
Seminoma with raised AFP	2	1	(50)	12, 29
Differentiated teratoma	1	0	0	13
Total	34	7	206	

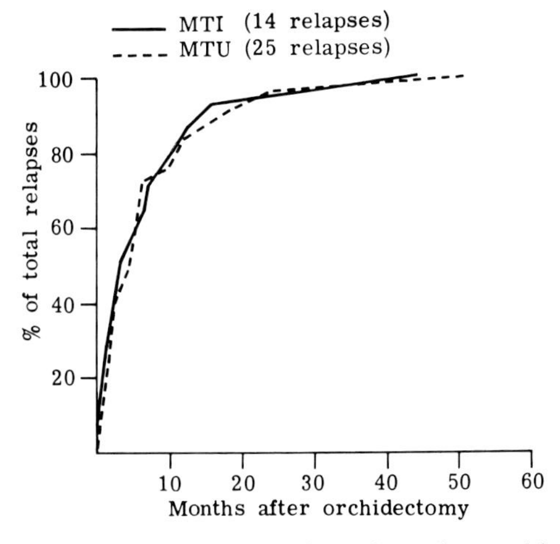

Figure 16.1. Time from orchiectomy to relapse in patients with clinical stage I nonseminomatous germ cell testicular tumors receiving lymph node irradiation. (Royal Marsden Hospital, 1963–1979.)

Table 16.4.
Clinical stage I nonseminoma testis, surveillance after orchiectomy only: details of relapsing patients. (the Royal Marsden Hospital, 1979–1981)

Total Relapses	Time Between Orchiectomy and Relapse	Site(s) of relapse			Disease Status of Relapses
		Abdominal Nodes	Abdominal Nodes + Lung	Markers only	
	(months)				
7	2, 2, 3, 5, 5, 5, 10	4	1	2	Six disease-free at 5, 11, 24, 25, 29 and 30 months; one on chemotherapy at 4 months

Figure 16.2 shows an example of four patients in whom serum α-fetoprotein levels cleared rapidly after orchiectomy and one patient in whom there was persistent elevation. Figure 16.3 shows serum marker levels in 19 patients in whom preorchiectomy blood samples were obtained, in 15 (79%) one or both markers were elevated indicating that preoperative elevation of serum marker level *per se* is not a significant prognostic factor, although it is not possible at this stage to say whether

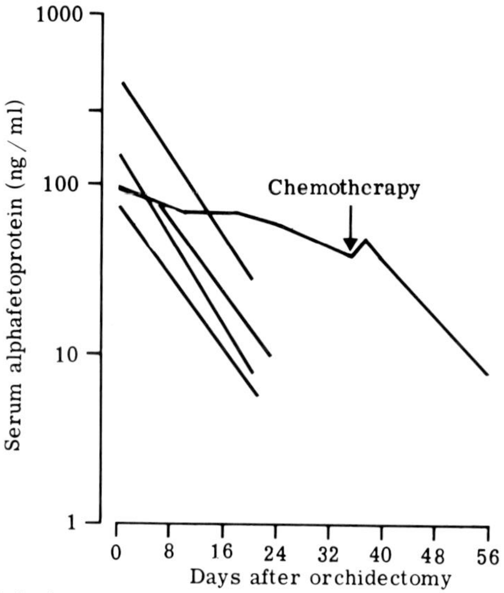

Figure 16.2. Clinical stage I nonseminomatous germ cell tumor of the testis: evolution of serum α-fetoprotein after orchiectomy showing complete clearance ($T\frac{1}{2}$, 5–6 days) and one example of slow incomplete clearance ($T\frac{1}{2}$ ~ 30 days).

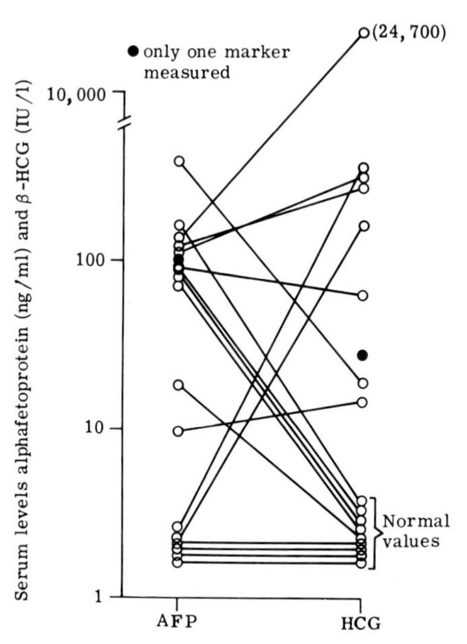

Figure 16.3. Blood marker levels immediately prior to orchiectomy in patients with clinical stage I nonseminomatous germ cell tumors of the testis entered into surveillance study.

marker titre will predict for subsequent relapse. One patient with a preorchiectomy β-HCG titre of 24,700 IU/l showed rapid normalization of marker levels following orchiectomy and at 12 months remains free of disease without further treatment. Overall in the study, 34 patients have been followed for a minimum period of 1 year since orchiectomy; of this group, seven (20.6%) have relapsed. All relapses have been detected when the patients had limited volume disease, and the six who have completed chemotherapy are in complete remission.

Conclusions

More data are needed before the prognostic significance of histology, serum markers, intratumor vascular invasion, lymphatic permeation and local extent of the primary tumor can be assessed. However, the preliminary results indicate that, as expected, only a minority of patients investigated with currently available clinical staging procedures harbor occult metastases and most are likely to be cured by orchiectomy alone. Patients who relapse can be successfully reclaimed with chemotherapy which is progressively becoming more acceptable and less toxic (see below). As discussed below, in patients with small volume metastases it may be possible to omit bleomycin and use etoposide and cisplatin alone. If this proves to be practicable the major toxic component of the presently used combination will have been removed without loss of therapeutic effect. Furthermore, non-nephrotoxic platinum analogues (see below) offer the prospect of developing a low toxicity drug combination compatible with recovery of spermatogensis and with no risk of long-term toxic sequelae.

These preliminary data suggest that the routine application of local treatment methods directed at occult metastases in draining lymph nodes may be inessential. If these observations are sustained by further experience, it would be unjustifiable to argue that radical lymph node dissection is valuable either as a therapeutic procedure or as a staging method.

MANAGEMENT OF PATIENTS WITH METASTATIC DISEASE

The important influence of tumor volume on the outcome of treatment with chemotherapy for testicular nonseminoma is illustrated in Figures 16.4 and 16.5. Figure 16.4 shows disease-free survival rate in relation to the size of retroperitoneal lymph nodes and Figure 16.5 shows survival in relation to the size of lung metastases. Figure 16.6 shows the survival results in 110 previously untreated patients with metastatic disease seen between 1976 and 1981 (minimum follow-up 12 months), and subdivided into two broad categories, small volume metastatic disease and large volume metastatic disease. Treatment included vinblastine and bleomycin (1976–1978), cisplatin, vinblastine and bleomycin (PVB) (1978–1980) and bleomycin, etoposide and cisplatin ± vinblastine (since 1980). The significant difference in survival characteristics between small volume and large volume disease groups provides a useful conceptual basis for considering future management.

In 1979, vinblastine in the cisplatinum, vinblastine, bleomycin combi-

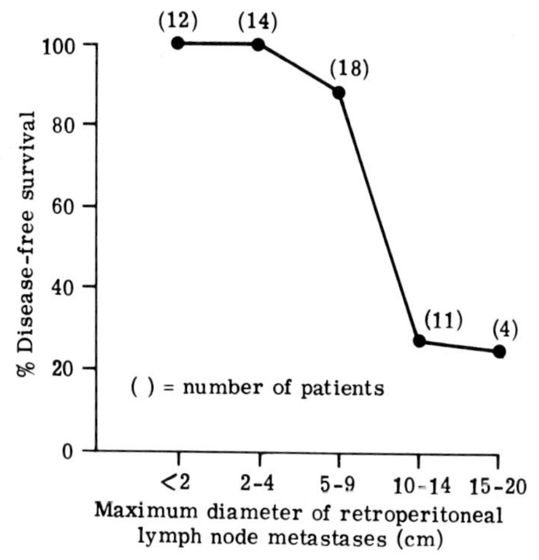

Figure 16.4. Relation between size of metastases and outcome of treatment in advanced (stages II, III and IV (L_1 + L_2) nonseminomatous germ cell tumors of the testis. (Royal Marsden Hospital 1976–1980.)

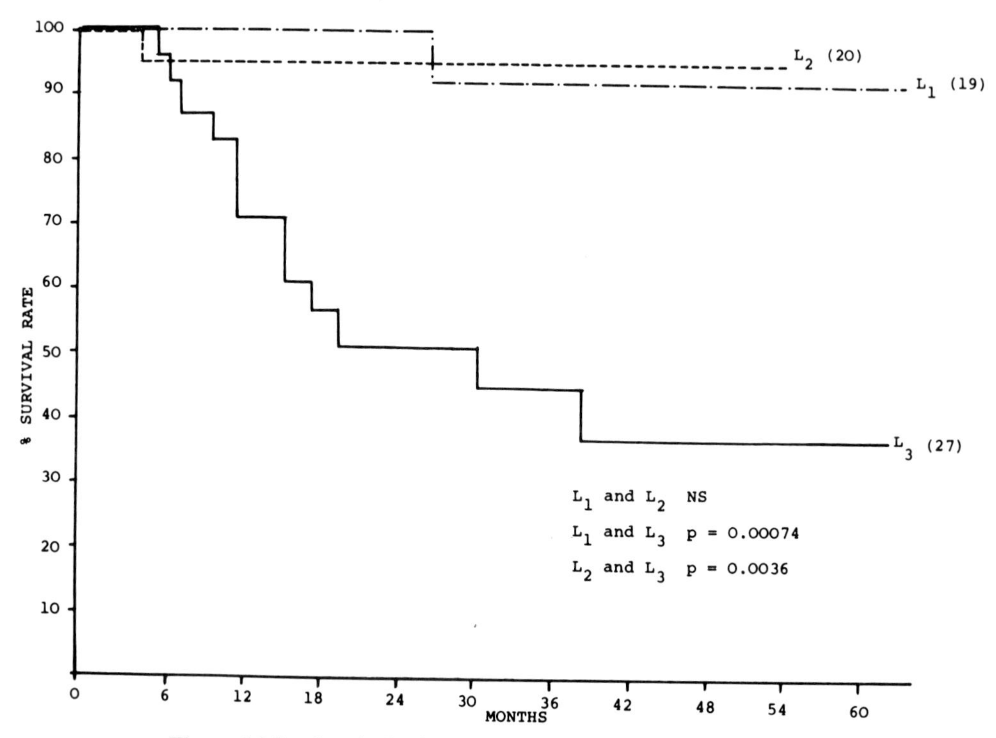

Figure 16.5. Survival of previously untreated patients with nonseminomatous germ cell testicular tumors showing the influence of the size of lung metastases on the outcome of chemotherapy.

nation[4] was replaced by epotoside (VP16) on the basis of the single agent activity of the latter drug in testicular nonseminoma,[2, 5, 9, 15] and in an attempt to reduce the toxicity of the PVB combination. Encouraged by the activity of the combination in a small group of patients treated for relapse after radiotherapy, PVB was abandoned in favor of bleomycin, etoposide and cisplatin (BEP) as first line treatment in 1980. Drug doses and administration is as follows: bleomycin 30 mg intravenously, days 2, 9 and 16; cisplatin 20 mg/m^2 intravenously infused over 6 hours, days 1–5; etoposide 120 mg/m^2 intravenously days 1–3. Cycles are repeated every 21 days and patients reassessed after four cycles. If disease was initially bulky or if normalization of serum markers was slow, a further two cycles was given. Of the whole group of 26 patients (Table 16.5), eight had six cycles, 17 had four cycles, and one patient had two cycles of chemotherapy. Selected patients proceeded to surgical resection of residual masses after four or six cycles of chemotherapy. If there is histologic evidence of residual malignancy, chemotherapy is continued after surgery. Until September 1981 patients were considered for radiotherapy after chemotherapy. Of the 22 patients shown in Table 16.6, 10 had postchemotherapy radiotherapy. Preliminary results of the BEP combination are summarized in Tables 16.5 and 16.6. As shown, more than 80% of patients are alive and disease-free. In the previously untreated group (Table 16.6) 5/5 patients with small volume disease are in complete remission and 8/9 patients with bulky disease are alive and disease-free. The major toxicity of the combination is myelosuppression. This is usually not severe, but in 29% of patients it has been necessary to increase the interval between the beginning of one cycle and the next from 3 to 4 weeks. However, this has not influenced therapeutic outcome. A detailed study of the toxicity of the combination is in progress.

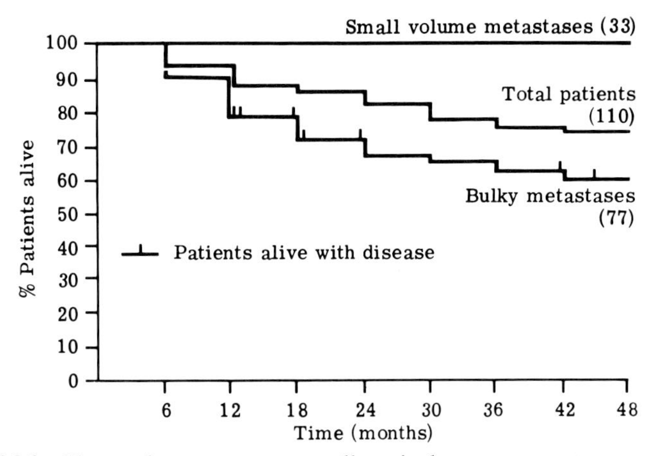

Figure 16.6. Nonseminomatous germ cell testicular tumors: outcome of treatment in relation to tumor volume (Royal Marsden Hospital, 1976–1981.)

Table 16.5. Bleomycin, etoposide (VP16-213) and cisplatin (BEP) for metastatic germ cell tumors[a]

Total Patients	Alive Disease-Free	Dead of Intercurrent Disease	Alive with Disease	Dead of Tumor
26[b]	22 (84.6%)	1	1	2

[a] Follow-up 9–31 months (median 12.5 months).

[b] Includes one ovarian yolk sac tumor (alive and disease free 12 months), and two patients with seminoma (disease free 10, 10 and 15 months).

The major longer term complications of the BEP combination are related to bleomycin. These include pulmonary toxicity, a proportion of patients develop Raynaud's syndrome, Lhermitte's syndrome, impairment of fine sensation, finger thickening, stiffness and tenderness. Although these complications have generally not resulted in severe functional disability, it is desirable to avoid them if possible. In view of the activity of epotoside and cisplatin as single agents a phase 2 study of these two drugs in combination has been initiated in patients with limited disease.

CIS-DIAMMINE-1, 1-CYCLOBUTANE, DICARBOXYLATE PLATINUM II (CBDCA)

Phase 1 studies with the platinum analogue CBDCA have shown that the drug is less nephrotoxic than cisplatin and that it may be given without hydration.[1] CBDCA is associated with emesis although this appears quantitatively less than is the case with cisplatin. Preliminary data indicate activity in ovarian carcinoma but only scanty data are yet available in germ cell malignancy. Because of the excellent results being obtained with currently available schedules in testicular tumors it is difficult to test new drugs in previously untreated patients. CBDCA shows a comparable activity to cisplatin in nonseminoma germ cell xenografts (Table 16.7). If CBDCA is cross-resistant with cisplatin, clinical studies confined to patients relapsing after first line chemotherapy are unlikely to demonstrate the potential activity of the drug in untreated patients. For this reason a phase 2 study has been initiated in patients with poor risk nonseminoma (disseminated bulky metastases and liver involvement). In this study CBDCA is employed as initial treatment, with serum markers and measureable disease as monitors before the patient proceeds to orthodox chemotherapy.

Table 16.6.
Bleomycin, epotoside (VP16-213) and cisplatin (BEP) for metastatic nonseminomatous germ cell testicular tumors

Stage Category	No Prior Radiotherapy	Prior Radiotherapy
Small volume[a]	5[b]/5	2/3
Large volume[c]	8/9	3/5
Total Patients	13/14[d]	5/8[e]

[a] Small volume includes stages Im, IIA and B, IIIA and B, IVA and B, L_1, L_2.
[b] Number disease-free over total patients treated.
[c] Large volume includes stages IIC, IIIC, IVL_3, IVC and IVH_+
[d] Follow-up 9–15 months (median 12 months)
[e] Follow-up 10–28 months (median 26 months)

Table 16.7.
Ranking of five cytotoxic drugs against four testicular germ cell tumor xenografts

Drugs	Growth delay at 1/10 the maximum tolerated dose (LD_{10}) (Days)
Cisplatin	12
CBDCA	12
Bleomycin	5
Vinblastine	3.5

Despite the overall improvement in the management of testicular nonseminomas, patients with disseminated bulky metastases have fared less well. In an attempt to improve treatment results in this subgroup a combination of bleomycin, etoposide, vinblastine and cisplatin (BEVIP) has been under investigation in a phase 2 study, under the auspices of the Medical Research Council Testicular Tumour Working Party. Preliminary data from the Royal Marsden Hospital series are shown in Table 16.8. It is premature to assess the value of the four-drug combination in relation to BEP or PVB. As expected, the major toxicity is myelosuppression, which is frequently severe.

RADIOTHERAPY AS AN ADJUVANT TO CHEMOTHERAPY IN PATIENTS WITH BULKY DISEASE

Between 1976 and 1982, as described elsewhere in detail,[10] radiotherapy was used following chemotherapy in selected patients. The objective was to sterilize residual malignancy in bulky tumor masses. The survival of this patient population is shown in Figure 16.7. In the absence of a randomized prospective study it is not possible to establish whether radiotherapy contributes to a reduction in the histology-positive rate in resected masses or to disease-free survival. Since available patient numbers prohibited such a study, postchemotherapy radiotherapy was discontinued in 1981 in favor of a policy of chemotherapy and selective surgery.

Table 16.8.
Outcome of treatment with bleomycin, etoposide, vinblastine and cisplatin (BE-VIP) for high risk patients with disseminated nonseminomatous testicular tumors (the Royal Marsden Hospital, 1979–1981)

Total Patients	Alive, Disease Free		Dead of Disease
		months	
10	5	(12, 13, 24, 29, 31)	5

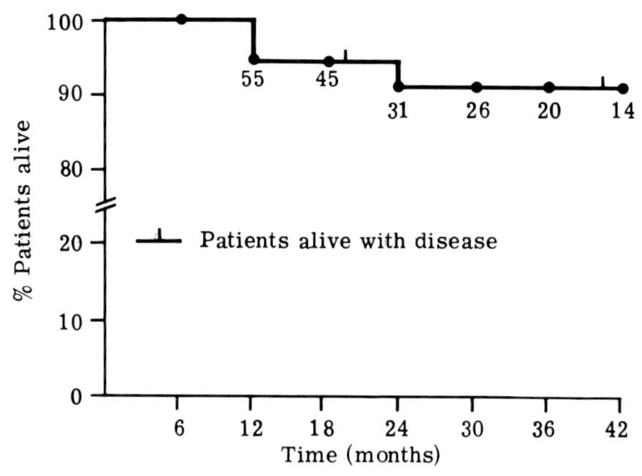

Figure 16.7. Nonseminomatous germ cell testicular tumors: outcome of treatment in patients receiving postchemotherapy involved-field irradiation (Royal Marsden Hospital, 1976–1980.)

The combined chemo-radiotherapy experience demonstrated that a sequence of chemotherapy followed by radiotherapy was not associated with toxicity. As discussed below, only 9% of patients with negative markers at the time of surgery for residual masses had histologic evidence of malignancy. The possible contribution of radiotherapy will be investigated by comparing previous experience with the results of surgery in patients having chemotherapy alone.

SURGERY FOR MASSES REMAINING FOLLOWING CHEMOTHERAPY

As shown in Table 16.9, of 41 patients undergoing surgery for residual tumor masses 9 (22%) have shown histologic evidence of active malignancy. Almost half the patient population showed evidence of differentiated teratoma. Of the total group, seven patients had raised markers at the time of surgery and six of these showed residual cancer. Only 3/34 (9%) of patients with negative serum markers had histologically positive masses. Bilateral node resection is associated with retrograde ejaculation and, since many patients are cured by the time they come to surgery, it would clearly be desirable to avoid an intervention wherever possible. In an attempt to predict the likelihood of residual tumor, the histology of resected tissue has been related to the size and x-ray density of the residual mass (expressed as CT number or Hounsfield units). Attempts are also being made to demonstrate residual malignancy using radioiodinated monoclonal antiteratoma antibodies. As shown in Table 16.10 the size of the residual mass appears to be a good indicator of whether or not there will be histologic evidence of residual cancer. Masses less than 4 cm in maximum diameter have been consistently negative. Since a proportion of these patients received radiotherapy after chemotherapy, the validity of the observations for patients receiving chemotherapy alone will need

Table 16.9.
Nonseminomatous testicular germ cell tumors: histology of masses resected after chemotherapy ± radiotherapy (the Royal Marsden Hospital, 1976–1981)[a]

Total Patients	Necrosis or Fibrosis	Differentiated Teratoma	Residual Malignancy
41	12 (29.3%)	20 (48.8%)	9 (21.9%)

[a] Data from Hendry *et al.*, 1981.[6]

Table 16.10.
Size of residual mass or histology in testicular nonseminoma patients undergoing surgery after chemotherapy ± radiotherapy (the Royal Marsden Hospital, 1976–1981)[a]

Histology	Size of Residual Mass	
	<4 cm Maximum Diameter	>4 cm
Necrosis/fibrosis	8	4
Differentiated teratoma	5	15
Malignancy	0	9

[a] Data from Hendry *et al.* 1981.

to be established. Of considerable interest is the potential value of CT number. As shown in Figure 16.8, patients with differentiated teratoma show a lower mean CT number than patients who have residual malignancy. The present evidence suggests that patients who have masses more than 4 cm in diameter with a high mean CT number should proceed to surgery since the risk of residual malignancy is high. Patients with large masses and a low CT number are likely to have differentiated teratoma. Since the natural history of differentiated teratoma left *in situ* is not established, surgery is advocated, although the timing and extent of the procedure may, in due course, be influenced by the findings discussed above.

CONCLUSIONS AND FUTURE PROSPECTS

The management of nonseminomatous germ cell testicular tumors remains a rapidly evolving field in which it is necessary to shed the prejudices of earlier treatment approaches. There is an overwhelming case for centralizing the management of these uncommon tumors into specialist units so that they can receive the attention of a team experienced in their management and where the necessary attention to detail can be assured. It is insufficient to justify the application of treatment methods such as radical lymph node dissection in stage I disease on the basis of the possible failure of patients to attend for regular follow-up. In our

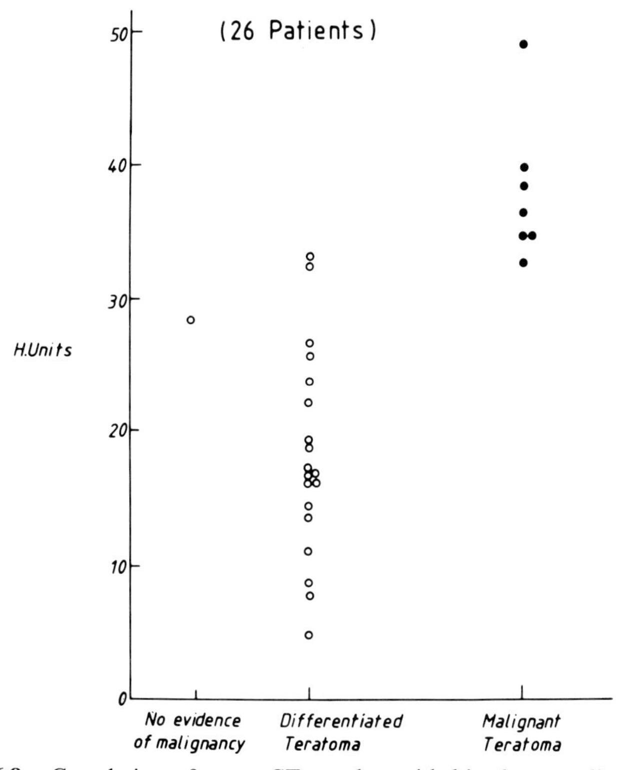

Figure 16.8. Correlation of mean CT number with histology: malignant teratoma. (Data adapted from Husband, Hawkes & Peckham, 1982.[8])

experience regular attendance in the surveillance study has not proved a problem so long as patients fully comprehend what it is the clinicians are trying to achieve. On present evidence it appears that this noninvasive treatment policy can be uniformly successful. In advanced-stage disease, testicular tumors offer the prime example in oncology of a clinical situation where it is possible to move progressively toward less toxic treatment schedules without loss of treatment effectiveness, hence, concentrating specifically on normal tissue rather than tumor response. This is not an unimportant consideration in patients presenting for treatment in their 20s and 30s.

REFERENCES

1. Calvert, A. H., Harland, S. J., Newell, D. R., Siddik, Z. H., Jones, A., McElwain, T. J., Raju, S., Wiltshaw, E., Smith, I. E., Peckham, M. J., Baker, J., and Harrap, K. R. Early clinical studies with *cis*-diammine-1, 1-cyclobutane dicarboxylate platinum II. AACR Abstracts (In press), 1982.
2. Cavelli, F., Klepp, O., Renard, J., Rohrt, M., and Alberto, P. A phase II study of oral VP-16-213 in nonseminomatous testicular cancer. *Eur. J. Cancer 17:*245–249, 1981.
3. Donohue, J. P., Einhorn, L. H., and Perez, J. M. Improved management of nonseminomatous testis tumors. *Cancer 42:*2903–2908, 1978.
4. Einhorn, L. H., and Donohue, J. P. *Cis*-diammine-dichloroplatinum, vinblastine and bleomycin combination chemotherapy in disseminated testicular cancer. *Ann. Intern. Med. 87:*293–298, 1977.
5. Fitzharris, B. M., Kaye, S. B., Saverymuttu, S., Newlands, E. S., Barrett, A., Peckham, M. J., and McElwain, T. J. VP16-213 as a single agent in advanced testicular tumors. *Eur. J. Can. 16:*1193–1197, 1980.
6. Hendry, W. F., Goldstraw, P., Husband, J. E., Barrett, A., McElwain, T. J., and Peckham, M. J. Elective delayed excision of bulky para-aortic lymph node metastases in advanced nonseminoma germ cell tumours of testis. *Br. J. Urol. 53:*648–653, 1981.
7. Heyderman, E. Immunoperoxidase technique in histopathology: application, methods and controls. *J. Clin. Pathol. 32:*971–978, 1979.
8. Husband, J. E., Hawkes, D., and Peckham, M. J. CT estimations of mean attenuation values and tumor volume in testicular tumors: a comparison with operative findings and histology. *Radiology* (In press), 1982.
9. Newlands, E. S., and Bagshawe, K. D. Epipodophyllin derivative (VP16-213) in malignant teratomas and choriocarcinomas. *Lancet 2:*87, 1977.
10. Peckham, M. J., and Barrett, A. Radiotherapy in testicular teratoma. In *The Management of Testicular Tumours*, pp. 174–201, Edited by M. J. Peckham. Edward Arnold, London, 1981.
11. Peckham, M. J., Hendry, W. F., McElwain, T. J., and Calman, F. M. B. The multimodality management of testicular teratomas. In *Adjuvant Therapy of Cancer, Proceedings of the International Conference on the Adjuvant Therapy of Cancer*, pp. 305–320, edited by S. E. Salmon and S. E. Jones. North-Holland, Amsterdam, 1977.
12. Peckham, M. J., Barrett, A., McElwain, T. J., Hendry, W. F., and Raghavan, D. Nonseminoma germ cell tumours (malignant teratoma) of the testis. Results of treatment and an analysis of prognostic factors. *Br. J. Urol. 53:*162–172, 1981.
13. Raghavan, D., Peckham, M. J., Heyderman, E., Tobias, J. S., and Austin, D. E. Prognostic factors in clinical stage I nonseminomatous germ cell tumours of the testis. *Br. J. Cancer 45:*167–173, 1982.
14. Skinner, D. G., and Scardino, P. T. Relevance of biochemical tumor markers and lymphadenectomy in the management of nonseminomatous testis tumors: current perspective. *Trans. Am. Assoc. Genitourin. Surg. 87:*293–298, 1979.
15. Williams, S. D., Einhorn, L. H., Greco, F. A., Oldham, R., and Fletcher, R. VP-16-213 salvage therapy for refractory germinal neoplasms. *Cancer 46:*2154–2158, 1980.

17

Randomized Clinical Trials and Cooperative Studies in Testicular Cancer

Nasser Javadpour, M.D., F.A.C.S.

Currently, the major problem in evaluating the survival of patients with urologic cancer is the lack of controlled clinical trials. The majority of the reported series comparing the various treatment modalities are either retrospective and/or lack controls. Therefore, one cannot interpret the data with certainty.

The objective of this chapter is to review certain existing randomized clinical trials and point out the need for newer ones in order to obtain critical answers to the clinical problems of patients with testicular cancer in a reliable fashion. Because of the paucity of information concerning the necessity and actual execution of prospective randomized clinical trials in urologic literatures, I shall start with a brief introduction.

Over the last several decades it has been recognized that in a complicated clinical setting, such as cancer, the superiority of a given treatment over another should be solved by a prospective concomitant randomized clinical trial. It has also been established that retrospective studies have biases against which large sample size is no protection. The fact that randomized studies are expensive, tedious and may need a long time or a large number of patients to answer certain critical clinical questions should not deter the clinicians from performing such trials in appropriate centers or participate in interinstitutional controlled investigations. An example of the necessity of randomized clinical trials is obvious from the following occurrence in clinical trials of immunotherapy of cancer including urologic cancer. In October 1977 the National Cancer Institute (NCI) sponsored a symposium on immunotherapy from various medical centers. In this symposium, as with almost all retrospective studies, the majority of the investigators reported the effectiveness of immunotherapy in different cancers. However, NCI sponsored another symposium in April 1980 (3 years later) and encouraged that only the results of randomized studies be presented. Suffice it to say that there were hardly any positive effective immunotherapies in these controlled clinical trials. Therefore, at the conclusion of the symposium it was clear that retrospective studies can only be suggestive and often will not stand the test of time or a randomized study. The discordance between randomized studies and noncontrolled studies are due to multiple factors including patient selection, biases of the institutions, the enthusiastic approach of the investigators and a host of other variables beyond the control of the investigators. Since it is absolutely essential to understand the objective of a prospective randomized study, before I discuss the current ongoing prospective randomized clinical trials, I should like to briefly discuss the requirements of a clinical trial with adequate control.

REQUIREMENTS OF RANDOMIZED STUDIES

The protocol is a written description of important question(s) for the study to answer. The protocol serves as a guideline for eligible patients, design of the study, defining complications or toxicities, time and number of patients necessary, the end point and method of randomization and stratification. A well designed protocol should include the following[1, 2] (Table 17.1):

Clear Objectives

The question(s) asked should be well defined, realistic and critical to the care of cancer patients. A vague, diffuse, poorly designed protocol leads to diffuse and ambiguous results. It is also important to attempt to ask reasonably limited questions. It is an error to attempt to answer many questions in a protocol because of the number of patients involved and other variables. One important consideration of the questions to be addressed is the potential impact that the question will have on the actual medical practice.

Design of the Protocol

The multimodality protocols are generally difficult to design and execute. However, a careful planning including limitations on the number

Table 17.1.
Subject headings for a protocol[2]

Introduction and rationale
Objectives
Patient eligibility
Design of protocol
Therapy groups
Procedures in event of toxicity and complication
Required clinical and laboratory data
Criteria for evaluating the effect of treatment
Statistical considerations
Informed consent
Data forms
References
Study chairperson and collaborators

of the study arms, realistic span of time and patient number usually help to answer limited, but significant, medical questions. In addition to limiting the number of questions in a given protocol, the diagnostic, therapeutic and prognostic procedures should not be so complex as to invite violation from the protocol. Violation of the protocol is a serious matter that will off-balance the results and interpretations of the protocol. The design of the protocol should also be able to attract the attention and cooperation of the participants.

Controls

Randomization is the most reliable method for constructing the groups to be compared. In randomization, the bias of low risk patient receiving surgery, therefore the surgical arm of the protocol, is naturally going to be superior regardless the merit of surgery itself is not a problem. The second advantage of randomization is to balance the factors known or unknown to the investigator concerning the results and prognosis. Many alternatives have been utilized including historic control, retrospective concomitant, patients treated in other institutions, patient refusal of treatment. Randomization is occasionally abused and based on the day of the week or the odd or even number of the age as to when the patient gets a surgical or medical treatment. Such a selection is biased because, if on a certain day of the week the patient is going to be randomized to surgery, a medical physician will refer the patient for admission on that day, or the admitting physician will not admit the patient based on even or odd number of age according to his belief, therefore entering bias in the study. The randomization procedure should be prepared by a competent and qualified statistician familiar with the randomized protocol.

Patient Selection

The selection of the patients to be randomized in a protocol is an important consideration that should lead to a definite answer. The type of patients to whom our conclusions apply are determined by the eligibility criteria of the protocol. The patient eligibility criteria should be explained in detail.

Treatment Program

The treatment program should be clearly defined. Care should be taken that all the arms of the protocol represent acceptable, ethical and most efficacious current treatment. It is not accepted to deprive any patient from a needed therapy. Surgical technique, portals, dose schedule of radiotherapy or chemotherapy must be clearly stated in the protocol. The number of patients necessary for the particular study depends on the statistical analysis of the various arms of the protocol comparing the differences in regard to the end point.[1, 2]

End Point

The end point of a protocol indicates the criteria which are necessary to terminate the study or to consider the achievement of the protocol. The ideal end point in cancer patients is cure, or tumor-free survival with acceptable quality of life. A number of protocols may also consider tumor size, partial regression or complete regression or certain subjective end points.

Informed Consent

An informed consent is necessary for every patient entering a randomized protocol. The patient should clearly understand that although the entry is by random, however, nobody knows which arm is the most effective therapeutic alternative. The therapeutic alternatives and their complications should be thoroughly discussed for patients. Patients should be given choices as to accept or reject the protocol. If the patient rejects participation in the protocol, he should be accepted off of the protocol for conventional therapy.

Miscellaneous

Data collections, references, study chairman, collaborating participants should be clearly stated in the protocol.

In conclusion, a protocol should reflect important medical questions likely to affect the practice of medicine. In my experience of conducting randomized studies, one of the hallmarks of a randomized study is the excellent care that is rendered to a patient on such protocols. The study objective should be defined and the treatment arms to which the patients are randomized must be practical (do-able) and acceptable treatment. The objectives and end points of the study as well as patient eligibility must be spelled out. Finally, proper informed consent in which the risks of different therapies and the off-protocol alternatives be discussed with patients. The compilations of protocols that are not concluded should not be taken as facts and utilized for the cancer patients who are not on the study. In light of this introduction, I would attempt to review the existing randomized protocols for stage I, II and III testicular cancers. Although a number of these protocols are ongoing or have just started, they give overall ongoing attempts to answer certain important questions. It should also be emphasized that there are a number of geographic differences between certain groups of the investigators. Such differences are clear as we will discuss the various protocols, *i.e.* the Danish randomized protocol for stage I NSTT is only designed for an observation arm *versus* radiotherapy alone and no arm for lymphadenectomy, perhaps due to the lack of expertise in performing such tedious operations. On the other hand the philosophy that prevails in the United States as the diminished role of radiotherapy in treatment of nonseminomatous testicular cancer (NSTT) has lead certain existing protocol for stage I NSTT to not consider radiotherapy. Obviously another important factor in executing a three-arm study is the large number of the patients necessary for such studies.

RANDOMIZED PROTOCOLS FOR STAGE I

Retroperitoneal lymphadenectomy has been the treatment of choice in stage I and stage II (IIA and IIB) of testicular cancer in the United States. This operation, when performed properly, has resulted in an approximately 96% tumor-free 2-year survival for the stage I and low stage II. The mortality and morbidity of this procedure has been accepted and young patients with testicular cancer tolerate the operation well. However, in certain European countries the treatment of choice for stage I and low stage II is radiotherapy—claiming to reach survival rates of equivalent to those of lymphadenectomy patients. There has been no prospective randomized clinical trials to compare lymphadenectomy, radiation therapy or just observing the patients with clinical stage I testicular cancer. A number of investigators have recently raised concern about the necessity of any treatment in stage I nonseminomatous testicular cancer. At the present time there are three randomized clinical trials for stage I testicular cancer.

Memorial-Sloan Kettering Randomized Trial

This study is comparing the efficacy of retroperitoneal lymphadenectomy with no treatment after a radical orchiectomy in clinical stage I nonseminomatous testicular cancer[3] (Fig. 17.1). Patients with clinical stage I nonseminomatous testicular cancer, excluding pure choriocarcinoma, are randomized in this protocol. The diagnosis of stage I testicular tumor is based on negative serum α-fetoprotein (AFP), HCG, CEA, LDH, intravenous pyelogram (IVP), lymphangiogram, abdominal CT and chest radiography. All these patients are followed on a monthly basis for 2 years and any patient who manifests clinical evidence of tumor progression will be treated with the conventional therapeutic modalities. The result of this study should provide important information as to the role of retroperitoneal lymphadenectomy.

The Danish Testicular Tumor Protocol for Stage I NSTT

The incidence of testicular cancer has been reported as doubling in Denmark over the past several decades. The Danish Cancer Society has collaborated an intergroup study for stage I, II and III testicular cancer in a randomized fashion.[4] Stage I nonseminomatous testicular cancer patients are randomized to radiotherapy (4000 rads) and an observation arm (Fig. 17.2). The clinical staging is based on the conventional modalities for staging including serum AFP and HCG. There is no lymphadenectomy arm in this study due to the prevailing views in Denmark that radiotherapy is the treatment of choice. However, they have indicated that if there will be no significant difference between radiotherapy and observation arms the inference will be that probably lymphadenectomy

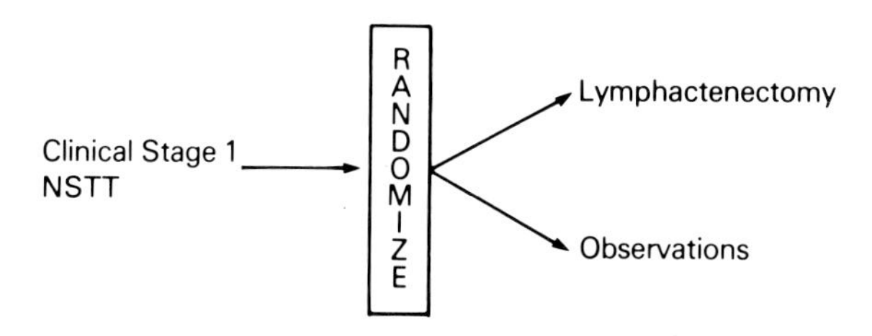

Figure 17.1. Randomized clinical trial of Memorial-Sloan Kettering for stage I testicular cancer. *NSTT*, nonseminomatous testicular cancer.

will be of no benefit in stage I testicular cancer. This assumption is open to question.

North California Oncology Group Phase III Study of Retroperitoneal Node Dissection *versus* Irradiation

In this study, the patients with clinical stage I NSTT are randomized to retroperitoneal lymph node dissection or radiation therapy to the retroperitoneal lymph nodes[5] (Fig. 17.3). Radiation therapy consists of 4500 rads that is given over a period of 6 weeks at 5 fractions/week. This study compares the effect of radiotherapy *versus* lymphadenectomy in a control fashion. The results of this study would have answered the important question whether radiotherapy or lymphadenectomy is more effective in stage I NSTT. This study did not attract patients and had to be terminated.[6]

RANDOMIZED PROTOCOLS FOR STAGE II

There are several available ongoing clinical trials for stage II testicular cancer as follows:

The Danish Testicular Tumor Protocol for Stage II NSTT

The Danish testicular cancer group randomizes the patients with NSTT that are clinically stage II after 3 cycles of platinum, vinblastine and bleomycin (PVB) to receive 4000 rads or to an observation arm. This study is aimed at determining the efficacy of chemotherapy with or without radiotherapy. Due to lack of practice of lymphadenectomy, there

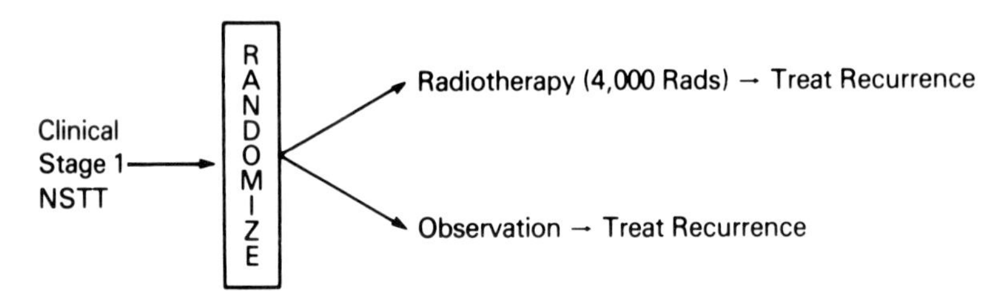

Figure 17.2. Randomized clinical trial of Danish testicular cancer group for stage I.

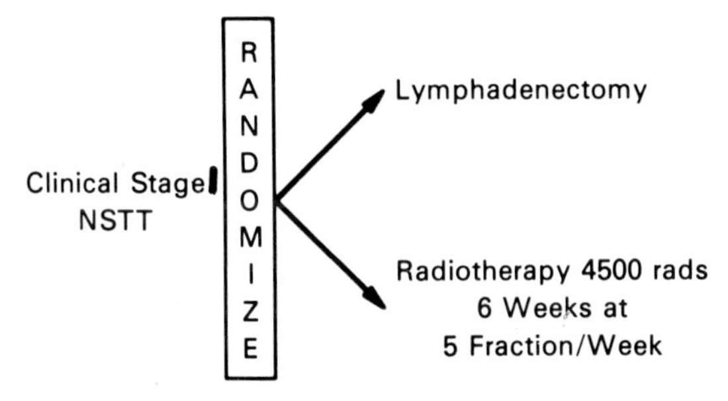

Figure 17.3. A randomized clinical trial of northern California oncology group for stage I NSTT.

is no lymphadenectomy arm in this study. (Fig. 17.4). The results of this study will indicate whether there is any role for radiation therapy in stage II as has been advocated by several groups.

Randomized Intergroup Study of NCI for stage II Testicular Cancer

This protocol randomized patients with pathologic stage II NSTT who have had complete resection of their tumor by initial orchiectomy followed by a retroperitoneal lymphadenectomy[7,8] (Fig. 17.5). Stage II patients with resectable retroperitoneal tumor (stage IIA, IIB and IIC) are randomly assigned to either an adjuvant chemotherapy arm or observation arm. There are two chemotherapy protocols available for this particular study[7,8]: (1) Combinations of platinum, vinblastine and bleomycin (PVB) as described by Einhorn and co-workers,[9] and (2) combinations of PVB plus cyclophosphamide (Cytoxan) and actinomycin (VAB VI) as described by Golbey and associates.[10]

This study has been activated for the past year and still accepts patients. The study will answer major critical questions as to the role of adjuvant chemotherapy in patients with clinically stage II testicular cancer who have undergone surgical resection with postoperative negative tumor markers.

Adjuvant Phase III Radiotherapy, Lymphadenectomy and Chemotherapy with Bleomycin, vinblastine and cisplatin for Stage I and II NSTT

This study is being conducted by the Southeast Cancer Study Group.[11] Patients with pathologic stage I or II NSTT documented by retroperitoneal dissection are randomized to radiotherapy followed by bleomycin (Bleo), vinblastine (VBL), cisplatin (DDP) or only radiotherapy to the retroperitoneal lymph nodes (Fig. 17.6). Although currently over 100

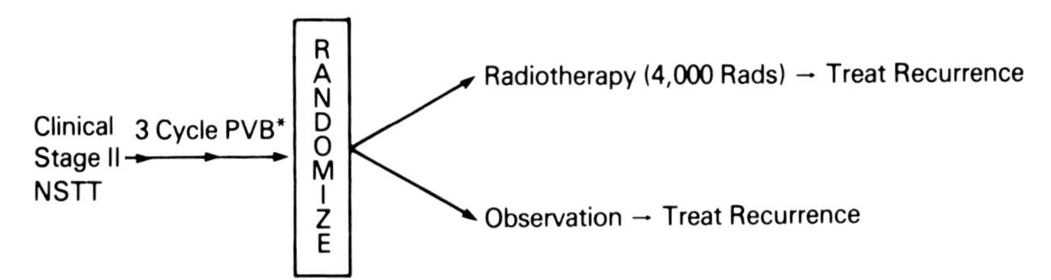

Figure 17.4. Randomized clinical trial of Danish testicular cancer group for stage II. *PVB*, platinum, vinblastine and bleomycin.

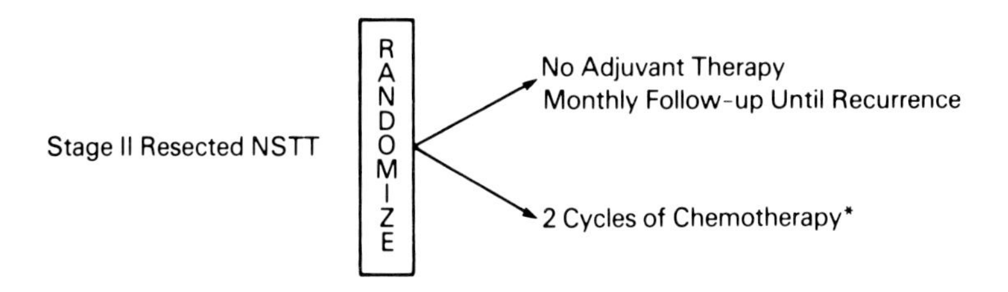

*There are 2 Protocols for the Selection of Chemotherapy 1) PVB
2) Cytoxan and Actinomycin D in Addition to PVB.

Figure 17.5. Randomized intergroup testicular cancer study for stage II NSTT.

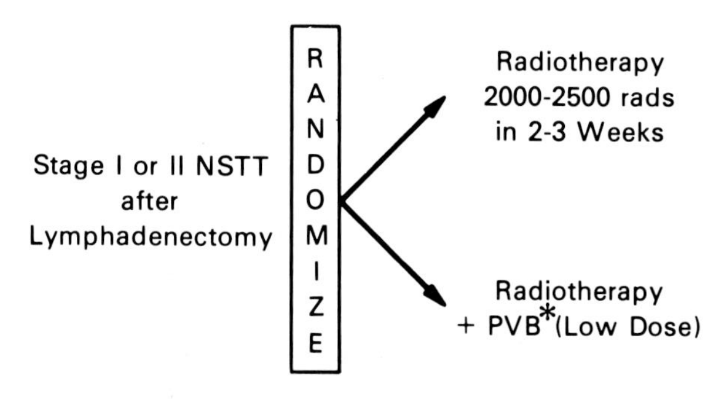

Figure 17.6. A randomized clinical trial of Southeastern cancer study group.

patients have entered into this protocol, the final results are not as yet available. This study will compare the disease-free interval and survival of patients with stage I and II NSTT who received radiotherapy with or without chemotherapy.

RANDOMIZED PROTOCOLS FOR STAGE III

It appears that chemotherapy is the treatment of choice for stage III testicular tumor. A 70–90% tumor-free survival has been achieved in nonbulky, low volume stage III testicular cancer, but the survival of patients with stage III bulky tumor with visceral metastases has been unfavorable. The next major question is whether a maintenance chemotherapy is necessary for stage III testicular cancer although the latter has been previously answered by Einhorn and associates.[9] Nevertheless, the Danish testicular group has embarked on such a study.

The Danish Testicular Cancer Study Group for Stage III

This collaborative group also has a randomized protocol for Stage III NSTT[4] (Fig. 17.7). The protocol for stage III is to treat the patients with 6 cycles of PVB then randomize the patients into a 4-month maintenance of actinomycin and vinblastine *versus* a 12-month maintenance of this combination. Although the result of this protocol is not available at the time of this writing, it appears from the other studies that the maintenance chemotherapy will have a very limited value in prolonging the survival of these patients.

NCI Randomized Study for Bulky Stage III

Chemotherapy has been shown to be more effective in experimental animal tumors when the size of the tumor is small. In man cytoreductive surgery has been advocated in a number of cancers including testicular, ovarian and certain renal cancer. In spite of effective chemotherapy for testicular cancer, the prognosis of patients with massive bulky disseminated testicular cancer is not favorable. The features of bulky testicular cancer rendering it a suitable model for cytoreductive surgery include availability of effective chemotherapeutic agents, do-able cytoreductive surgery, specific tumor markers and other objective modalities to detect the residual tumor.[12, 13] To date, no randomized trial has been performed to test whether the results of effective chemotherapy can be enhanced by cytoreductive surgery in patients with disseminated bulky cancer not curable by either chemotherapy or surgery alone. In 1976 the Surgical Oncology Branch and Medicine Branch, NCI, started a prospective randomized trial of cytoreductive surgery in patients with disseminated massive, bulky testicular cancer with a very poor prognosis (Fig. 17.8). In this protocol 39 patients with bulky stage III untreated nonseminomatous testicular cancer were randomized to cytoreductive surgery followed by chemotherapy or to chemotherapy alone.[14] All patients had documented histologic diagnoses. Cytoreductive surgery consisted of removal of the major bulk disease from the abdomen and/or thorax. Chemotherapy consisted of three intensive 21-day induction cycles with cyclophosphamide (CYT) 100 mg/m^2, vinblastine, 4 mg/m^2, actinomycin-D, 1 mg/m^2 I.V. on day 1; cisplatin (DDP), 100 mg/m^2 I.V. on day 7; and bleomycin (Bleo), 15 μ/m^2 I.V. infusion on days 1–5. Patients also received 2 nonintensive induction cycles with lower doses of CYT (100 mg/m^2 by mouth days 1–8) and DDP (25 mg/m^2) and Bleo (15 μ/m^2 on day 1) as well as 18 cycles of maintenance chemotherapy without any Bleo and DDP only on alternate cycles. For patients receiving initial chemotherapy alone, the complete remission rate was 7/19 (37%), partial remission rate was 8/19 (42%) and no response was 4/19 (21%). Three patients in this group were rendered a complete remission by excision of a mature teratoma. Patients randomized to surgery had 70–90% of the tumor resected prior to chemotherapy. There was one surgical death and one patient was not evaluable. Following chemotherapy, the complete remission rate was 8/18 (44%), partial remission was 7/18 (39%), and no

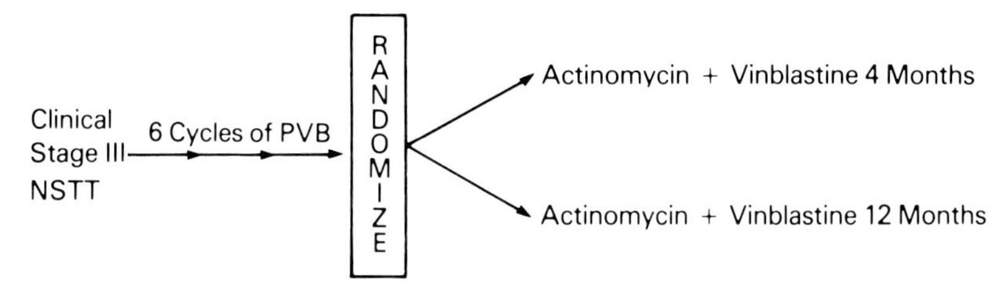

Figure 17.7. Randomized clinical trial of Danish testicular cancer group for stage III.

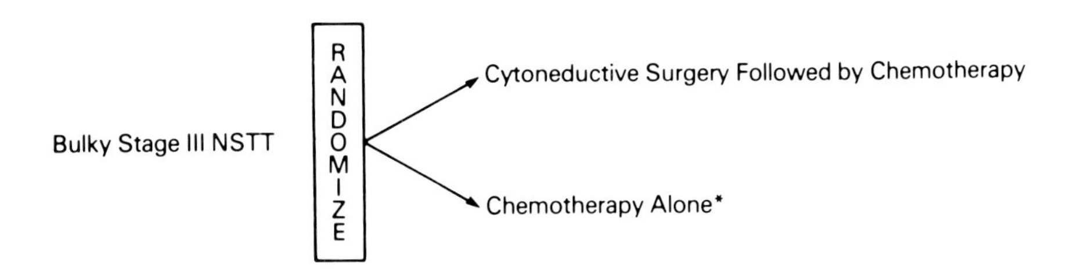

Figure 17.8. Randomized clinical trial of NCI for bulky disseminated stage III NSTT.

response was 3/18 (17%). Life table analysis failed to disclose any statistically significant differences in survival between the two groups. Regardless of therapy, patients receiving a complete remission had long survival as there has been only one relapse. This randomized trial demonstrates that while cytoreductive surgery is technically feasible in untreated bulky stage III testicular cancer patients, there is no improvement in response to subsequent chemotherapy or in survival compared to initial treatment with chemotherapy alone. Also, it is apparent that patients with massive bulky metastatic testicular cancer have poor prognosis in spite of effective chemotherapy. Therefore, we have begun a randomized clinical trial including newer chemotherapeutic agents and autologous bone marrow rescue for these subsets of testicular cancer with multiple poor prognostic criteria (Fig. 17.9).

Other Protocols in Testicular Cancer

Although the current chemotherapeutic agents have produced a dramatic improvement in survival of patients with disseminated testicular cancer, these agents may cause substantial cachectogenic effects. For this reason Samuels and co-workers[15] have studied this problem in a randomized clinical trial and I would like to present the summary of their paper.

Thirty evaluable patients with stage III metastatic testicular cancer were prospectively randomized to receive intravenous hyperalimentation (IVH) starting on day 1 of hospitalization (Fig. 17.10). There were 16 IVH patients and 14 control patients and a total of 88 evaluable trials. The IVH patients received 35 kcal/kg/day as 25% dextrose with 4.25% amino acids, while controls received 3 liters/day of 5% dextrose in 0.5 normal saline when gastrointestinal side effects from chemotherapy impaired the normal ingestion of food and fluids, usually by treatment day 3 or 4. Chemotherapy was started on hospital day 2, and consisted of vinblastine plus bleomycin, with a second randomization to low-dose cisplatin, 75 mg/m^2, with the first and third courses. Four courses were programmed for each patient; IVH successfully blunted weight loss from the gastrointestinal side effects of chemotherapy. The controls showed a mean weight loss per trial of 4.89 kg, in comparison to 1.67 kg/trial for

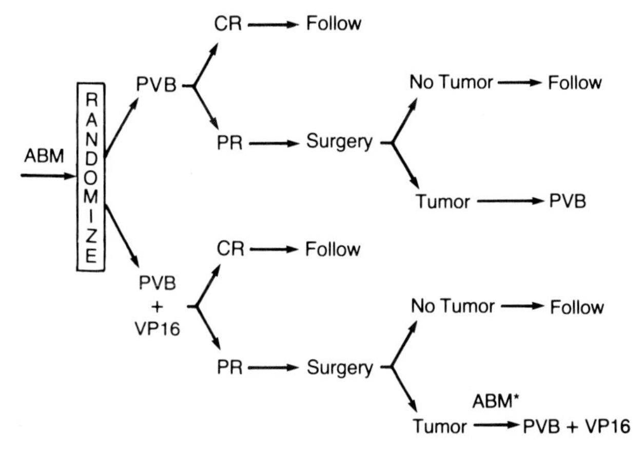

Figure 17.9. Bulky stage III testicular cancer. *ABM*, autologous bone marrow.

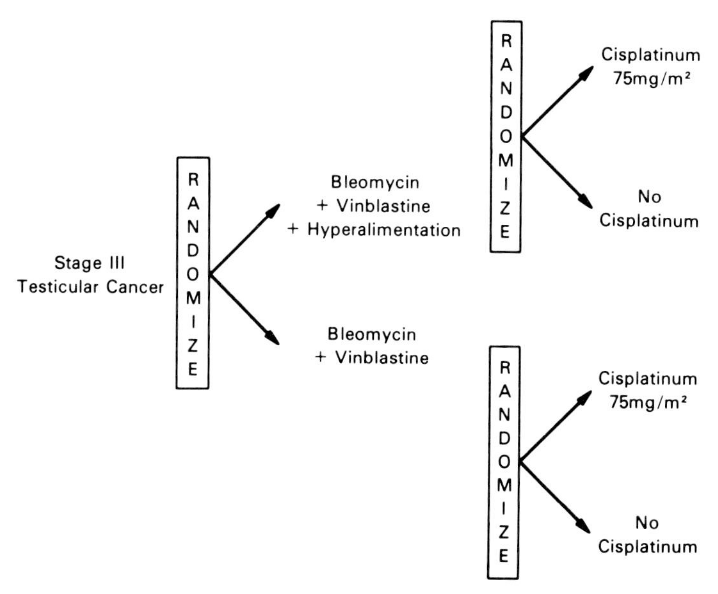

Figure 17.10. A randomized clinical trial of intravenous hyperalimentation (IVH) in disseminated testicular cancer.

the IVH patients ($p < 0.001$). However, other serious side effects were not lessened. Granulocytopenia was severe in both groups. The mean leukopenia nadir, nadir day and recovery day also showed no significant clinical differences. The control patients developed two bacteriologically proven septicemias with prompt recovery in both cases, while the IVH group developed five cases of bacteriologically proven septicemia and two of pneumonia. The one infection death was from *Klebsiella pneumoniae* pneumonia, which appeared on treatment day 4 and produced death day 8. The increased number of life-threatening infections in the IVH group was significant ($p = 0.047$). Only one septicemia was catheter related. Seventy-two percent of the IVH patients were hyperglycemic during the early part of the trials and this may have been an important etiological factor. The mean duration of IVH was 48 days for noninfected patients and 18 days for infected. The complete response rate for the IVH patients was 63% while the controls showed a 79% complete response rate ($p = 0.29$). Likewise, the addition of low-dose cisplatin did not significantly improve the initial complete response rate. With the addition of surgery for residual disease and secondary salvage chemotherapy, the complete response and probable cure rates are in excess of 75% for the entire population. During the study, a bowel perforation from tumor occurred in an IVH patient with liver metastases and we were able to continue chemotherapy and induce a complete remission that continues beyond 2 years. In addition, three control patients who suffered high weight loss after initial chemotherapy, were changed to IVH and two have remained in stable complete remission beyond the 2-year risk period. These investigators have concluded that aggressive meaningful chemotherapy was made possible by the addition of IVH in these select patients. However, in the testis cancer patients receiving vinblastine, bleomycin, and cisplatin, IVH should be restricted to those who present with a significant weight

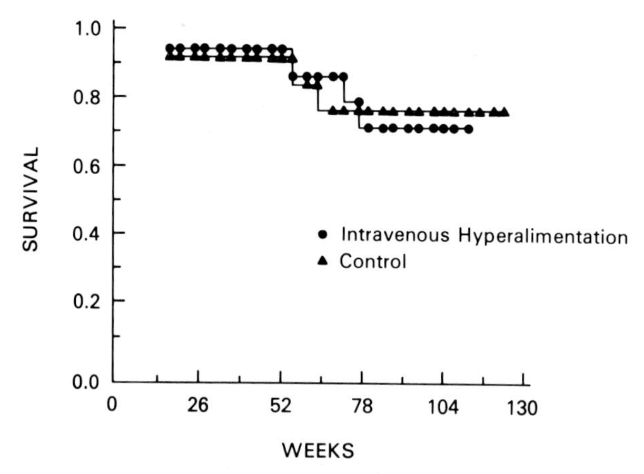

Figure 17.11. Survival of randomized clinical trial of metastatic testicular cancer intravenous hyperalimentation (IVH) *versus* control.

loss or who fail to regain lost weight during rest periods between courses. Also, there is no statistically significant difference in survival between the IVH and control group[15] ($p < 0.5$, Fig. 17.11).

FUTURE PERSPECTIVES

There has been a substantial progress in treating testicular cancer. These advances have been in the finding of newer chemotherapeutic regimens, tumor markers, and better modalities of detecting tumor. However, the major problem in evaluating survival of these patients has been lack of prospective randomized clinical trials. Almost all published series at the time of this writing, in which the various treatments in testicular cancer are compared, are either retrospective or lack controls. Therefore, one cannot interpret the data with certainty. The time has come to perform more controlled clinical trials and address the question what is the best minimal treatment for patients with testicular tumor with the least complications and an acceptable quality of life. Since the treatment modalities including surgery, chemotherapy or radiotherapy carry certain mortality and morbidities we need to know the exact efficacy of these therapeutic modalities in various stages in patients with testicular cancer. We also need to establish other reliable prognostic indicators in addition to tumor cell type, stage, tumor volume and visceral involvement. The prognostic value of the elevated tumor marker not related to tumor volume should also be determined in a controlled setting.

Finally, although there are a number of ongoing prospective randomized clinical trials, more controlled studies are needed to answer controversial clinical problems such as the role of various therapeutic modalities in seminoma patients with or without elevated serum HCG. Hopefully, the successful executions of the ongoing control trials and starting new ones will solve the existing controversies in reliable fashion, therefore avoiding the problems of retrospective studies and establishing firm guidelines in therapy of these patients.

REFERENCES

1. Byar, D. P. Statistical procedure in cancer. In *Recent Advances in Urologic Oncology*, pp. 1–19, edited by N. Javadpour. Williams & Wilkins, Baltimore, 1982.
2. Simon, R. Design of prospective clinical trials. In *Principles and Management of Urologic Cancer*, pp. 291–319, edited by N. Javadpour. Williams & Wilkins, Baltimore, 1982.
3. Whitmore, W. F., and Golbey, R. B. (Personal communications) 1980.
4. Schultz, H. P. (Personal communications) 1980.
5. Carter, S. K. Phase III study of retroperitoneal node surgery *versus* irradiation for stage I nonseminomatous testicular cancer. *Compilation of Cancer Therapy Protocols*, p. 164. National Institutes of Health, Bethesda, Md., April 1980.
6. Carter, S. K. (Personal communications) 1980.
7. Dewys, W. D. Surgery with or without VAB-V chemotherapy for stage II nonseminomatous, nonchoriocarcinomatous testicular germ cell tumors. *Compilation of Cancer Therapy Protocols Summaries*, p. 168. National Institutes of Health, Bethesda, Md., April 1980.
8. Dewys, W. D. Surgery with or without PVB chemotherapy for stage II nonseminomatous, nonchoriocarcinomatous testicular cancer germ cell tumors. *Compilation of Cancer Therapy Protocols Summaries*, p. 169, National Institutes of Health, Bethesda, Md., April 1980.
9. Einhorn, L. H., and Donohue, J. P. *Cis*-diamine dichloroplatinum, vinblastine and bleomycin combination chemotherapy in disseminated testicular cancer. *Ann. Intern. Med. 87:*293–98, 1977.
10. Golbey, R. B., Reynolds, T. F., and Vugrin, D. Chemotherapy of metastatic germ cell tumors. *Semin. Oncol. 6:*82–86, 1979.
11. Durant, J. R. Adjuvant phase III radiotherapy, lymphadenectomy and chemotherapy with Bleo, vinblastine, *cis*-platinum for nonseminomatous germ cell testicular tumors. *Compilation of Cancer Therapy Protocols Summaries*, p. 166, National Institutes of Health, Bethesda, Md., April 1980.
12. Donohue, J. P., Einhorn, L. H., and Williams, S. D. Cytoreductive surgery for metastatic testis cancer: considerations of time and extent. *J. Urol. 123:*876, 1980.
13. Javadpour, N. The National Cancer Institute experience with testicular cancer. *J. Urol. 120:*651, 1978.
14. Javadpour, N., Ozals, R. F., Anderson, T., Barlock, A., and Young, R. C. A randomized trial of cytoreductive surgery followed by chemotherapy *versus* chemotherapy alone in bulky stage III testicular cancer with poor prognosis. *Cancer 50:*2004, 1982.
15. Samuels, M. Intravenous hyperalimentation in stage III metastatic testicular cancer. *Cancer* Treat. Rept.*65:*615, 1981.

18

Final Comments

One of the prerogatives of an editor is to exercise the opportunity for final commentary. Irresistible as the notion of a "parting shot" may be, it is of much less value if exercised alone. At the outset, I promised each contributor the chance to summarize his views in a few words.

True to its name, the reader has now the opportunity of an international perspective from a diversity of authoritative viewpoints. Each contributor is a major worker in the field and is widely respected for his views. No final summary chapter would be fair or complete without the input of each contributor.

In bringing down the curtain on this volume, we raise the curtain once more for a brief encore. It is of special interest to have a glimpse down the vista of the future as viewed from the past. Each contributor has great personal experience and, on behalf of the readership, I thank them for what now follows. Here is a summary view of, not so much where we are but, where we see ourselves going. I hope to have the chance to read this every 5 years for several decades at least. I wonder if I will be as pleased then as I am now.

John P. Donohue

At the present we are passing out of what might be described as the "light microscope era" in the pathological diagnosis of testis tumors, and the introduction of more elaborate laboratory techniques, such as electron microscopy and immunocytochemistry, is altering our perspectives. The same is true of the very dramatic changes that have taken place in the last few years in the clinical field, especially since the introduction of primary chemotherapy. Yet much exciting work remains to be done by workers in many disparate disciplines, whose efforts can only be expected to yield optimum results if they can be concentrated in major referral centers and if clinical trials can be organized at national and international levels.

The current histopathological classifications need to be clarified and brought up to date, with adequate correlation of light and electron microscopical appearances with serum and tissue marker studies and also with accurate follow-up information. Fresh tumor tissue must be made available to basic scientists for fundamental research into the malignant process, using such techniques as tissue culture, etc. Also, experimental models have their place. Serum samples from tumor patients need to be frozen and banked so that retrospective analysis, and identification, of as yet unidentified marker substances will be possible. Many genetic and environmental factors remain to be assessed and, in the clinicopathological field, the "high risk" groups of patients with atypical germ cells in their testicular tubules (such as cryptorchids and infertile men) must be clearly identified and then treated.

Roger C. B. Pugh

A question that urologists frequently ask is whether the seminoma that they have just excised is "anaplastic" or not. Although I used to be rather enthusiastic about distinguishing anaplastic from classical seminomas, I must admit that my faith in the existence of the anaplastic variant as a crisply defined morphologic entity has waned to some degree. This, I suppose, follows my own inability to employ consistently reliable diagnostic criteria and the knowledge that I know at least a few colleagues who have experienced similar difficulties with this lesions. This, by the way, does not mean that one cannot identify seminomas that are histologically more disturbing than the classical type. What I would like to convey is that it is difficult to draw sharp lines in an area in which nature has produced an apparently fuzzy transition which, itself, requires more study. Actually, it is this more "worrisome" histologic variant that may yield evidence showing that some seminomas may transform into nonseminomatous germ cell tumors, this without postulating that the occurrence of such a switch implies a missed focus of, say, embryonal carcinoma in the primary tumor. In this regard, I was most interested in the report of Lange and Raghavan (Chapter 6), who appear to have produced a xenografted seminoma that manufactures α-fetoprotein, a product of the fetal yolk sac and interpreted as a marker of nonseminomatous germ cell cancer. The result of their experiment would support the possibility of seminomas converting to other germ cell types. That such conversion may occur is also borne out by the fact that the more atypical seminomas often resemble embryonal carcinoma very closely. I also recall examining seminomas that display somewhat provocative pseudoglandular patterns, hinting, as it were, at their nonseminomatous potential. There remains, I am sure, work to be done on the mixed seminomas and teratomas (the so-called "combined tumors"), with a view towards a careful study of the relationships between the different patterns. Presently, as far as the anaplastic seminoma is concerned, I tend to adopt the practice of those pathologists who, when confronted with one of these lesions, designate it a seminoma, but append a comment indicating their recognition of potentially important histological variation. Into this matrix, I suppose one should weave the occasional production of HCG by seminomas, but here too, I personally prefer to stipulate the presence of trophoblast in a separate statement, rather than by invoking a different, all-encompassing, diagnostic term.

Lucien E. Nochomovitz

Our manuscript, "Experimental Pathology," reviews the enigma of teratocarcinoma (from a somatic cell genetics perspective) by employing the stem cell model. In this model, the teratocarcinoma cell populations originate from stem cells that may be multipotential. Thus, stem cells may be seen to differentiate (assumed to be along normal developmental pathways) according to the environment (*i.e.* field). The stem cell (embryonal carcinoma, EC) is tumorigenic in most fields, whereas the differentiated cells have only a limited number of cell divisions and, therefore, are not tumorigenic. Rigorous cloning experiments have supported the model for mouse embryonal carcinoma. Several studies reported since the preparation of the manuscript now provide parallel support for human EC clones. Andrews *et al.*[1] and Avner *et al.*[2] have characterized presumptive human FC clones by morphological and immunological criteria. Both studies find differences in the antigen expression of human and mouse EC cell lines using monoclonal antibodies against various cell surface markers. Although the *in vitro* differentiation is limited, different combinations of markers are expressed by human and mouse EC cells and their immediate derivatives. Andrews *et al.* attempted repeated immunoselection cycles and cloning cycles in an attempt to establish cells that have undergone differentiation. Their inability to obtain such cells is consistent with the stem cell model. However, much more analysis may be performed in this area and I think that there will be many surprises.

The clinician has been aware of this proposed model for 30 years and pathological classification is based on this concept. However, hard support from human data has been slow coming. Potential pathological sampling errors preclude true testing of the observations that differentiated cells are not tumorigenic. The difficulties of *in vitro* cell growth have, until recently, hampered experimental studies. The future promises new markers which are badly needed for patient surveillance as well as the potential for targeted imaging and therapy.

John F. Harris
Michael A. S. Jewett

Major advances have been made in identification of active chemotherapeutic agents for testicular tumors, giving urologists and medical oncologists the luxury of effective therapy even for patients with advanced stages of disease. As dramatically improved survival rates are achieved regularly in multiple centers, attention has now been turned to the achievement of similar survival rates with lesser amounts of therapy and, hence, morbidity.

Implicit in the selection of lesser amounts of therapy is the need for accurate clinical staging parameters. At the current time, even with the best noninvasive modalities, accurate depiction of retroperitoneal lymph node involvement can be achieved in only 75–80% of individuals. The question of whether this percentage of false-negative staging procedures will enable avoidance of retroperitoneal lymph node dissection, with salvage by systemic chemotherapy for those who fail, remains unanswered. Certainly, however, with refinement of staging techniques, retroperitoneal lymphadenectomy for patients with limited disease will be performed less frequently in the future.

The role of adjuvant chemotherapy in low stage disease remains unproven. Strong experimental evidence suggests that an active agent, such as actinomycin D, can diminish systemic recurrences when given early in the course of disease. However, any adjuvant therapy implies treatment of a large number of individuals to secure the benefit for a smaller number. One must weigh the risks of exposure of all patients to chemotherapeutic agents, the amount of benefit gained, and whether or not these agents prejudice successful salvage in those patients who subsequently recur. A randomized protocol, using two cycles of platinum-based polychemotherapy, is being studied in an adjuvant setting for stage II patients. My concerns for this protocol include exposure of all patients to cisplatin, the long-term effects of which have not been well studied, and the use of two cycles of the same agents and doses that must be utilized for a salvage protocol should relapse occur. With close follow-up, survival rates with adjuvant chemotherapy or salvage chemotherapy should both be greater than 90%, and again the question of exposing a large number of patients to a potentially toxic regimen to benefit a few will have to be weighed carefully.

The above questions represent minor variations on a theme. We now have the luxury of long-term survival, and cure, in the overwhelming percentage of patients who present with primary gonadal germ cell terms. New avenues of therapy, however, must be initiated for those patients with primary extragonadal germ cell tumors, whose survival is not nearly as favorable.

Jerome P. Richie

I continue to believe that retroperitoneal lymphadenectomy, with chemotherapy as necessary, is the best means of managing the retroperitoneal lymph nodes of most patients with nonseminomatous testicular cancer. As the data from the Universities of Minnesota, Indiana, and California-Los Angeles show, the long-term survival rates in patients with pathologic stages I–IIB disease exceed 95% for patients so treated, whereas the long-term survival rates for these same stages with radiation therapy averages 81–89%. In addition, lymphadenectomy does not cause serious radiation injury, nor does it cause cancer. As I wrote recently, I suspect the day is fast approaching when we will no longer be discussing the merits of routine retroperitoneal irradiation for low stage nonseminomatous testicular cancer. This should be particularly true for the so-called "sandwich" treatment (radiation-lymphadenectomy-radiation*), the merits of which have always escaped me, as it seems to me that the radiation serves to make the operation more difficult. I note that in the most recent report from Walter Reed, sandwich treatment cured 89% of patients with clinical stage I disease (approximately equivalent to pathologic stages I–IIB) and radiation therapy alone only 86%, both of which compare unfavorably with the recent results of operation cited earlier. Now that we have shown that a therapeutically sound lymphadenectomy can be done that permits the return of normal antegrade ejaculation in at least half the patients with low stage tumors, the operation looks even more appealing.

---

* One of my more sardonic associates has called attention to which of the treatments is considered the meat and which only the bread.

We have been watching with great interest that study being done by Michael J. Peckham and his colleagues in London. In essence, when they find a patient in whom the most sensitive and specific nonoperative staging techniques reveal no spread of the tumor beyond the testis and who is believed to be reliable enough to return regularly and often for follow-up, they offer him the option of receiving no treatment beyond orchiectomy unless and until he has a proven relapse. In May 1981, Peckham made a preliminary report on his results at the International Meeting on Germ Cell Tumors in London and said that 13 patients with undifferentiated malignant teratoma (MTU) (roughly equivalent to embryonal carcinoma) had been managed in this way up to that time. Four of them had had retroperitoneal recurrences (one also had pulmonary metastases), but all were apparently free of disease after chemotherapy. I confess that I am unsettled at leaving these patients untreated and relying on them for regular follow-up when I know, on the basis of our experience with 355 patients, that at least a quarter of those without nonoperative evidence of metastases do indeed have retroperitoneal tumor, another 10% will have pulmonary metastases without retroperitoneal tumor, and all too many cannot be relied on to adhere to a follow-up and treatment regimen even when they are told they still have proven cancer.

Is this the management of the future? We should know within a few years. In the meantime, I will persist in my conviction that retroperitoneal lymphadenectomy is the most cost-effective treatment with the fewest serious long-term side effects for most of these patients.

Elwin E. Fraley

The effective use of α-fetoprotein (AFP) and HCG as serum tumor markers in testicular cancer has now become a routine skill. Further progress in this field will be sporadic, depending more on alert bedside observation than on retrospective analyses of large populations of patients. The suggested prognostic importance of HCG in advanced seminoma will probably be obscured by more effective chemotherapy, and similarly, the use of apparent half-life calculations may diminish in importance; in prospective studies, where modern platinum-based chemotherapy has been used, marker decay has seemed to be a less useful tool. β-1 glycoprotein (SP-1), while common in the blood of patients with testicular cancer, and occasionally useful in our clinical experience, does not seem to be an important marker, despite the development of more sensitive assays. However, it does appear that placental alkaline phosphatase (P1AP) will have clinical importance as a new marker for seminoma, although more experience will be necessary to understand the nuances of application. There is some evidence that testicular P1AP has different physicochemical properties from P1AP of placental origin, and this may have important experimental and practical implications.

Monoclonal antibodies to testicular tumor antigens in mice and men are being produced by many groups and already have illustrated the heterogeneity of these tumors. We will hear much more about these efforts in the future. Radioimmunolocalization in man is still experimental and awaits the development of more specific and avid antibodies (perhaps monoclonal) and improved scanning technology. To date, our experience with this modality has been encouraging and there may yet be a role for eventual routine clinical application.

In a more clinical context, several important issues come to mind. The ultimate place of lymphadenectomy as a staging or therapeutic maneuver for stage I and possibly stage II disease requires continual re-evaluation. We must not lose ground, however, in our eagerness for change. Cytoreductive surgery now has an established role in management, but our criteria for selection and the timing of this procedure should be carefully re-examined. This surgery requires skill and boldness, and surgeons who perform it well are a resource to be developed and maintained at major medical centers. With respect to chemotherapy, we need to become more adept at determining high risk groups so that more intensive therapy can be applied earlier. In addition, the developmental studies in progress at centers such as the Royal Marsden Hospital, where a "watch" policy is employed in carefully selected patients, with close monitoring with tumor markers and CAT scans, will be of great interest, and may yield management approaches of lesser toxicity without loss of efficacy. The long-term toxicity of chemotherapy on renal and cardiovascular function, and the risk of second malignancies, could be important, and our management algorithms may thus require revision as these effects become known. Advances have been made in improving fertility after lymphadenectomy and we understand better the consequences of platinum-based chemotherapy on spermatogenesis. Further improvements can be expected by changing surgical boundaries and perhaps by protecting the gonads from the effects of cytotoxic agents by simultaneous hormonal manipulation. Despite the spectacular improvement in survival in patients with testicular cancer, it is not yet time to rest on our laurels.

Paul H. Lange
Derek Raghavan

Management of testes tumors has undergone many changes in the past decade. Survivals at the present time with both seminoma and nonseminomatous germinal tumors is approaching 100%. In my opinion, the proper management of seminoma is adequate irradiation to the lymph-bearing areas following an inguinal orchiectomy. These patients must be followed with monthly tumor markers. With nonseminomatous germinal tumors after inguinal orchiectomy, a bilateral retroperitoneal lymphadenectomy is necessary. This procedure is required for both staging, as well as cure.

Although still controversial, I have found that adjuvant chemotherapy has increased survival if given after a retroperitoneal lymphadenectomy. In Stage I disease one course of actinomycin D is given during the postoperative period, and then every 3 months for 1 year. Stage II patients are given a three-drug regimen consisting of cisplatin, vincristine, and bleomycin. After one course during the postoperative period, they are given as many maintenance courses over a period of time as deemed necessary. Those patients presenting with bulky disease are managed with chemotherapy preoperatively, followed by a bilateral retroperitoneal lymphadenectomy and then placed on a maintenance course of multiple-agent chemotherapy for as long as necessary. Stage III patients must be individualized depending on the extent of disease. Usually they are given one or more courses of chemotherapy prior to either a bilateral lymphadenectomy and/or a debulking procedure and then followed for an indefinite period with multiple chemotherapy agents. All stages are followed monthly with tumor markers, chest x-rays including chest tomography, and a thorough physical examination. Sonography, skinny needle biopsy and CAT scans are used when indicated.

William J. Staubitz

For more than 20 years we have regarded seminoma and nonseminoma as if they were two entirely distinct entities. Today, immunoperoxidase staining for tumor markers, on the one hand, and evidence from the mouse laboratory on the other, forces us to see them as different hues in a continuous spectrum. We should stop being surprised when a seminoma metastasises as a teratoma, and we should stop prescribing one form of treatment for seminoma, and another for nonseminoma. The old antithesis between node dissection and radiation has now been rendered irrevelant and out-of-date by the advance of combination chemotherapy. Far more interesting questions pose themselves: what is chemotherapy really doing—is it disciplining anaplastic tissue into something more differentiated? Is it merely killing off the more malignant parts? What good do we do by cutting out nonmalignant necrotic tissue? What is the role of radiotherapy—should it be an adjunct or an alternative, should it form one part of a cocktail of combination therapy, or kept in reserve?

Above all we must continue to ask some of the old questions, for they still need an answer: why do these young men still come up so late in the disease? Why is the diagnosis so often missed? Maybe the next step forward must come from the classroom, not the chemotherapy laboratory.

John Peter Blandy

Cisplatin-based chemotherapy will, with or without subsequent surgical excision of residual disease, produce disease-free status in around 80% of patients so treated. The relapse rate from complete remission is around 10% or slightly less and does not appear to be affected by maintenance chemotherapy. Thus, around 70% of patients with disseminated testicular cancer will be cured. In the cohort of patients not cured by initial therapy, salvage chemotherapy with cisplatin plus etopside (VP16) will allow a few more patients to be long term disease free survivors.

By manipulation of initial drug dosages and more experience with this regimen, acute toxicity has been reduced and, in experienced hands, the drug-related mortality should be quite low. There has been no chronic renal disease or lung disease and normal reproductive function will return in some patients. Neurotoxicity can be a long-term problem but appears to diminish with time. Premature coronary artery disease and the induction of second neoplasms continues to be a potential problem with little data available regarding their frequency.

In addition to the evaluation of VP16-containing therapy as first line, there are several other potentially fruitful areas of investigation. Highly desirable would be a reliable method initially to select which patients are destined not to be cured with standard therapy so they may be placed on trials of innovative treatment at the time of diagnosis of metastatic disease. Potential regimens include modification of dose, schedule of the drugs used in induction therapy, or the addition of other active agents. It is conceivable that high dose chemotherapy with autologous marrow rescue might also improve therapeutic results.

The fate of patients with disseminated testicular cancer is vastly improved from that of 10 years ago and it is likely that in the next decade the cure rate will be even higher with more precisely defined and lesser toxicity.

Stephen D. Williams
Lawrence H. Einhorn

There has been a substantial progress in testicular cancer. These advances have been in the finding of newer chemotherapeutic regimens, tumor markers, and better modalities of detecting tumor. However, the major problem in evaluating survival of these patients has been lack of prospective randomized clinical trials. Almost all published series at the time of this writing, in which the various treatments in testicular cancer are compared, are either retrospective or lack controls. Therefore, one cannot interpret the data with certainty. The time has come to perform controlled clinical trials and address the question: what is the best minimal treatment for patients with testicular tumor with the least complications and an acceptable quality of life? Since the treatment modalities including surgery, chemotherapy or radiotherapy carry certain mortality and morbidities, we need to know the exact efficacious role of these therapeutic modalities in various stages and other clinical settings of the patients with testicular cancer.

The role of lymphadenectomy in stage I nonseminomatous testicular cancer (NSTT) needs clarification. The exact role of radiation in stage I and II seminoma also is not clear. The most efficacious therapy in bulky stage II and stage III seminoma require more investigations. The optimal treatment stage II NSTT in terms of adjuvant therapy and stage III bulky tumor with poor prognostic features requires a better chemotherapeutic regimen with maximum efficacy and minimal toxicities are obvious.

Also, we need to establish the prognostic indicators in addition to tumor cell type, stage, tumor volume and visceral involvement. The prognostic value of the elevated tumor marker not related to tumor volume should also be determined in a controlled setting.

Also the adverse effects of orchiectomy, lymphadenectomy, intensive chemotherapy and radiotherapy on socioeconomic, emotional, sexual activity, masculinity and infertility of this young group of patients should be carefully considered. The occasional necessity of marriage counselling, psychiatric consultation and frequent assurances in certain patients must be a part of the overall objective of any study and improvement of quality of life resulting in a socially productive and happy individual.

Hopefully, the successful execution of the ongoing control trials and undertaking of other necessary protocols will solve the existing controversies in reliable fashion, therefore avoiding the problems of current retrospective studies.

Nasser Javadpour

Future prospects in the area of testis cancer are much brighter than with other urologic tumors where we have failed to make as much progress in the past decade. Thanks to the good advances in chemotherapy, testis tumor can be approached more conservatively initially and may require a very aggressive approach late in its course in some cases.

First, in the area of diagnosis, I foresee four areas of improvement. (1) Male self-examination will be more widely taught and better accepted by the lay public. Teaching films for physicians, paramedical personnel, and lay people will be distributed and promulgated so that patients will bring testicular masses to the physician's attention at an earlier stage. (2) Markers will be more sensitive and radioisotopic-tagged scans will also be applied in cases of difficult locations of serologic relapses. As of now, the sensitivity of biologic markers, such as α-fetoprotein and β-HCG are not quite what they will be in the future. (3) Computed axial tomography will continue to sharpen in its resolution and other mechanisms of imaging, such as nuclear magnetic resonance, will assist in the staging of retroperitoneal and mediastinal lymphadenopathy. (4) Needle aspiration cytology might be used together with various imaging guidance techniques. Some preliminary work with this in prostate cancer is already promising. It might well be possible to aspirate the primary nodal areas of drainage to further reduce the false negative rate which currently is no better than 20% even with the use of lymphography today.

If these improvements in diagnosis come to pass, as I expect they shall, clinical staging should become sensitive and specific enough to allow for primary observation in clinically negative (stage I) patients.

In terms of treatment, the role of staging retroperitoneal lymphadenectomy (RPLND) will greatly diminish and probably disappear entirely. This will be replaced by the modalities noted above, especially if fine needle aspiration of these nodes can be used to confirm or rule out tumor involvement, early combination chemotherapy can be given in position cases, thus obviating entirely the role of *staging* RPLND. Early evidence with short follow-up suggests this approach is feasible, at least in the setting of a tightly controlled single study with perfect follow-up.[3] Whether this can be applied to the vicissitudes of community care at large is quite another question.

However, the role of surgery will increase in the area of cytoreductive RPLND. Many patients presenting with advanced disease will still have persistent mass lesions in the chest, mediastinum, or retroperitoneum. These will need to be excised in order to guide further management. Those with persistent malignant elements will still be salvageable with good salvage chemotherapy, particularly if their mass lesion is completely resected. So on the one hand, clinical staging will become further refined and probably supplant surgical staging RPLND. On the other hand, primary chemotherapy for advanced disease will render many otherwise inoperable patients clearly operable for tissue diagnosis and therapy. These changes are already well under way.[4, 5]

Advanced seminoma, particularly disseminated disease, will be more often treated with primary chemotherapy, which seems to be extremely effective in this disease. Our experience with resected mass lesions after chemotherapy in patients with primary seminoma has revealed only necrosis in the tissue. There is such a high rate of sterilized tumor, that many centers will entirely forego surgical debulking postchemotherapy for seminoma. This seminoma group might be treated with radiotherapy to the residual lesion as one clinical trial in America has done to good effect.[6]

The chemosensitivity of germ cell tumors has dramatically changed our approach to both early and late stage disease. This may be harbinger of things to come with other urologic tumors.

John P. Donohue

REFERENCES

1. Andrews *et al. Int. J. Cancer 29:*523, 1982.
2. Avner *et al. J. Immunogenet. 8:*151, 1981.
3. Peckham, M. J., Barrett, A., Husband, J. E., Hendry, W. F. Orchidectomy alone in testicular stage I nonseminomatous germ cell tumors. Lancet *2:*678–680, 1982.
4. Donohue, J. P., Perez, J. M., and Einhorn, L. H. Improved management of nonseminomatous testis tumors. *J. Urol. 121:*425, 1979.
5. Donohue, J. P., Einhorn, L. H., and Williams, S. D. Cytoreductive surgery for metastatic testis cancer: considerations of timing and extent. *J. Urol. 123:*876, 1980.
6. Crawford, J., deKernion, J., Smith, R. Treatment of advanced seminoma—a SWOG study. *J. Urol.* (in press), 1983.

Index